A History of Burn Care

A History of Burn Care

Editors

Lars P. Kamolz
Bernd Hartmann

MDPI • Basel • Beijing • Wuhan • Barcelona • Belgrade • Manchester • Tokyo • Cluj • Tianjin

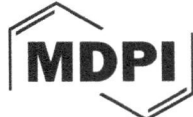

Editors
Lars P. Kamolz
Medical University Graz
Austria

Bernd Hartmann
Unfallkrankenhaus Berlin
Germany

Editorial Office
MDPI
St. Alban-Anlage 66
4052 Basel, Switzerland

This is a reprint of articles from the Special Issue published online in the open access journal *Medicina* (ISSN 1648-9144) (available at: https://www.mdpi.com/journal/medicina/special_issues/burn_care).

For citation purposes, cite each article independently as indicated on the article page online and as indicated below:

LastName, A.A.; LastName, B.B.; LastName, C.C. Article Title. *Journal Name* **Year**, *Volume Number*, Page Range.

ISBN 978-3-0365-1525-0 (Hbk)
ISBN 978-3-0365-1526-7 (PDF)

© 2021 by the authors. Articles in this book are Open Access and distributed under the Creative Commons Attribution (CC BY) license, which allows users to download, copy and build upon published articles, as long as the author and publisher are properly credited, which ensures maximum dissemination and a wider impact of our publications.

The book as a whole is distributed by MDPI under the terms and conditions of the Creative Commons license CC BY-NC-ND.

Contents

About the Editors vii

Lars-Peter Kamolz and Bernd Hartmann
A History of Burn Care
Reprinted from: *Medicina* **2021**, *57*, 541, doi:10.3390/medicina57060541 1

Christoph Wallner, Eric Moormann, Patricia Lulof, Marius Drysch, Marcus Lehnhardt and Björn Behr
Burn Care in the Greek and Roman Antiquity
Reprinted from: *Medicina* **2020**, *56*, 657, doi:10.3390/medicina56120657 3

Michael Giretzlehner, Isabell Ganitzer and Herbert Haller
Technical and Medical Aspects of Burn Size Assessment and Documentation
Reprinted from: *Medicina* **2021**, *57*, 242, doi:10.3390/medicina57030242 13

Michael Kohlhauser, Hanna Luze, Sebastian Philipp Nischwitz and Lars Peter Kamolz
Historical Evolution of Skin Grafting—A Journey through Time
Reprinted from: *Medicina* **2021**, *57*, 348, doi:10.3390/medicina57040348 29

Deepak K. Ozhathil, Michael W. Tay, Steven E. Wolf and Ludwik K. Branski
A Narrative Review of the History of Skin Grafting in Burn Care
Reprinted from: *Medicina* **2021**, *57*, 380, doi:10.3390/medicina57040380 43

Frederik Schlottmann, Vesna Bucan, Peter M. Vogt and Nicco Krezdorn
A Short History of Skin Grafting in Burns: From the Gold Standard of Autologous Skin Grafting to the Possibilities of Allogeneic Skin Grafting with Immunomodulatory Approaches
Reprinted from: *Medicina* **2021**, *57*, 225, doi:10.3390/medicina57030225 71

Wolfram Heitzmann, Paul Christian Fuchs and Jennifer Lynn Schiefer
Historical Perspectives on the Development of Current Standards of Care for
Enzymatic Debridement
Reprinted from: *Medicina* **2020**, *56*, 706, doi:10.3390/medicina56120706 87

Dorothee Boehm and Henrik Menke
A History of Fluid Management—From "One Size Fits All" to an Individualized Fluid Therapy in Burn Resuscitation
Reprinted from: *Medicina* **2021**, *57*, 187, doi:10.3390/medicina57020187 95

Ioannis-Fivos Megas, Justus P. Beier and Gerrit Grieb
The History of Carbon Monoxide Intoxication
Reprinted from: *Medicina* **2021**, *57*, 400, doi:10.3390/medicina57050400 105

Christian Smolle, Joerg Lindenmann, Lars Kamolz and Freyja-Maria Smolle-Juettner
The History and Development of Hyperbaric Oxygenation (HBO) in Thermal Burn Injury
Reprinted from: *Medicina* **2021**, *57*, 49, doi:10.3390/medicina57010049 113

Arij El Khatib and Marc G. Jeschke
Contemporary Aspects of Burn Care
Reprinted from: *Medicina* **2021**, *57*, 386, doi:10.3390/medicina57040386 139

Herbert Leopold Haller, Matthias Rapp, Daniel Popp, Sebastian Philipp Nischwitz and Lars Peter Kamolz
Made in Germany: A Quality Indicator Not Only in the Automobile Industry But Also When It Comes to Skin Replacement: How an Automobile Textile Research Institute Developed a New Skin Substitute
Reprinted from: *Medicina* **2021**, *57*, 143, doi:10.3390/medicina57020143 . . . . **157**

Herbert L. Haller, Sigrid E. Blome-Eberwein, Ludwik K. Branski, Joshua S. Carson, Roselle E. Crombie, William L. Hickerson, Lars Peter Kamolz, Booker T. King, Sebastian P. Nischwitz, Daniel Popp, Jeffrey W. Shupp and Steven E. Wolf
Porcine Xenograft and Epidermal Fully Synthetic Skin Substitutes in the Treatment of Partial-Thickness Burns: A Literature Review
Reprinted from: *Medicina* **2021**, *57*, 432, doi:10.3390/medicina57050432 . . . . **173**

About the Editors

Lars P. Kamolz M.D., M.Sc.; (1) Division of Plastic, Aesthetic and Reconstructive Surgery, Department of Surgery, Medical University Graz, Austria (2) COREMED – Cooperative Center for Regenerative Medicine, JOANNEUM RESEARCH Forschungsgesellschaft mbH, Graz, Austria, lars.kamolz@medunigraz.at

Bernd Hartmann M.D.; Director: Burn Center and Plastic Surgery, Unfallkrankenhaus Berlin, Berlin, Germany.

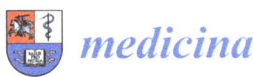

Editorial
A History of Burn Care

Lars-Peter Kamolz [1,2,*] and Bernd Hartmann [3]

[1] Division of Plastic, Aesthetic and Reconstructive Surgery, Department of Surgery, Medical University Graz, 8036 Graz, Austria
[2] COREMED—Cooperative Center for Regenerative Medicine, Joanneum Research Forschungsgesellschaft mbH, 8010 Graz, Austria
[3] Burn Center and Plastic Surgery, Unfallkrankenhaus Berlin, 12683 Berlin, Germany; bernd.hartmann@ukb.de
* Correspondence: lars.kamolz@medunigraz.at

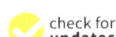

Citation: Kamolz, L.-P.; Hartmann, B. A History of Burn Care. *Medicina* 2021, 57, 541. https://doi.org/10.3390/medicina57060541

Received: 24 May 2021
Accepted: 27 May 2021
Published: 28 May 2021

Publisher's Note: MDPI stays neutral with regard to jurisdictional claims in published maps and institutional affiliations.

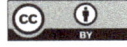

Copyright: © 2021 by the authors. Licensee MDPI, Basel, Switzerland. This article is an open access article distributed under the terms and conditions of the Creative Commons Attribution (CC BY) license (https://creativecommons.org/licenses/by/4.0/).

Burn injuries are still one of the most common and devastating injuries in humans and the treatment of major burns remains a major challenge for physicians worldwide. Modern burn care involves many components from initial first aid, burn size and burn depth assessment, fluid resuscitation, wound care, excision and grafting/coverage, infection control and nutritional support.

Progress in each of these areas has contributed significantly to the overall enhanced survival of burn victims over the past decades.

In this Special Issue we look back at how the treatment of burns has evolved over the past decades and hundreds of years. Most major advances in burn care occurred in the last 50 years, spurred on by wars and great fires. The use of systemic antibiotics and topical anti-infective agents greatly reduced sepsis-related mortality. This, along with the improvement of new surgical and skin-grafting techniques, allowed the earlier excision and coverage of deep burns which resulted in greatly improved survival rates and better functional and aesthetic outcomes. Advancements concerning objective burn assessment paved the way for a more accurate fluid resuscitation, minimising the effects of shock and avoiding fluid over-resuscitation.

This article aims to explore the history of burn care to identify milestones and step-changes in each of these areas in the patient's care and burn care-related research. The advancement of burn care has been closely associated with our deeper understanding of its pathophysiology; we have now come to understand the impact that burn injuries have in multiple fields of current medical science i.e., in metabolism and circulation, electrolyte balance and nutrition, immunology and infection, inflammation, pulmonary function and wound healing. Despite this, many challenges still remain and the focus of burn care in the future will be to overcome the existing problems of burn-related injuries (e.g., burns in the elderly, extensive burn injuries, shortening healing times and, therefore, lengths of hospital stay, and to improve scarring). It is hoped that new technologies and advances in wound care will achieve faster wound coverage with minimal scarring.

We invite you to read the articles of "A History of Burn Care" in order to learn from the past and to be fit for the future in burn care.

Funding: This research received no external funding.

Conflicts of Interest: The authors declare no conflict of interest.

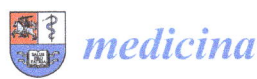 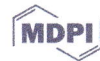

Review

Burn Care in the Greek and Roman Antiquity

Christoph Wallner [1,2,*], Eric Moormann [3], Patricia Lulof [2], Marius Drysch [1], Marcus Lehnhardt [1] and Björn Behr [1]

1. Department of Plastic Surgery, BG University Hospital Bergmannsheil, Ruhr University Bochum, Bürkle-de-la-Camp Platz 1, 44789 Bochum, Germany; marius.drysch@rub.de (M.D.); marcus.lehnhardt@rub.de (M.L.); bjorn.behr@rub.de (B.B.)
2. Department of Archaeology, Amsterdam Centre of Ancient Studies and Archaeology-ACASA, University of Amsterdam, Turfdraagsterpad 9, 1012 XT Amsterdam, The Netherlands; P.S.Lulof@uva.nl
3. Department of History, Art History and Classics, Radboud University, Erasmusplein 1, 6525 HT Nijmegen, The Netherlands; e.moormann@let.ru.nl
* Correspondence: Christoph.wallner@bergmannsheil.de

Received: 13 October 2020; Accepted: 26 November 2020; Published: 28 November 2020

Abstract: The last century brought about more rapid new developments in the treatment of burns, which significantly lowered the mortality of burn injuries. However, burns were already treated in antiquity, where the threshold from spirituality to scientific medicine originated. The existing literature on burn treatment is very limited and there are many cross-references, some of them incorrect. The aim of this work by an interdisciplinary team of historians and physicians is to offer a more precise reproduction of the burn treatment of Greek and Roman antiquity using original texts in context and with a modern scientific background. There are many sources from ancient doctors on the subject of burn treatment, as well as the treatment of burned-out wounds and frostbite, which have not yet been mentioned. The literature research also showed an understanding of scientific contexts in ancient medicine, such as antiseptics or rheology. Interestingly, there was a change in burn medicine from everyday Greek medicine to Roman military medicine with other burn patterns. The care of patients using analgetics and the therapy of burn shock arose from the literature. The ancient world is considered to be the foundation of medicine, but it is believed to have been based mainly on shamanism rather than science. However, already more than two millennia ago, burns were correctly assessed and treated according to today's scientific standards and scientific relationships were recognized.

Keywords: burn; care; antiquity; phytotherapy; ancient medicine

1. Introduction

Over the past centuries but especially in recent decades, the advances in burn care have led to a massive improvement of clinical care and therefore to a decrease in mortality of burn patients [1]. While innovations in modern medicine reduce the mortality of those with severe burns to less than 5%, new challenges arise from, for example, multi-drug resistant microorganisms. Burn patients with large wound areas and relatively long mechanical ventilation are particularly susceptible to these germs and exposed to them without protection. While modern concepts fail, very old methods of treating burn injuries are used, which, like medical honey, overcome multi-drug resistant microorganisms [2,3]. The use of medicinal honey in the treatment of wounds was first recorded in ancient times. On the one hand, through the writing of medical treatments but also through the technological progress of the time—there was a medical revolution in antiquity. In this article, we want to focus on the treatment of burns in the Greek and Roman antiquity. There is little translated literature available from Greek and Roman antiquity about the treatment of burns. We therefore see a great opportunity in summarizing the existing medical literature as well as in translating unnoticed texts on the therapy of burn injuries from this time.

To include a relevant body of modern medical literature, a search on pubmed with the MeSH ""Burns/history" [MAJR]" was performed on 26 September 2020 including 144 results, of which 12 results included the era of the Greek and Roman antiquity. For the classical literature review, texts of Hippocrates of Kos, Galen of Pergamon, the Alexandrian school (Heracleides of Tarentum, Sostratos, Herophilos of Chalkedon, Praxagoras of Kos and others), Pedanios Dioscurides, and Aulus Cornelius Celsus were considered. In addition, "Der Kleine Pauly" as the standard reference work of antiquity served as the basis for the extended search.

1.1. Animal Products

On pubmed, only a small number of references to the medical treatment of burns in antiquity and an even smaller number referring to Roman and Greek antiquity was found. Interestingly, animal products have been a main source for the local treatment of burns. In early antiquity, Egyptians used goats milk and milk from women who had given birth to a son [1]. It has been shown in recent literature that milk not only has antibacterial and antiviral properties but also pro-regenerative capacity [2–4]. This might have been the observation in early antiquity leading to the long tradition in Roman antiquity, middle ages and modern times of using milk and derived products like butter or oil for the treatment of wounds in general. According to modern knowledge, fresh milk in particular has a bactericidal and antiseptic effect due to the milk compounds lactoferrin and β-casein [2,5–7].

The earliest account of using parts of a dead animal is recorded in the Papyrus of Ebers 1500 BC, by using a warmed frog in oil and rubbed onto a burned surface [8]. Around 430 BC, Hippocrates reported using pig lard as a treatment option for burns and referred to a better appearance of scars [9] (p. 367 et sqq.):

> *To soften you must employ the following medications–more so in winter than in summer–medications for softening, which also make the scars neat. Pound this internal pulpy material of the squill, or pine bark with fresh lard, squill and a little olive oil. Whitest wax and fresh clean grease. Or squill white olive oil, verdigris, squill and resin: let there be two parts of the aged lard and of the other components as much as seems appropriate. Melt fresh grease, pour it off into another cup, grind galena very fine, sift, mix the two together and boil stirring at first; boil until when dripped on to the shavings of nettle-tree wood and red ochre: anoint with this, then boil leaves of cuckoo-pint in wine and olive oil, appl them to the burn and bind them in place with a bandage.*

Already in Egyptian literature, the treatment of burns with honey and grease was documented on the Papyrus Edwin Smith around 1500 BC [10] (see Figure 1). In ancient Greece, honey (known as "nectar of Gods") was also mixed with vinegar, alum, sodium, carbonate and bile. This was known as *enheme*—to desiccate a wound and prevent suppuration [11]. Celsus, around 30 AD, proposed honey combined with bran as a topical remedy for burn wounds. The *Materia Medica* by Pedanios Dioscurides, a Greek physician in the Roman army, consists of five books, and is considered the most important and influential ancient work on medicines (origin see Figure 1). Dioscorides designated honey as the treatment of choice for the treatment of rotten and hollow ulcers [12] (bk.1). He recommended to change the dressings on a frequent basis. Interestingly, indigenous people of Australia and the Americas also used honey as a treatment for wounds. Today, it is scientifically acknowledged that honey, with its antibacterial properties—mostly through its glucose oxidase, methylglyoxal and bee defensin-1, anti-inflammatory, antioxidant and pro-regenerative capacity, reduces infections on burns and accelerates the healing [13,14].

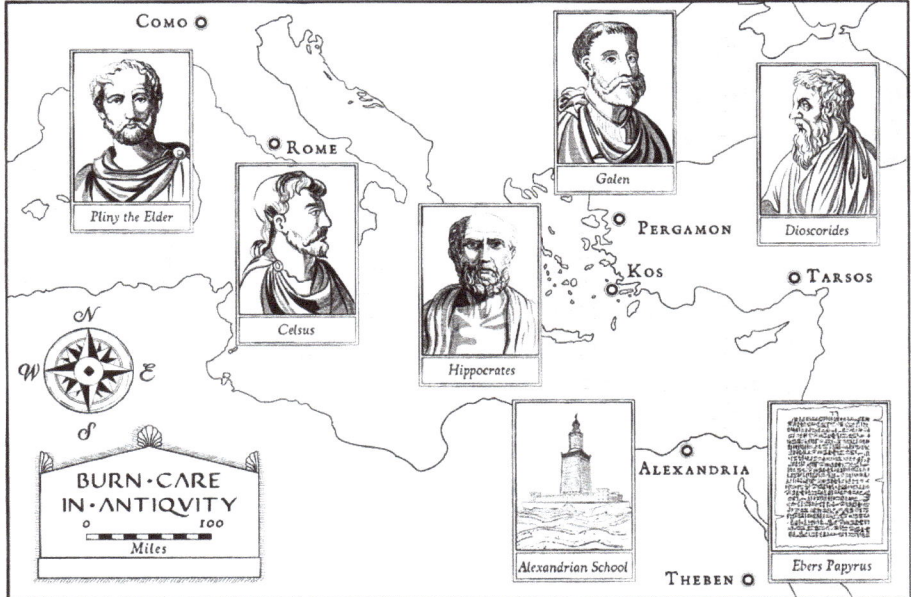

Figure 1. Origin of the various sources for the treatment of burns in ancient times: The Ebers Papyrus is one of the earliest medical records ever (1500 BC) and already contains the treatment of burns. While Hippocrates was active in ancient Greece around 400 BC, in Hellenism, the scientific elite gathered in the Alexandrian School at the mouth of the Nile. In the early Roman Empire, Pliny the Elder, Disorides, and Celsus had a major impact on medical progress. Around 150 AD, Galen led another surge in medical research. All of them contributed substantially to the treatment of burns.

Dioscorides wrote about using a conch shell and burned leather from shoes as treatments for burn wounds [12] (bk.2; paragraph 8/51):

The roasted trumpet snails, they are even more caustic. If you burn them in a raw pot filled with salt, they make a good means for brushing your teeth and as a poultice for burns. But you have to let the remedy burn as hard as a broken glass; after the burn wound has scarred, it falls off by itself.

The leather of old shoe soles, burned and finely pounded, heals as Envelope burns, decubitus and the pressure of shoes caused inflammation.

He also wrote down various recipes of cattle droppings for the treatment of purulent burns. This has been used in conjunction with rose oil and honey for inflamed burn wounds [12] (bk.2; paragraph 98). At this point, it must be mentioned that many substances have been tried that, from today's perspective, have a negative effect on wound treatment; however, in combination with antiseptic substances such as rose oil or honey, these ingredients were wrongly identified as good wound topicals. Interestingly, cow dung was identified to be antiseptic through its methanol, hydro alcohol and aqueous compounds [15].

1.2. Plant-Based Products

Around the year 3000 BC, an unknown Sumerian physician documented several plant-based remedies. The Papyrus of Ebers described, around 1500 BC, the topical application of lemon stripes on burn wounds. A new insight revitalizes the findings of Hippocrates that suggest vinegar is an effective treatment of burns to avoid infection. Acetic acid is capable of treating particularly pseudomonal wound infections and can break down biofilms [16,17]. Hippocrates was also known to use red wine with similar effects to treat burn wounds [9] (p. 367 et sqq.). In the first century AD, Celsus described the use of wine and myrrh as a burn lotion, which is known to have bacteriostatic properties [18]. Celsus also commented on inflammation in his book *De medicina* [19] (bk.5; Chapter 2):

> *The following subdue inflammation: alum, both split alum called schiston, and alum brine; quince oil, orpiment, verdigris, copper ore, blacking.*

Today, myrrh is scientifically proven to treat complicated wounds and ulcers, especially in very moist wounds. It is similarly effective against most Gram-negative strains, Gram-positive strains and even yeast compared to modern antibiotics [20]. In 430 BC, Hippocrates used bitumen mixed with resin to treat advanced cases of burns. It has been shown that resin of certain plants leads to increased angiogenesis in an animal burn study [21]. Resin of most plants is antibacterial as it is well known to interfere with reproduction of parasitic microbes. E. faecalis was most sensitive and S. typhi was resistant to *myrrh*. The extracts of O. turpethum were active against all tested strains in which B. subtilis and S. aureus were the most sensitive [22].

With the Roman expansion, the treatment of war injuries attracted the interest of many physician. Gaius Plinius Secundus recommends using garlic (raw or cooked) onto burn wounds, as the alliin contained in it, later discovered, has an antibiotic effect (Plinius, XX, 51: Suspiriosis coctum, aliqui crudum id dedere).

Dioscorides alluded that oil from the immature *Olea europaea* called *Omphakion* can be used as an ointment and heals wounds. Recent studies showed increased wound contraction and wound tensile strength when treated with extracts of *Olea europaea* [23]. In modern day studies, olive oil exhibited substantial wound healing efficacy in chronic wounds [24]. However, the antimicrobial capacity is limited [25]. Dioscorides also reported using incense *Boswellia sacra* or *Asphodelus racemosusin* in multiple ways and was one of the first to mention frostbites [12] (bk.1; paragraph 81) [12] (bk.2; paragraph 199):

> *It has the power to warm up, to astringent, to drive away the darkenings on the pupils, to fill in the hollow areas of the wounds and to scar them, to glue up bloody wounds, to hold back all blood flow, including that from the brain. Rubbed and spread on charpie with milk, it soothes the malignant ulcers around the anus and the other parts; In the beginning, spreading it with vinegar and pitch, it drives away the warts and lichen. With pork or goose lard he also heals burned-out ulcers and frost damage. He cures bad grind together with nitrum (soda), paronychia with honey, bruised ears spread with pitch, against the other ear complaints he helps with sweet wine. It heals inflammation of the breasts from birth as an ointment with cimolic earth and rose oil.*

> *If oil (Asphodelus racemosusin) is heated in a fire in the hollowed-out roots, it helps with burns and ulcerated chilblains . . .*

After the burnout of wounds developed its long tradition in the Roman army, the treatment of burned-out wounds was described in the texts accordingly. Dioscorides wrote about treating burned-out wounds with bark from the pine [12] (bk.1; paragraph 86), which contains antiseptic alkaloids, as modern research has shown [26,27]:

> *The pine is a well-known tree; that belongs to the same species spruce, which is different in appearance from it.*

> *The bark of both is contracting; when sprinkled on top of it, it is a good remedy for Wolf, and likewise with black lead and manna for granulation growths and burned-out wounds.*

However, he also writes clearly about burns and their treatment with grinded blossoms of the *Cistus creticus* and pickled olives to avoid blistering with [12] (bk.1; paragraph 126/138):

For themselves as an envelope, they hold up eating ulcers. With wax ointment, they heal burns and old wounds.

Canned, finely pounded olives are used as a poultice for burns with fire, preventing blistering and cleaning dirty wounds.

He also differentiated superficial and deep burn wounds and suggests to put fig together barley flour onto sun burns [12] (bk.1; paragraph 183). Barley flour might have antiseptic and wound healing properties due to a high level of antioxidants [28].

1.3. Chemical Products

Without knowing about germ theory, silver was used in ancient folklore medicine. Silver was used for water storage and water disinfection [29]. In 350 BC, Alexander the Great only drank water from silver vessels. When a more precise definition of the wounds was lacking, silver nitrate was used by Roman physicians as a remedy [29,30]. It has not yet been proven whether this was also used for burns. Silver is shown to be highly effective against Pseudomonas, Streptococcus and Staphylococcus [30]. Due to the introduction of silver sulfadiazine in the 1960s, silver was the standard topical antimicrobial for burn wounds for decades. In the past decade, however, silver sulfadiazine has been superseded by other more effective agents [31,32].

Dioscorides mixed sulfur together with Carthamus corymbosus to avoid spots of sunburns [12] (bk.3; paragraph 9). He also described how the Phyrigian stone was applied to the wound to remove eschar and was combined with wax ointment to heal burn wounds [12] (bk.5; paragraph 140).

1.4. Aspects of Patient Care

Hippocrates mentioned the importance of aseptic conditions when treating burn wounds as well as the proper supply of fluids per os diluted with honey. He also described septicemia after burn injury [9] (p. 367 et sqq.):

In this condition acute fever and increased pulse rate occurred" ... "In major burns, spasm or tetanus are poor prognostic signs" ... "Rigors with delirium lead to death."

For analgesia and wound cleaning, Hippocrates applied sea water to the wound. It is also described that he used red wine to clean the wound. As described before, Hippocrates and Galen used vinegar for antiseptic burn treatment, but its evaporation and cooling effect was an effective local analectic [1]. Celsus documented the use of various analgesic plants, including poppy seeds with the alkaloids morphine, codeine, and papaverine they contain. Overdose was described by Gaius Plinius Secundus and Dioscorides [33] (bk.20; p. 198 et sqq.). Analgesics for operations performed at the time may also have been used to treat burns. These include hemp, deadly nightshade and mandrake [12] (bk.4; 69 et sqq.). In modern anesthesia and consequently burn medicine, opioids have become as indispensable as strong analgesics. Synthetic derivatives of morphine, such as sufentanil, are used in everyday operations and anesthesiology. In 2018, 388.2 tons of morphine was produced and either consumed or processed into derivatives; 1.5 tons of fentanyl, which is about 100 times stronger than morphine, was consumed in 2018 [34] (p. 30).

In his fifth book *De Medicina*, Celsus explained the differentiation and properties of different debris associated with inflammation and the application of vinegar [19] (bk.5, Chapter 26). He also mentioned the surgical excision of contracted scars in burn wounds [19] (bk.5, Chapter 26).

Dioscorides had also referred to pediatric burn injuries and developed recipes specifically for children [12] (bk.4; paragraph 71):

(Solanum nigrum) ... spread with rose ointment, it is a good remedy for children who suffer from sunburn.

Celsus provided the first description of the four cardinal signs of inflammation "rubor", "calor", "tumor" and "dolor", which are applicable for burn wounds too. Galen of Pergamon added the "functio laesa" around 150 AD.

1.5. Summa Summarum

Through our review of modern literature on ancient Mediterranean medicine, we found a lot of cross-referencing with a small number of reliable translations. Some descriptions only mention a spiritual or alternative medical therapy of burns in this time period [35]. The translation of ancient texts could shed new light on the treatment of burns in ancient times with a huge variety of strategies to treat burn wounds, to control infections but also to treat the patient during a burn-associated shock. Ancient medicine has to be viewed in the context of non-written, passed down and thus actually non-existent medicine, before the transition of medicine into the Middle Ages happened with the accompanying loss of established and successful therapies. Many of them, i.e., the medical honey, silver and plant extracts, have been reintroduced into modern evidence-based medicine in the past 100 years.

We assume that ancient Greek medicine developed based on observation and so, for the first time in history, it represents evidence-based medicine. There seem to be many references to local therapeutics with little religious reference, whereas in ancient Egypt, gods were mostly invoked and therapeutics were used generically.

However, when translating Dioscorides Materia medica, it can be seen that some recommended recipes (using ingredients that are today identified as harmful like livestock manure) were only able to work together with other antiseptic ingredients, for example, rose oil.

Interestingly, the clinical pictures and applications vary from the Greek sources described as everyday injuries to the military medicine described in the Roman sources. This is elucidated, for example, through the burning out of gunshot wounds and their treatment as well as frostbites, which were described in the Caesarean Germanic or British wars. Thousands of years later, the First and Second World Wars in particular, significantly revolutionized wound treatment through innovations such as penicillin, modern surgery and anesthesia.

1.6. Legacy of the Ancient World

In the centuries that followed, it was not only a lack of development in the treatment of burns that happened but also a retrograde doctrine took place assuming that suppuration was essential and helpful to healing, as proposed by Galen. Avicenna also propagated the pre-Hippocratic aphorism that diseases that cannot be cured by iron are cured by fire. It took as long as until the late Middle Ages until medical professionals as barbers reintroduced the principles of Hippocrates' "antiseptic" treatment of burns [36]. Despite modern medical research, burn medicine is facing new challenges such as multi-drug resistant microbes and, in view of the increasing comorbidities, wounds that are difficult to treat. Today's burn medicine is rediscovering ancient recipes to face these challenges.

2. Conclusions

In summary, ancient medicine gave birth to scientific thinking and acted as the beginning of evidence-based medicine. There was a lively exchange and correspondence between the different schools. The meetings between active physicians in centers (e.g., Alexandria) as well as the adoption of concepts over generations in the whole Mediterranean area is documented [37]. Burn medicine stands, pars pro toto, for the development, testing and application of this newly emerging thinking. Unlike before, the favor of the gods was no longer relied on in curing various diseases, but observations of nature were implemented and further developed in the context of critical assessment for a successful medical treatment.

Author Contributions: Conceptualization, C.W., P.L., and E.M.; methodology, C.W.; validation, C.W., E.M., B.B., M.D., M.L. and P.L.; formal analysis; investigation, C.W., P.L., E.M.; resources, C.W., M.L., P.L., E.M.; data curation, C.W., M.D.; writing—original draft preparation, C.W., E.M., B.B., M.D., M.L. and P.L.; writing—review and editing, C.W., E.M., B.B., M.D., M.L. and P.L.; visualization, C.W.; supervision, C.W.; project administration, C.W. All authors have read and agreed to the published version of the manuscript.

Funding: This research received no external funding.

Acknowledgments: We thank Ira Vershina for the illustration (Figure 1).

Conflicts of Interest: The authors declare no conflict of interest.

References

1. Pinnegar, M.D.; Pinnegar, F.C. History of burn care. *Burns* **1986**, *12*, 508–517. Available online: https://linkinghub.elsevier.com/retrieve/pii/0305417986900793. [CrossRef]
2. Florisa, R.; Recio, I.; Berkhout, B.; Visser, S. Antibacterial and Antiviral Effects of Milk Proteins and Derivatives Thereof. *Curr. Pharm. Des.* **2003**, *9*, 1257–1275. Available online: http://www.eurekaselect.com/openurl/content.php?genre=article&issn=1381-6128&volume=9&issue=16&spage=1257 (accessed on 18 October 2020). [CrossRef] [PubMed]
3. Zimecki, M.; Artym, J. [Therapeutic properties of proteins and peptides from colostrum and milk]. *Postepy Hig. Med. Dosw.* **2005**, *59*, 309–323. Available online: http://www.ncbi.nlm.nih.gov/pubmed/15995598 (accessed on 15 October 2020).
4. Dalli, J.; Chiang, N.; Serhan, C.N. Identification of 14-series sulfido-conjugated mediators that promote resolution of infection and organ protection. *Proc. Natl. Acad. Sci. USA* **2014**, *111*, E4753–E4761. [CrossRef] [PubMed]
5. Ohashi, A.; Murata, E.; Yamamoto, K.; Majima, E.; Sano, E.; Le, Q.; Katunuma, N. New functions of lactoferrin and β-casein in mammalian milk as cysteine protease inhibitors. Biochem. *Biophys. Res. Commun.* **2003**, *306*, 98–103. [CrossRef]
6. Hanssen, F.S. The bactericidal property of milk. *Br. J. Exp. Pathol.* **1924**, *5*, 271.
7. Harati, K.; Behr, B.; Wallner, C.; Daigeler, A.; Hirsch, T.; Jacobsen, F.; Renner, M.; Harati, A.; Lehnhardt, M.; Becerikli, M. Anti-proliferative activity of epigallocatechin-3-gallate and silibinin on soft tissue sarcoma cells. *Mol. Med. Rep.* **2017**, *15*, 103–110. [CrossRef]
8. Ebers, G. Papyros Ebers: Das Hermetische Buch über die Arzneimittel der alten Ägypter in hieratischer Schrift. Available online: https://digi.ub.uni-heidelberg.de/diglit/ebers1875bd2/0001 (accessed on 15 October 2020).
9. Potter, P. *Hippocrates Volume 8*; Harvard University Press: Cambridge, UK, 1995.
10. von Deines, H.; Grapow, H. *Grundriss der Medizin der alten Ägypter*; Akademie: Berlin, Germany, 1959.
11. Rogalska, T. Healing the Bee's Knees—On Honey and Wound Healing. *JAMA Dermatol.* **2016**, *152*, 275. [CrossRef]
12. Dioscorides, P. De Materia Medica. Available online: https://www.wdl.org/en/item/10632/ (accessed on 15 October 2020).
13. Yaghoobi, R.; Kazerouni, A.; Kazerouni, O. Evidence for Clinical Use of Honey in Wound Healing as an Anti-bacterial, Anti-inflammatory Anti-oxidant and Anti-viral Agent: A Review. *Jundishapur J. Nat. Pharm. Prod.* **2013**, *8*, 100–104. Available online: http://www.ncbi.nlm.nih.gov/pubmed/24624197 (accessed on 15 October 2020). [CrossRef]
14. Kwakman, P.H.S.; Zaat, S.A.J. Antibacterial components of honey. *IUBMB Life* **2012**, *64*, 48–55. [CrossRef]
15. Thenmozhi, S.; Mageswari, M.; Chinnamani, S. Antimicrobial activity of animal waste (Cow dung). *World J. Sci. Res.* **2018**, *3*, 37–41.
16. Nagoba, B.S.; Selkar, S.P.; Wadher, B.J.; Gandhi, R.C. Acetic acid treatment of pseudomonal wound infections—A review. *J. Infect. Public Health* **2013**, *6*, 410–415. Available online: https://linkinghub.elsevier.com/retrieve/pii/S1876034113000956 (accessed on 15 October 2020). [CrossRef] [PubMed]
17. Youn, C.K.; Jun, Y.; Jo, E.-R.; Jang, S.-J.; Song, H.; I Cho, S. Comparative efficacies of topical antiseptic eardrops against biofilms from methicillin-resistant Staphylococcus aureus and quinolone-resistant Pseudomonas aeruginosa. *J. Laryngol. Otol.* **2018**, *132*, 519–522. Available online: https://www.cambridge.org/core/product/identifier/S0022215118000932/type/journal_article (accessed on 15 October 2020). [CrossRef] [PubMed]

18. Majno, G. *The Healing Hand: Man and Wound in the Ancient World*; Harvard University Press: Cambridge, MA, USA, 1991.
19. Celsus, A.C. De Medicina. Available online: https://www.amazon.com/Medicina-Latin-Celsus/dp/3849671410 (accessed on 15 October 2020).
20. Elzayat, E.M.; Auda, S.H.; Alanazi, F.K.; Al-Agamy, M.H. Evaluation of wound healing activity of henna, pomegranate and myrrh herbal ointment blend. *Saudi Pharm. J.* **2018**, *26*, 733–738. Available online: https://linkinghub.elsevier.com/retrieve/pii/S1319016418300409 (accessed on 17 October 2020). [CrossRef]
21. Haghdoost, F.; Mahdavi, M.M.B.; Zandifar, A.; Sanei, M.H.; Zolfaghari, B.; Javanmard, S.H. Pistacia atlantica Resin Has a Dose-Dependent Effect on Angiogenesis and Skin Burn Wound Healing in Rat. Evidence-Based Complement. *Altern. Med.* **2013**, *2013*, 1–8. Available online: http://www.hindawi.com/journals/ecam/2013/893425/ (accessed on 25 October 2020).
22. Shuaib, M.; Ali, A.; Ali, M.; Panda, B.P.; Ahmad, M.I. Antibacterial activity of resin rich plant extracts. *J. Pharm. Bioallied Sci.* **2013**, *5*, 265. Available online: http://www.jpbsonline.org/text.asp?2013/5/4/265/120073 (accessed on 17 October 2020). [CrossRef]
23. Koca-Caliskan, U.; Süntar, I.; Akkol, E.K.; Yilmazer, D.; Alper, M.; Yılmazer, D. Wound Repair Potential of Olea europaea L. Leaf Extracts Revealed by In Vivo Experimental Models and Comparative Evaluation of the Extracts' Antioxidant Activity. *J. Med. Food* **2011**, *14*, 140–146. [CrossRef]
24. Vitsos, A.; Tsagarousianos, C.; Vergos, O.; Stithos, D.; Mathioudakis, D.; Vitsos, I.; Zouni, P.; Kakolyri, A.; Loupa, C.V.; Kyriazi, M.; et al. Efficacy of a Ceratothoa oestroides Olive Oil Extract in Patients With Chronic Ulcers: A Pilot Study. *Int. J. Low. Extrem. Wounds* **2019**, *18*, 309–316. [CrossRef]
25. Warnke, P.H.; Lott, A.J.; Sherry, E.; Wiltfang, J.; Podschun, R. The ongoing battle against multi-resistant strains: In-vitro inhibition of hospital-acquired MRSA, VRE, Pseudomonas, ESBL *E. coli* and Klebsiella species in the presence of plant-derived antiseptic oils. *J. Cranio Maxillofacial Surg.* **2013**, *41*, 321–326. Available online: https://linkinghub.elsevier.com/retrieve/pii/S1010518212002272 (accessed on 17 October 2020). [CrossRef]
26. De Armas, E.; Sarracent, Y.; Marrero, E.; Fernández, O.; Branford-White, C. Efficacy of Rhizophora mangle aqueous bark extract (RMABE) in the treatment of aphthous ulcers: A pilot study. *Curr. Med. Res. Opin.* **2005**, *21*, 1711–1715. [CrossRef]
27. Gonzales, M.V.M.; Tolentino, A.G. Extraction and isolation of the alkaloids from the Samanea saman (Acacia) bark: Its antiseptic potential. *IInternational J. Sci. Technol. Res.* **2014**, *3*, 119–124.
28. Holtekjølen, A.; Bævre, A.; Rødbotten, M.; Berg, H.; Knutsen, S.H. Antioxidant properties and sensory profiles of breads containing barley flour. *Food Chem.* **2008**, *110*, 414–421. [CrossRef] [PubMed]
29. Melaiye, A.; Youngs, W.J. Silver and its application as an antimicrobial agent. *Expert Opin. Ther. Pat.* **2005**, *15*, 125–130. [CrossRef]
30. White, R.J. An historical overview of the use of silver in wound management. *Br. J. Community Nurs.* **2001**, *6*, 3–8. [CrossRef]
31. Heyneman, A.; Hoeksema, H.; Vandekerckhove, D.; Pirayesh, A.; Monstrey, S. The role of silver sulphadiazine in the conservative treatment of partial thickness burn wounds: A systematic review. *Burns* **2016**, *42*, 1377–1386. Available online: http://www.ncbi.nlm.nih.gov/pubmed/27126813 (accessed on 25 October 2020). [CrossRef]
32. Wasiak, J.; Cleland, H.; Campbell, F.; Spinks, A. Dressings for superficial and partial thickness burns. *Cochrane Database Syst. Rev.* **2013**. Available online: http://www.ncbi.nlm.nih.gov/pubmed/23543513 (accessed on 25 October 2020). [CrossRef]
33. Schnell, A.; Hoffleit, D.; Waelkens, C.; Winter, T.N.; Achar, N.; Efremov, Y.N.; Davenhall, A.C.; Elliott, I.; Pawsey, S.F.; Haramundanis, K.; et al. Plinius Secundus. *Biogr. Encycl. Astron.* **2007**, *XX.* 77AD, 916. [CrossRef]
34. United Nations. *Narcotic Drugs Estimated World Requirements for 2020 Statistics for 2018*; United Nations: New York, NY, USA, 2019. Available online: https://www.incb.org/documents/Narcotic-Drugs/Technical-Publications/2019/Narcotic_Drugs_Technical_Publication_2019_web.pdf (accessed on 25 October 2020).
35. Hussain, A.; Choukairi, F. To cool or not to cool: Evolution of the treatment of burns in the 18th century. *Int. J. Surg.* **2013**, *11*, 503–506. Available online: https://linkinghub.elsevier.com/retrieve/pii/S1743919113001076 (accessed on 25 October 2020). [CrossRef]

36. Polycratis, G.S. Conclusions on Hippocratic Behaviour in the Treatment of Wounds and Burns. 1987. Available online: http://www.medbc.com/annals/review/vol_1/num_1/text/vol1n1p9.htm (accessed on 30 September 2020).
37. Blumenthal, H. Alexandria as a Centre of Greek Philosophy in Later Classical Antiquity. *Ill. Classic. Stud.* **1993**, *18*, 307–325. Available online: http://www.jstor.org/stable/23064453 (accessed on 25 October 2020).

Publisher's Note: MDPI stays neutral with regard to jurisdictional claims in published maps and institutional affiliations.

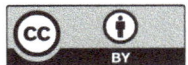

© 2020 by the authors. Licensee MDPI, Basel, Switzerland. This article is an open access article distributed under the terms and conditions of the Creative Commons Attribution (CC BY) license (http://creativecommons.org/licenses/by/4.0/).

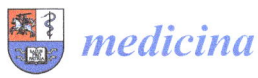

Review

Technical and Medical Aspects of Burn Size Assessment and Documentation

Michael Giretzlehner [1,*], Isabell Ganitzer [1] and Herbert Haller [2]

[1] Research Unit for Medical Informatics, RISC Software GmbH, Johannes Kepler University Linz, Upper Austrian Research GmbH, A-4232 Hagenberg, Austria; isabell.ganitzer@risc-software.at
[2] Trauma Hospital Berlin, Trauma Hospital Linz (ret), HLMedConsult, A-4020 Leonding, Austria; herberthaller@gmail.com
* Correspondence: michael.giretzlehner@risc.uni-linz.ac.at

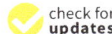

Citation: Giretzlehner, M.; Ganitzer, I.; Haller, H. Technical and Medical Aspects of Burn Size Assessment and Documentation. *Medicina* 2021, 57, 242. https://doi.org/10.3390/medicina57030242

Academic Editor: Edgaras Stankevičius

Received: 28 December 2020
Accepted: 2 March 2021
Published: 5 March 2021

Publisher's Note: MDPI stays neutral with regard to jurisdictional claims in published maps and institutional affiliations.

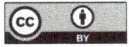

Copyright: © 2021 by the authors. Licensee MDPI, Basel, Switzerland. This article is an open access article distributed under the terms and conditions of the Creative Commons Attribution (CC BY) license (https://creativecommons.org/licenses/by/4.0/).

Abstract: In burn medicine, the percentage of the burned body surface area (TBSA-B) to the total body surface area (TBSA) is a crucial parameter to ensure adequate treatment and therapy. Inaccurate estimations of the burn extent can lead to wrong medical decisions resulting in considerable consequences for patients. These include, for instance, over-resuscitation, complications due to fluid aggregation from burn edema, or non-optimal distribution of patients. Due to the frequent inaccurate TBSA-B estimation in practice, objective methods allowing for precise assessments are required. Over time, various methods have been established whose development has been influenced by contemporary technical standards. This article provides an overview of the history of burn size estimation and describes existing methods with a critical view of their benefits and limitations. Traditional methods that are still of great practical relevance were developed from the middle of the 20th century. These include the "Lund Browder Chart", the "Rule of Nines", and the "Rule of Palms". These methods have in common that they assume specific values for different body parts' surface as a proportion of the TBSA. Due to the missing consideration of differences regarding sex, age, weight, height, and body shape, these methods have practical limitations. Due to intensive medical research, it has been possible to develop three-dimensional computer-based systems that consider patients' body characteristics and allow a very realistic burn size assessment. To ensure high-quality burn treatment, comprehensive documentation of the treatment process, and wound healing is essential. Although traditional paper-based documentation is still used in practice, it no longer meets modern requirements. Instead, adequate documentation is ensured by electronic documentation systems. An illustrative software already being used worldwide is "BurnCase 3D". It allows for an accurate burn size assessment and a complete medical documentation.

Keywords: burn size assessment; three-dimensional; estimation accuracy; medical documentation; consequences of inaccurate assessment

1. Introduction

An accurate assessment of both the burn depth and the burn extent is essential for adequate and successful treatment. In order to determine the burn depth, German-speaking countries differentiate between so-called burn degrees correlating with an increasing depth of a burn of the skin [1,2]:

"First-Degree" burns affect the epidermis and lead to redness and severe pain but do not cause cell death.

"Second-Degree" burns are distinguished between "second-degree superficial" (2a) and "second-degree deep" (2b). Whereas the first type involves damage to the epidermis and the superficial dermis, with blisters, a rosy and recapillarizing wound base, severe pain, and firmly anchored hair, the second type is characterized by injuries to the deep dermis and skin appendages. The wound is comparatively pale and has little or no recapillarization, and the pain receptors are partially destroyed, the pain perception of the patient is reduced, and the hairs are easy to remove.

"Third-Degree" burns lead to complete epidermal and dermal destruction and are accompanied by hair absence and a dry, white, leathery hard wound base without pain.

Historically, a "fourth-degree" burn was also distinguished. In this type of burn, charring occurs, and in addition to the epidermis and dermis, other layers are destroyed, such as the subcutaneous fatty tissue, muscles, tendons, bones, or joints.

In comparison, English-speaking countries classify the burn depth into "superficial", "superficial partial thickness" burn (equal to second-degree superficial), "deep partial thickness" burn (equal to second-degree deep), and "full thickness" burn (equal to a third-degree or fourth-degree) [2]. Clinical evaluations are never reliable, and "the accuracy of bedside depth assessment is widely considered to be far from optimal" [3] (p. 762).

While in clinical practice, an assessment of burn depth based on these classifications tends to be difficult, a classification based on healing time is usually of higher practical value [3]. Usually, burns healing within one week are categorized as "first-degree" or "superficial" burns; those healing within two weeks are referred to as "second-degree superficial" or "superficial partial thickness" burns. If healing occurs within three weeks or more, the burns are classified as "second-degree deep" or "deep partial thickness" burns, while burns taking even longer to heal but still heal spontaneously from the skin's appendages are classified in the same group. "Full thickness" burns do not heal from regenerative tissue in the wound but the margins [3]. An exact classification of which burn degree correlates with healing time is not given. It is challenging to differentiate between partial deep or 2b burns and full thickness or third-degree burns.

As described above, in addition to the depth of a burn injury, the burn extent is the second important criterion to be assessed to determine adequate treatment methods. The latter is defined as the percentage of the burned body surface area (TBSA-B) to the total body surface area (TBSA), whereby first-degree burns are excluded. According to different studies, an accurate determination of the extent of a burn injury often proves to be challenging in practice. In most cases, TBSA-B is overestimated [2].

Although both burn depth and burn extent are important criteria in burn medicine, the scope of this paper is limited to the assessment and documentation of burn extent.

2. Consequences of Inaccurate TBSA-B Assessment

Inaccurate TBSA-B estimations can lead to considerable consequences. The most important ones are described in the following.

2.1. Over-Resuscitation

Underhill [4] first published the suggestion to treat burns with fluids intravenously in 1930. A significant advance in the shock treatment of burn injuries was achieved with feasible fluid resuscitation rules based on the "Parkland formula", also known as the "Baxter Parkland formula". Baxter and Shires proposed it in 1968 [5]. In 1979, a conference sponsored by the "National Institutes of Health" (NIH) was concluded with a recommendation to resuscitate burn patients with as little fluid as possible to maintain organ perfusion. Accordingly, the initial fluid therapy in the first 24 h should consist of isotonic crystalloid with a volume between 2 and 4 mL/kg/TBSA-B and should be titrated to ensure the urinary output of 30–50 mL/h [6].

Abdominal compartments drew attention because most burn centers used fluid volumes for resuscitation, some of which were significantly above the calculated 4 mL/kg/TBSA-B. Several possible reasons for this are described below.

First of all, there was a trend to optimizing resuscitation to "supranormal values" [7] (p. 416). Small fluid boluses were administered until the cardiac output stopped increasing. According to the motto "the more, the better", this procedure allowed the application of very high volumes. While the initial findings appeared promising, supranormal values did not yield improved results in a multicenter study [8]. Sympathetic activation by vasoconstrictive substances like catecholamine or angiotensin 2 raises central venous pressure (CVP) and releases arterial natriuretic peptide (ANP). Release appears in the early phase of the burn injury when pain increases blood pressure and triggers tachycardia. ANP mediates the "shredding" of the glycocalyx responsible for hindering vessels from leakage [9,10]. The application of additional fluid can aggravate the "shredding" [11]. Damage to the glycocalyx can cause capillary leakage, which later requires higher amounts of fluid [12]. Low volume and high volume responders could be identified after the first four hours. The difference started after two hours and remained unchanged [13]. Once initiated, "fluid begets more fluid" [12] (p. 234). Urinary control alone fails to hinder severe capillary leakage, as fluid goes into the interstitial tissue, which does not necessarily cause higher blood pressure or higher urine output. Friedrich et al. [14] demonstrated this, examining supra-Baxter resuscitation, and did not observe any difference in 24-h urine output between groups with high and low resuscitation volume. Similarly, Engrav et al. [15] found that there is no rise in average urine output despite increased fluid administration. Regan and Hotwagner [16] recommended the goal of 1 mL/kg per hour for pediatrics below 30 kg and 0.5 mL/kg per hour for those weighing more than 30 kg.

The initial overestimation of TBSA-B enhances all previous effects. Over-resuscitation due to overestimation frequently happens in the course of primary transport, when urine output is not measured, and it often occurs in emergency departments. Overestimation leads to over-resuscitation, and this contributes to capillary damage and edema. The consequences of burn edema can lead to severe complications, which cannot be reversed easily later.

2.2. Complications Because of Fluid Aggregation from Burn Edema

While frequently occurring consequences of burn edema, including pulmonary dysfunction and increased intraabdominal and intercompartmental complications, are well described [17], mortality resulting from high-volume resuscitation has not been scientifically proven. However, from abdominal compartments in burns, Strang et al. [18] described an average mortality rate of 74.8%. To the authors' best knowledge, local complications, such as reduced take rates of dermatomes, have not been investigated by adequate studies up to date, although it is common surgical knowledge [19]. However, it was proved that low volume resuscitation mitigates the probability of multiple organ dysfunction syndromes (MODS) and improves lung function in the early stages [20]. Besides, "suboptimal fluid resuscitation in burn patients leads to greater burn depth and extension of the shock period" [21] (p. 293).

2.3. Missing Accuracy in Studies

It is widely accepted that scientific approaches to burn treatment rely on an accurate TBSA-B assessment. Aiming at establishing standards for burn treatment, various international initiatives have been started. Without being exhaustive, these include, for example, the "One Burn One Standard" (OBOS) initiative of the "American Burn Association" (ABA) Committee for the "Organization and Delivery of Burn Care" (ODBC) [22], the "One World, One Burn Rehabilitation Standard" of the "International Society for Burn Injuries" (ISBI) [23], or the standardization initiatives of the German Society for Burn Medicine [1].

The need for standards has been well demonstrated, for example, in the study "Inflammation and the Host Response to Injury" [24]. The development of a standard operating procedure was considered relevant for the study to provide high-quality clinical outcome measures in burn treatment as a basis for further evaluation of genetic and proteomic alterations and their influence on inflammation [25]. As in other studies, the TBSA-B assessment in this study relies on the "Lund Browder Chart" and does not consider inherent errors such as over- and underestimation or inter-rater errors, i.e., two investigators estimating the size of one and the same burn differently. Even in an expert environment where TBSA-B assessments are carried out, the method's validity and error-based data are essential for further conclusions. As pointed out by Nichter et al. [26] and Wachtel et al. [27], an inter-rater error of 10% can affect the results and significance of studies. Errors like these can easily be avoided and modified using electronic media.

2.4. Non-Optimal Distribution of Patients

2.4.1. Distribution to Burn Centers

In deciding whether patients should be transferred to burn centers, the size of a burn injury is the most crucial factor. It is initially evaluated either preclinically or in the emergency room, in surroundings usually not accustomed to the burn treatment. In many cases it deviates significantly from the subsequent TBSA-B evaluation in a burn center [28,29]. Goverman et al. [30] showed that as a result of the initial burn assessment, 59% of pediatric patients of an average age of 4.1 years were given significantly more fluid than according to the later evaluation in the burn center would have been required. Furthermore, this study's authors reported an overestimation of burn size in 94% of all transferred children, with an average TBSA-B overestimation of 339% by referring hospitals. Reasons for this might be the lacking experience of non-trained medical personnel and the unavailability of special technical equipment [31,32]. Since the "Lund Browder Chart", which usually results in an overestimation of burn size, was the basis for the assessment, the reported overestimation rate might be higher. However, according to ABA rules, specific percentages of TBSA-B indicate patient transfers to burn centers; hence, an overestimation could result not only in excessive use of resources but also in avoidable costs for transportation [33].

2.4.2. Distribution of Patients in Mass Casualty Situations

In the case of mass casualty situations, the capacity utilization of burn centers is of crucial importance. Therefore, the distribution of burn patients needs to be carefully managed. Inaccurate burn size estimations can lead to non-optimal treatment decisions and complications. Failed distribution to burn centers can hinder treatment for those patients who urgently need it.

3. Methods for Burn Size Estimation

Due to the frequently occurring inaccurate estimation of the burn size in practice and the associated far-reaching consequences for patients and medical resources, objective methods allowing for a more accurate burn size assessment are required. Over time, various methods have been established, whose development has been influenced by contemporary technical standards. The following is an extract of burn size estimation history and shows methods proven in practice or with high practical potential. Figure 1 shows this extract of TBSA-B determination methods as a timeline.

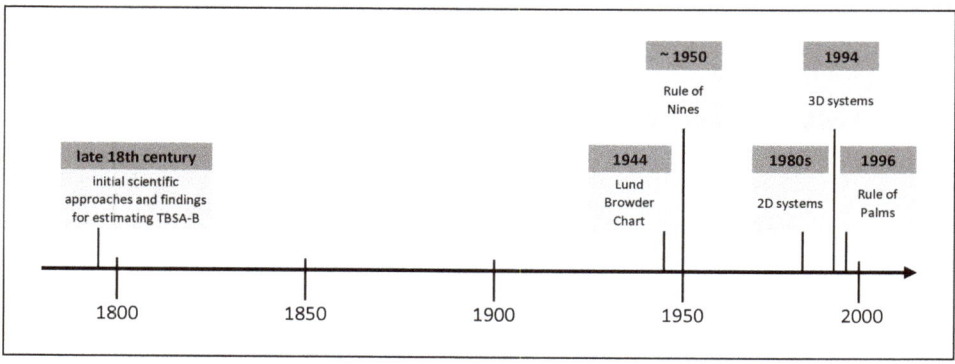

Figure 1. Timeline of methods for TBSA-B determination described in this article.

3.1. Initial Scientific Approaches and Findings for Estimating TBSA-B

Documented knowledge about the link between the severity of burns and the survival probability begun in Europe in the late 18th century with Richter's report in the year 1788. Schjerning gave a rough description of this connection in 1884. The correlation of burn size and mortality was questioned at that time, for example, by Liman [34]. Based on Meeh's calculations in 1879, Weidenfeld from the University of Vienna established a constant ratio of well-defined body areas to the TBSA. He defined the ratio as proportions and not yet as percentages. Besides, Weidenfeld demonstrated the correlation between burn size and time of early death [34]. Riehl confirmed these findings in 1925 [35].

Without being aware of the work by Weidenfeld, Berkow recalculated the surface area of the body parts of five people with different physiques according to Dubois and Dubois [36]. He observed a mean error rate of 15% in Meeh's calculations and reported an average error below 5% in his owns. Further, Berkow found that children's body proportions differ from those of adults and suggested to take this into account. He proposed to name the method of calculating burn size as a percentage of the TBSA according to Weidenfeld and himself, but this was rejected [34].

In 1942, the scientifically based burn treatment became the focus of national interest, not only due to the ongoing World War but also because of the "coconut grove nightclub disaster". A Burn Research Service was established at Boston City Hospital, and a "National Committee for Burn and Trauma Research" begun its work. TBSA-B determination and the feasibility of a high-quality method became increasingly important. Treating burn shock on the basis of TBSA-B was suggested at the "National Research Council Conference" in 1942 [34].

3.2. Lund Browder Chart

Two years later, in 1944, C.C. Lund and N.C. Browder [37] from Harvard Medical School published the so-called "Lund Browder Chart" to improve the calculation of body proportions and to reduce errors. This chart was based on Boyd's [38] surface area calculations. Lund and Browder defined clear boundaries of body regions and considered different proportions during human growth. Even though many authors have modified the "Lund Browder Chart" [39,40], it has remained in use in its original form until the present.

3.2.1. Description

The "Lund Browder Chart" illustrates the human body's front and back in a graphic model and assigns different body proportions to different age groups. It shows the boundaries of specific body regions for which different percentages of TBSA are defined. For the calculation procedure, an adapted planimetry is used. Even though the "Lund Browder Chart" does not differentiate depending on sex, weight, height, or body shape, many authors consider it "the most accurate" method [41] (p. 58).

3.2.2. Estimation Accuracy and Criticism

Several authors reported an overestimation of burn extent when using the "Lund Browder Chart". This could be due to the fact that it is based on just a single physique. Different weight categories and body shapes are not taken into account, nor are changes in body proportions between the respective age groups [41,42].

Additionally, in comparison with 3D methods, burn size assessments using the "Lund Browder Chart" result in severe overestimations [42]. Overestimations tend to be more significant in small burns and smaller in more extensive burns [43]. When using the "Lund Browder Chart", underestimation of the extent of a burn injury is comparatively rare. It is particularly likely to occur in the case of very extensive burns, as the assessor may tend to estimate the healthy skin areas rather than the burned ones [41].

Furthermore, the use of the "Lund Browder Chart" often leads to high inter-rater errors. Such differences between assessors evaluating the same burn are often related to different environments (e.g., accident and emergency departments, preclinical evaluations, and burn centers), where several errors may occur. In many studies, large differences were found [28,29,44,45], with most of the preclinical evaluations being compared with the evaluation results of the burn centers, which in turn relied on the "Lund Browder Chart".

The challenge in the evaluation of the "Lund Browder Chart" lies in comparing it with objective measurements. Although not objective either, the "gold standard" for comparisons is typically an experienced senior surgeon at a burn center. Computer-aided planimetry can only improve the percentage of burns in identified areas without calculating the actual extent since the projection error is inherent in this method. However, computerized techniques, such as 3D measurements and stereogrammetry, can be appropriate. Another way to evaluate burns is to use paper squares [41]. Klippel [46] expressed doubts regarding the validity of the "Lund Browder Chart" since it has not been validated and is based on rather old data.

3.3. Rule of Nines

Continuing with the history of burn size estimation, another method still used in practice is the so-called "Rule of Nines", originating from a discussion between friends Wallace and Pulaski in 1949. At a symposium of the "National Burns Research Council" in Washington in 1950, Pulaski presented a slide of the "Rule of Nines" based on a collaboration with Tennison, leading to the fact that most American authors consider these two to be the original authors of the rule [34].

3.3.1. Description

In his publication in 1951, Wallace [47] assumed for different body parts the following proportions of the TBSA: arms 9% of the TBSA each, legs 18% each, chest and back 18% each, head and face 9%, neck 1%, and genital area 1%. Like the "Lund Browder Chart", the "Rule of Nines" ignores differences in sex, weight, height, and body shapes.

3.3.2. Estimation Accuracy and Criticism

Initially, the "Rule of Nines" was meant for preclinical application in the event of disasters and mass casualties. When using this rule, the burn extent is overestimated in many cases [27,48]. For example, Giretzlehner et al. [49] reported a mean overestimation rate of 138% using the "Rule of Nines" and the "Lund Browder Chart". Furthermore, overestimation mostly occurs in patients with an increased body mass index (BMI). For patients weighing more than 80 kg, it is more promising to apply a "Rule of Fives", and below 10 kg to apply a "Rule of Eights" [50]. Disregarding different body shapes usually results in an overestimation of extremity burns and underestimating upper body burns [51]. In comparison to the results of 3D scans, the back and the torso of normal-weighted patients are overrepresented by the "Rule of Nines" [52]. Additionally, a high inter-rater error can be expected [42].

3.4. Rule of Palms

The "Rule of Palms" by Rossiter et al. [53] relies on the original "Lund Browder Chart". It can be applied either alone or in combination with other methods such as the "Lund Browder Chart" to estimate the TBSA-B of a specific body region.

3.4.1. Description

In its simplest form, the "Rule of Palms" states that the patient's hand's surface accounts for approximately 1% of the TBSA. Due to different understandings on whether the palm should be calculated including or excluding fingers, this rule is used inconsistently in practice [53]. It is mainly applied to measure the size of reasonably small burn injuries [34].

3.4.2. Estimation Accuracy and Criticism

Usually, the "Rule of Palms" results in an overestimation of the actual burn extent. Fundamental differences are depending on sex and age. Assuming normal BMI, the palm of a man represents an average of 0.81% and the palm of a woman 0.67% [53] of the TBSA. The isolated palm without fingers amounts to 0.52% for males and 0.43% for females [53]. In children aged between one and 13 years, the palm with fingers accounts for 0.92% and the palm without fingers for 0.52% on average [54].

The BMI influences the "Rule of Palms" since the palm's actual area does not change to the same extent as the TBSA with a BMI above 30 [55] in neither men nor women. Butz et al. [56] described the percentage of the palmar surface area of the TBSA depending on the BMI. In average weight persons with a BMI from 18.5 to 24.9, values between 0.87% and 0.91% in women and between 0.95% and 0.99% in men were reported. In persons with a BMI of 40 and higher, the values ranged between 0.67% and 0.70% for females and between 0.68% and 0.72% for males.

In the practical application of the "Rule of Palms", the degree of overestimation varies. For example, Hintermüller [31] found an average overestimation of 70.88% of the actual area, with seven wounds overestimated in the range from 41.55% to 173.08%. The "Rule of Palms" could be a reason for the substantial overestimation of up to 100% in the emergency departments as it was described by Laing et al. [57]. An explicit dependency on the specialization and grade of assessors in emergency departments was described. Estimations were between 7% and 133% too high, even though applying a "Lund Browder Chart", possibly due to the "Rule of Palms" to assist in "Lund Browder Chart" evaluation. Besides, Cone [58] described a mean overestimation rate of 75% when referring physicians. When combining the "Chinese Rule of Nines" with the "Rule of Palms", Sheng et al. [59] reported an overestimation in the range from 12% to 30% in 17 wounds evaluated by four surgeons.

Summing up, a palm does not result in exactly 1% of the TBSA. Not least because of the inaccurate definition and different usage in practice, a high overestimation rate can be expected when applying the "Rule of Palms". Furthermore, a low inter-rater reliability can be expected [42].

3.5. Two-Dimensional Computer-Aided Systems

In the course of technical advances, the development and implementation of IT-based systems started at the beginning of the 1980s. Wachtel et al. [60] and Nichter et al. [26] were among the first to employ electronic systems.

3.5.1. Description

Two-dimensional (2D) computer models rely on simple human body drawings on a computer screen. These models do not consider the human body's three-dimensionality, and in many applications, it is not possible to capture the lateral and other parts of the body. Moreover, 2D models usually do not depict individual differences in sex, weight, height, and body shape. Nevertheless, they are easy to handle but can only provide a rather rough overview of the burn type and the affected areas, particularly on the lateral parts of the body. In many cases, they miss the actual extent of the burned area.

The planimetry type can be distinguished between simple planimetry and adapted planimetry. While the former is related to a simple pixel count in a 2D image and is used in some electronic devices, the latter is a pixel count in a 2D image that is additionally corrected by a particular percentage recommended for a specific body region.

3.5.2. Sample Applications

An example of a 2D system is the smartphone application "Mersey Burns". The app was approved as a medical device by the "U.K. Medicines and Healthcare Regulatory Agency" [61,62], although the TBSA-B estimation error was not examined. The basis for the electronic calculations is a two-dimensional "Lund Browder Chart" [62].

Besides, "SAGE II" ("Surface Area Graphic Evaluation II") was developed by Parshley in 1987 and relies on an adapted planimetry of "Lund Browder". It uses 2D charts that can be adapted to age, weight, and height [63]. It is available online for free single evaluations or as a licensed version for multiple observations. Unfortunately, the web application is no longer running in modern web browsers. Other examples for adapted planimetry include the "Rule of Nines" [64], the "Rule of Fives" [51], the "Lund Browder Chart" [37], and related charts, and some computerized charts partly accommodated to the individual characteristics of the patient. Furthermore, most apps for smartphones rely on 2D calculations that are corrected by the percentages of "Lund Browder".

3.5.3. Quality of Estimation Reliability

In terms of estimation accuracy, 2D systems have the disadvantage that projection errors occur. When displaying a lateral burn, e.g., a burn in the lateral abdominal area, a 2D system would display the body in an anterior and posterior half. This results in a distortion and thus an incorrect calculation of the extent of the burn. Figure 2 shows an example where a quarter of the anterior trunk is affected. In the 2D perspective this would only be 0.25 of the body width. Using a 3D system, the same represents the arc length of 0.345, which is $\Delta = 27.54\%$ larger (Δ represents the difference in percentage).

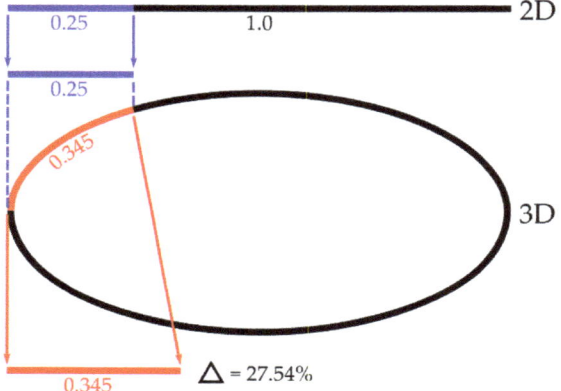

Figure 2. Comparison of 2D and 3D calculation of burned area.

3.6. Three-Dimensional Computer-Aided Systems

In 1994, Lee et al. were the first to develop and describe 3D (three-dimensional) systems [65,66]. The significant advantages of 3D models are the lateral areas' presence and the possibility of adapting to the patients' characteristics and better representing the real patient. Three-dimensional systems prevent the methodological error of reduction to a 2D drawing. Typically, 3D systems allow for an adaptation to sex, weight, height, and body shape. Available systems achieve a high validity in adults with a BMI below 30, but there are some limitations with very obese burn patients and unusual body proportions. The more accurate the model is, the more precise the adaptation to the individual body shape and body characteristics of the patient [67].

Systems based on individual measurements should provide an exact picture of the patient's body to be assessed, considering the individual body characteristics. A precise 3D scan appears to be a complete individual and accurate 3D model. However, due to the time-consuming process, they were mainly applied in studies, having deficiencies, and showing other methods' weaknesses [68].

Model-based systems use models that are modified to sex, height, weight, age, and body shape. Based on the measurements, the model is selected from a library either by the user or partially or fully computer-aided. As far as the computer system allows, the model is then adapted to the individual characteristics.

3.6.1. Three-Dimensional Images

3D images, together with a size objectification (e.g., a ruler, a fixed distance between photos, or a grid pattern [69]) have a high potential to accurately assess the extent of burns, particularly of small ones. Since the values are expressed in square centimeters, calculating the TBSA-B percentage requires a TBSA estimation formula. Therefore, this method is only suitable for small burn injuries [70].

3.6.2. Three-Dimensional Scans

Three-dimensional scans provide a good support to accurately determine TBSA-B since once calibrated, these systems indicate an area's absolute size.

Partial scans: One field of application of partial scans is the production of compression devices, e.g., for the head. The 3D scan of the face and scars replaces the traditional plaster cast method. 3D printers can produce compression devices. Unique algorithms must determine the degree of compression.

Total scans: In the case of burn injuries or unusual body proportions, the 3D scan requires a full body scan of each aspect. Since a scan is only able to determine the body surface, scans of the armpit, perineum, and others are also required. Thus, an average of eight scans is needed to precisely reconstruct a body [71]. The individual scans have to be combined into one whole-body scan image that requires evaluating the composition procedure. Three-dimensional scans from point clouds need to be stored in a model to evaluate changes on the surface. All surface points can be tracked over the timeline.

So far, no useful 3D scan has been published for whole-body scans in the context of burn injuries. "BurnCalc" shows the accuracy of 3D scans but does not indicate their application in the case of patients under ventilation and sedation. The storage in a point cloud does not track a specific spot of the surface over different scans [59].

3.6.3. Sample Applications

"3D Burn Vision" is a software (V1.0, University of Chicago, Chicago, CA, USA) developed at the University of Chicago and was sponsored by the EPRI ("Electric Power Research Institute", Washington, DC, USA). It offered many advanced functionalities, such as adapting to the individual body characteristics of the patient. It allowed for zoom and rotation, had a morph function, joints could be moved, the results could be stored in an electronic database and it enabled multiple observations [63]. "3D Burn Vision" allowed for a documentation of burn degrees and the area of allografts and autografts. Several use concepts could not be realized due to funding [42].

The research project "BurnCase 3D" allows for 3D registration and documentation of burn patients. It was initiated as a student project in the year 2001 and is currently operated by RISC Software GmbH (V2.6, RISC Software GmbH, Hagenberg, Austria) that is 80% a subsidiary of the Johannes Kepler University in Linz and 20% owned by Upper Austrian Research. For an annual fee, members can use the full functionality, influence the ongoing project and receive support. The software and database run on modern Windows versions and can be used as a standalone version or as a server with multiple clients serving different departments or even hospital networks.

The development of "BurnCase 3D" was supported by numerous medical partners. It is the basis for implementing a new software framework for application-oriented research in the documentation and treatment of burns. This framework is being developed within the ongoing international follow-up research project "SenseBurn" ("EUREKA-2 Eurostars"). The latter is characterized by numerous qualities that allow for easy and accurate estimation and burn injuries documentation:

Platform independence: The development resulted in software that runs on Android, iOS, Windows, Linux, MacOS, and directly in a web browser without requiring installation.

Patient-Specific 3D models: The creation and adaptation of patient-specific 3D models for different body shapes and proportions were realized with hand-crafted expansion vectors deforming a 3D model from a uniform model collection. These unified 3D models allow for continuous documentation, even if body proportions require a different base model. Personalized models considerably increase documentation quality.

Pose adaptation: The implementation of an automated pose adaptation of the model was realized to facilitate efficient clinical routine use. For this purpose, the joints' location and position are extracted from a single RGB image using machine learning algorithms. Due to the exact match of pose and shape of the 3D model, the wound surfaces' transfer is possible with minimal effort and high accuracy.

Exact transmission of wound areas without artifacts: With the development of a new method for wound annotation independent of the mesh resolution of the 3D model, it is now possible for the first time to document tiny areas or slight changes over time.

New possibilities: The implementation of new algorithms such as machine learning provides the opportunity to use future technologies.

Nichter et al. already implemented graphics tablets for drawing burns in 1984 [26]. Technological advances decreased the size of computers and monitors, providing more power than the large ones of earlier times. As a result, many applications were created to perform TBSA calculations based on the principles described later [32,62]. More recently, platform-independent TBSA calculators have been developed as apps for smartphones and tablets.

Another system is "BurnCalc" that was developed by Sheng et al. [59]. It allows for 3D scanning, 3D reconstruction, and interactive TBSA-B calculation. It is a high-tech approach demonstrating the high accuracy of 3D systems. However, its feasibility has not been proven in clinical application.

The programs and apps described above can guide burn treatment, but their implementation is limited because of medical device regulations and the lack of certifications as a medical product by the Food and Drug Administration (FDA) or/and the European Community.

3.6.4. Quality of Estimation Reliability

Different results of calculators can be explained by different methods used. Usually, 3D systems show a little inter-rater error and a high intraclass correlation.

Hintermüller [31] compared an electronic 2D system ("Mersey Burns") with an electronic 3D system ("BurnCase 3D"). As the results showed, "Mersey Burns" was associated with a mean overestimation rate of 32.16% to the ground truth. "BurnCase 3D" showed an overall difference to the ground truth of −4.53%. Thus, in terms of accuracy, the 3D system outperformed the 2D method. Goldberg et al. [72] reported similar results.

Parvizi et al. [67] demonstrated the high reliability and validity of "BurnCase 3D". In their validation study, artificial burn wounds of known size were applied to different ages and sex models. The study showed an average overestimation rate of burn extent of 0.4% in the pediatric model, 2.8% in the female model, and 1.5% in the male model.

Hintermüller [31] concluded that IT systems could help minimize potential errors or deviations from the actual burn extent, mostly when the less experienced medical staff performs the assessment.

As already pointed out, overestimation of the burn extent often leads to over-resuscitation, which in turn is a frequent cause of complications such as burn edema or capillary damage. Since 3D systems allow a very accurate calculation of the burn extent, their application can reduce such complications.

Adaptations of conventional methods such as the "Rule of Nines" or the "Lund Browder Chart" were developed to meet the challenge of varying body proportions during growth. Nevertheless, the developments led to inaccurate results in measuring TBSA-B, often with overestimation of burn extent or low inter-rater reliability [73].

Haller et al. [42] scored the extent to which different TBSA-B assessment methods meet future requirements in burn care. Traditional manual methods have the advantage that they are easy to use and require little equipment. However, compared to electronic

3D systems, they do not consider differences in individual physiology and are therefore less accurate.

Computer-based systems can still be prone to a methodological error, which occurs when transferring a 3D surface to a 2D model. The percentage assigned for a specific area by "Lund Browder" is not accurate for an individual. Nevertheless, inter-rater error is lower than manual and brain work, both in 2D and 3D systems [31,60,67,74].

4. Documentation

4.1. Medical Documentation

Any documentation aims to make the documented facts available. In most cases, such documentations focus on gathering data itself rather than making existing data available.

Documentation requirements are far beyond traditional paper-based documentation, even if converted into computer-based forms. Experts have well defined the required medical features for wound documentation. Even if there is plenty of literature dealing with chronic wounds [75,76], we found no validated standards for burn wound documentation of all necessary aspects.

From a medical point of view, the requirements to ensure modern and up-to-date wound documentation should be adapted to burn wounds and at least consist of:

- Medical history and general status of the patient with all its features;
- Recent and frequent photographic documentation to evaluate changes in the wound;
- Wound assessment with all its features;
- Course of healing;
- Documentation of therapeutic measures and their efficacy;
- Results of follow-ups;
- Traceability and verification of authors.

4.2. Standards Required for Data Analysis

Due to a possibly low number of cases, it is beneficial to analyze multiple burn centers' collected data. A shared merged datastore is necessary considering data security concerns. Merging data from multiple sources is a significant challenge because institutions use different software tools, different types of data storage structures, different conventions, unequal periods, and different levels of data aggregation. Commonly accepted data standards and compliant implementation of all parties' systems are necessary [77]. Solutions to get standardized data of different institutions might be the usage of a standardized documentation system like "BurnCase 3D" or the transforming of each single data collection to a unique one.

4.3. Existing Documentation Systems

Although paper-based documentation has significant shortcomings compared to electronic wound documentation [78], many institutions still use paper forms (or free-text electronic forms). The literature shows that most clinical systems do not meet the known requirements for successful burn documentation.

Many existing documentation systems use predefined terms without indicating their sources or have deficiencies in capturing a patient's complete medical history due to the lack of standards. Besides, most of them do not include the ability to perform statistical analysis of the collected data simultaneously, and only a few systems can collect data via mobile devices [79].

4.3.1. Electronic Documentation

Paper-based wound documentation is no valid alternative. Up-to-date wound documentation brings up more challenges and requirements.

Electronic documentation systems proved qualitative and quantitative advantages in several studies. They enhance documentation quality, reduce documentation errors, and result in positive attitudes among medical staff. Advantages like better availability and evaluability of the collected data, the more direct exchange of information (for consultation of experts), easier access to resources, and creation of new medical knowledge were described by Törnvall et al. [78] and Kinnunen et al. [75].

Electronic documentation does not necessarily generate scientifically useful data. Even though free-text documentation has flexible terms, dynamic expressions, and more effective recording through dictation, it also has serious shortcomings. Due to linguistic diversity and the lack of structure, there is no possibility to check the quality and completeness of the documentation. Additionally, free-text documentation often assumes besides text other implicit information, and data analysis beyond single patients is complicated and error-prone [80].

Thus, to ensure an optimal basis for data evaluation, a documentation system should provide structured data for selection and avoid free-text documentation. Structured recording allows for an exact recording of facts of defined scopes, such as the complete patient, an exceptional condition, or a single examination. Although the information given might sometimes be less comprehensive than in free-text documentation [80], the quality of structured data is superior due to uniform terminology.

Specifically, for the documentation of burn injuries, a relatively comprehensive documentation system has been developed. "BurnCase 3D" provides a library of 3D models, which can be adapted to sex, age, height, and weight. This system replaces estimation by automatically calculating the burned surface area (TBSA-B) regardless of body shape. The 3D model can be moved, rotated, and scaled. Users can transfer burn wounds from superimposed photos to the 3D model. "BurnCase 3D" enables full documentation of the entire treatment process from initial assessment to the outcome. Parvizi et al. [67] proved "BurnCase 3D" as a valid and reliable tool for TBSA-B determination and documentation.

From the perspective of medical care management, a significant advantage of 3D systems such as "Burncase 3D" is the accurate documentation of the wound healing process over time, so that the course of treatment can be monitored and appropriate follow-up treatment measures can be taken.

For significant improvements in modern burn care, it is essential to optimize TBSA-B methods and have complete comparable documentation sets.

4.3.2. Mobile Documentation

Mobile devices change the paradigm of data acquisition. Smartphones and tablets facilitate the remote exchange of medical information to assist diagnosis and treatment [81]. These devices are operated on different software platforms (e.g., Android, iOS, and Windows). A modern, state-of-the-art computer documentation system must be able to handle different operating systems. A platform-independent (e.g., HTML5-based) solution is required for this reason.

4.3.3. Photo Documentation

Recent and frequent photographic documentation is necessary to evaluate changes in the wound. Changing staff requires up to date information to avoid unnecessary pain and disturbing dressing changes. For scientific evaluation of the wound, photographic documentation is essential. Infrared and multispectral imaging are examples for particular photographic applications.

Assignment of photos to an actual body localization must be intuitive to be beneficial. High-quality photographs stored in a PACS (picture archiving and communication system) with an automated assignment to all available data (e.g., patient body region and burn condition, date) is necessary to be useful in medical routine. Burn documentation must be able to interact with PACS in the most automated way.

5. Conclusions

The article shows up the consequences of inaccurate TBSA-B assessment, which underlines the importance of appropriate methods. During the last century, several approaches have been developed to meet the requirements and enhance the burn size determination.

Several traditional methods like the "Lund Browder Chart", the "Rule of Nines", or the "Rule of Palms" are still of high practical relevance due to their simplicity and availability. Literature has shown some limitations of those methods; therefore, it is important to be aware of them.

In accordance with the technical achievements, modern computer-aided methods have proven to be superior to conventional methods. Computer-aided assessment and documentation systems have the potential to enable the way to a holistic structured and standardized documentation, which is essential to create new medical evidence, which brings the burn treatment a step forward.

To enable an even more comprehensive determination and documentation of burn injuries, 3D systems could be combined with various methods for determining the burn depth in the future. Examples of the latter are already existing methods such as laser Doppler or multispectral analysis. In the authors' view, such combinations could enable a wide range of new possibilities in burn medicine.

Author Contributions: Conceptualization, M.G., I.G. and H.H.; methodology, M.G., I.G. and H.H.; validation, M.G., I.G. and H.H.; investigation, M.G., I.G. and H.H.; resources, M.G., I.G. and H.H.; writing—original draft preparation, I.G.; writing—review and editing, M.G., I.G. and H.H.; visualization, I.G.; supervision, H.H.; project administration, M.G.; funding acquisition, M.G. All authors have read and agreed to the published version of the manuscript.

Funding: The research project BurnCase 3D was supported by the strategic economic- and research program "Innovatives OÖ 2020" of the province of Upper Austria. RISC Software GmbH is Member of UAR (Upper Austrian Research) Innovation Network. The research project SenseBurn received funding from the Eurostars-2 joint program with cofunding from the European Union Horizon 2020 research and innovation program.

Institutional Review Board Statement: Not applicable.

Informed Consent Statement: Not applicable.

Conflicts of Interest: Michael Giretzlehner and Isabell Ganitzer are employed at RISC Software GmbH, the developer of BurnCase 3D.

Abbreviations

2D	two-dimensional
3D	three-dimensional
ABA	American Burn Association
ANP	arterial natriuretic peptide
BMI	body mass index
CVP	central venous pressure
EPRI	Electric Power Research Institute
FDA	Food and Drug Administration
ISBI	International Society for Burn Injuries
IT	information technology
MODS	multiple organ dysfunction syndromes
NIH	National Institutes of Health (United States)
OBOS	One Burn One Standard
ODBC	Committee for the Organization and Delivery of Burn Care
PACS	picture archiving and communication system
RISC	Research Institute for Symbolic Computation
SAGE II	Surface Area Graphic Evaluation II
TBSA	total body surface area
TBSA-B	percentage of the total body surface area burned

References

1. Deutsche Gesellschaft für Verbrennungsmedizin (DGV). Leitlinie Behandlung Thermischer Verletzungen des Erwachsenen. Klasse: S2k. AWMF-Register-Nr.: 044-001 2018. Available online: https://www.verbrennungsmedizin.de/files/dgv_files/pdf/leitlinien/044-001l_S2k_Thermische__Verletzungen_Erwachsene_2018-10.pdf#page=4 (accessed on 30 November 2020).
2. Haller, H. Verbrennungstiefe und Ausmaß. In *Verbrennungen*; Springer: Berlin/Heidelberg, Germany, 2009; pp. 159–167.
3. Monstrey, S.; Hoeksema, H.; Verbelen, J.; Pirayesh, A.; Blondeel, P. Assessment of Burn Depth and Burn Wound Healing Potential. *Burns* 2008, 34, 761–769. [CrossRef]
4. Underhill, F.P. The Significance of Anhydremia in Extensive Superficial Burns. *JAMA* 1930, 95, 852. [CrossRef]
5. Baxter, C.R.; Shires, T. Physiological response to crystalloid resuscitation of severe burns. *Ann. N. Y. Acad. Sci.* 1968, 150, 874–894. [CrossRef] [PubMed]
6. Schwartz, S.I. Supportive Therapy in Burn Care. Consensus Summary on Fluid Resuscitation. *J. Trauma* 1979, 19, 876–877.
7. Velmahos, G.C.; Demetriades, D.; Shoemaker, W.C.; Chan, L.S.; Tatevossian, R.; Wo, C.C.; Vassiliu, P.; Cornwell, E.E.; Murray, J.A.; Roth, B.; et al. Endpoints of Resuscitation of Critically Injured Patients: Normal or Supranormal? *Ann. Surg.* 2000, 232, 409–418. [CrossRef]
8. Rhee, P. Shock, Electrolytes, and Fluid. In *Textbook of Oral and Maxillofacial Surgery*, 19th ed.; Elsevier Inc.: Amsterdam, The Netherlands, 2012; ISBN 9781437715606.
9. Bruegger, D.; Schwartz, L.; Chappell, D.; Jacob, M.; Rehm, M.; Vogeser, M.; Christ, F.; Reichart, B.; Becker, B.F. Release of Atrial Natriuretic Peptide Precedes Shedding of the Endothelial Glycocalyx Equally in Patients Undergoing On- and off-Pump Coronary Artery Bypass Surgery. *Basic Res. Cardiol.* 2011, 106, 1111–1121. [CrossRef] [PubMed]
10. Jacob, M.; Chappell, D. Mythen Und Fakten Der Perioperativen Infusionstherapie. *Deutsch* 2009, 358–376.
11. Lobo, D.N.; Stanga, Z.; Aloysius, M.M.; Wicks, C.; Nunes, Q.M.; Ingram, K.L.; Risch, L.; Allison, S.P. Effect of Volume Loading with 1 Liter Intravenous Infusions of 0.9% Saline, 4% Succinylated Gelatine (Gelofusine) and 6% Hydroxyethyl Starch (Voluven) on Blood Volume and Endocrine Responses: A Randomized, Three-Way Crossover Study in Healthy Volunteers. *Crit. Care Med.* 2010, 38, 464–470. [CrossRef] [PubMed]
12. Chung, K.K.; Wolf, S.E.; Cancio, L.C.; Alvarado, R.; Jones, J.A.; McCorcle, J.; King, B.T.; Barillo, D.J.; Renz, E.M.; Blackbourne, L.H. Resuscitation of Severely Burned Military Casualties: Fluid Begets More Fluid. *J. Trauma Inj. Infect. Crit. Care* 2009, 67, 231–237. [CrossRef] [PubMed]
13. Cancio, L.C.; Chávez, S.; Alvarado-Ortega, M.; Barillo, D.J.; Walker, S.C.; McManus, A.T.; Goodwin, C.W. Predicting Increased Fluid Requirements during the Resuscitation of Thermally Injured Patients. *J. Trauma* 2004, 56, 404–413. [CrossRef]
14. Friedrich, J.B.; Sullivan, S.R.; Engrav, L.H.; Round, K.A.; Blayney, C.B.; Carrougher, G.J.; Heimbach, D.M.; Honari, S.; Klein, M.B.; Gibran, N.S. Is Supra-Baxter Resuscitation in Burn Patients a New Phenomenon? *Burns* 2004, 30, 464–466. [CrossRef] [PubMed]
15. Engrav, L.H.; Heimbach, D.M.; Rivara, F.P.; Kerr, K.F.; Osler, T.; Pham, T.N.; Sharar, S.R.; Esselman, P.C.; Bulger, E.M.; Carrougher, G.J.; et al. Harborview Burns—1974 to 2009. *PLoS ONE* 2012, 7, e40086. [CrossRef] [PubMed]
16. Regan, A.; Hotwagner, D.T. Burn Fluid Management. In *StatPearls*; StatPearls Publishing: Treasure Island, FL, USA, 2020.
17. Cartotto, R.; Zhou, A. Fluid Creep: The Pendulum Hasn't Swung Back Yet! *J. Burn Care Res.* 2010, 31, 551–558. [CrossRef]
18. Strang, S.G.; Van Lieshout, E.M.M.; Breederveld, R.S.; Van Waes, O.J.F. A Systematic Review on Intra-Abdominal Pressure in Severely Burned Patients. *Burns* 2014, 40, 9–16. [CrossRef] [PubMed]
19. Browning, J.A.; Cindass, R. Burn Debridement, Grafting, and Reconstruction. In *StatPearls*; StatPearls Publishing: Treasure Island, FL, USA, 2020.
20. Zhang, J.; Xiang, F.; Tong, D.; Luo, Q.; Yuan, Z.; Yan, H.; Li, X.; Chen, J.; Peng, D.; Luo, G.; et al. Comparative study on the effect of restrictive fluid management strategy on the early pulmonary function of patients with severe burn. *Zhonghua Shao Shang Za Zhi* 2012, 28, 165–169.
21. Guilabert, P.; Usúa, G.; Martín, N.; Abarca, L.; Barret, J.P.; Colomina, M.J. Fluid Resuscitation Management in Patients with Burns: Update. *Br. J. Anaesth.* 2016, 117, 284–296. [CrossRef]
22. Hickerson, W.L.; Ryan, C.M.; Conlon, K.M.; Harrington, D.T.; Foster, K.; Schwartz, S.; Iyer, N.; Jeschke, M.; Haller, H.L.; Faucher, L.D.; et al. What's in a Name? Recent Key Projects of the Committee on Organization and Delivery of Burn Care. *J. Burn Care Res.* 2015, 36, 619–625. [CrossRef] [PubMed]
23. Serghiou, M.A.; Niszczak, J.; Parry, I.; Li-Tsang, C.W.P.; Van den Kerckhove, E.; Smailes, S.; Edgar, D. One World One Burn Rehabilitation Standard. *Burns* 2016, 42, 1047–1058. [CrossRef]
24. West, M.A.; Moore, E.E.; Shapiro, M.B.; Nathens, A.B.; Cuschieri, J.; Johnson, J.L.; Harbrecht, B.G.; Minei, J.P.; Bankey, P.E.; Maier, R.V. Inflammation and the Host Response to Injury, a Large-Scale Collaborative Project: Patient-Oriented Research Core—Standard Operating Procedures for Clinical Care VII—Guidelines for Antibiotic Administration in Severely Injured Patients. *J. Trauma Inj. Infect. Crit. Care* 2008, 65, 1511–1519. [CrossRef] [PubMed]
25. Silver, G.M.; Klein, M.B.; Herndon, D.N.; Gamelli, R.L.; Gibran, N.S.; Altstein, L.; McDonald-Smith, G.P.; Tompkins, R.G.; Hunt, J.L.; The Inflammation and the Host Response to Trauma, Collaborative Research Program. Standard Operating Procedures for the Clinical Management of Patients Enrolled in a Prospective Study of Inflammation and the Host Response to Thermal Injury. *J. Burn Care Res.* 2007, 28, 222–230. [CrossRef]
26. Nichter, L.S.; Williams, J.; Bryant, C.A.; Edlich, R.F. Improving the Accuracy of Burn-Surface Estimation. *Plast. Reconstr. Surg.* 1985, 76, 428–433. [CrossRef]

27. Wachtel, T.L.; Berry, C.C.; Wachtel, E.E.; Frank, H.A. The Inter-Rater Reliability of Estimating the Size of Burns from Various Burn Area Chart Drawings. *Burn. J. Int. Soc. Burn Inj.* **2000**, *26*, 156–170. [CrossRef]
28. Berkebile, B.L.; Goldfarb, I.W.; Slater, H. Comparison of Burn Size Estimates Between Prehospital Reports and Burn Center Evaluations. *J. Burn Care Rehabil.* **1986**, *7*, 411–412. [CrossRef] [PubMed]
29. Hammond, J.S.; Ward, C.G. Transfers from Emergency Room to Burn Center: Errors in Burn Size Estimate. *J. Trauma* **1987**, *27*, 1161–1165. [CrossRef] [PubMed]
30. Goverman, J.; Bittner, E.A.; Friedstat, J.S.; Moore, M.; Nozari, A.; Ibrahim, A.E.; Sarhane, K.A.; Chang, P.H.; Sheridan, R.L.; Fagan, S.P. Discrepancy in Initial Pediatric Burn Estimates and Its Impact on Fluid Resuscitation. *J. Burn Care Res.* **2015**, *36*, 574–579. [CrossRef] [PubMed]
31. Hintermüller, C. *Estimation of Total Burn Surface Area: A Comparison of Four Different Methods*; Paracelsus Medical University: Salzburg, Austria, 2016.
32. Wurzer, P.; Parvizi, D.; Lumenta, D.B.; Giretzlehner, M.; Branski, L.K.; Finnerty, C.C.; Herndon, D.N.; Tuca, A.; Rappl, T.; Smolle, C.; et al. Smartphone Applications in Burns. *Burns* **2015**, *41*, 977–989. [CrossRef]
33. Vercruysse, G.A.; Ingram, W.L.; Feliciano, D.V. Overutilization of Regional Burn Centers for Pediatric Patientsa Healthcare System Problem That Should Be Corrected. *Am. J. Surg.* **2011**, *202*, 802–809. [CrossRef]
34. Klasen, H.J. Chapter I: Classification of burns. In *History of Burns*; Erasmus Publishing: Rotterdam, The Netherlands, 2004; pp. 21–66. ISBN 90 5235 168 6.
35. Riehl, G. Zur Therapie Schwerer Verbrennungen. *Wien Klin Wochenschr.* **1925**, *37*, 833–834.
36. Dubois, D.; Dubois, E. A Formula to Estimate the Approximate Surface Area If Height and Weight Be Known. *Arch. Intern. Med.* **1916**, *17*, 863–871. [CrossRef]
37. Lund, C.C.; Browder, N.C. The Estimation of Areas of Burns. *Surg. Gynecol. Obstet.* **1944**, *79*, 352–358.
38. Boyd, E. *The Growth of the Surface Area of the Human Body*; University of Minnesota Press: Minnesota, MN, USA, 1935.
39. Neaman, K.C.; Andres, L.A.; McClure, A.M.; Burton, M.E.; Kemmeter, P.R.; Ford, R.D. A New Method for Estimation of Involved BSAs for Obese and Normal-Weight Patients with Burn Injury. *J. Burn Care Res.* **2011**, *32*, 421–428. [CrossRef] [PubMed]
40. Wilson, G.R.; Fowler, C.A.; Housden, P.L. A New Burn Area Assessment Chart. *Burns* **1987**, *13*, 401–405. [CrossRef]
41. Miminas, D.A. A Critical Evaluation of the Lund and Browder Chart. *Wounds* **2007**, *3*, 58–68.
42. Haller, H.L.; Giretzlehner, M.; Thumfart, S. Burn Size Estimation, Challenges, and Novel Technology. In *Handbook of Burns Volume 1: Acute Burn Care*; Jeschke, M.G., Kamolz, L.-P., Sjöberg, F., Wolf, S.E., Eds.; Springer International Publishing: Cham, Switzerland, 2020; pp. 181–197. ISBN 978-3-030-18940-2.
43. Collis, N.; Smith, G.; Fenton, O.M. Accuracy of Burn Size Estimation and Subsequent Fluid Resuscitation Prior to Arrival at the Yorkshire Regional Burns Unit. A Three Year Retrospective Study. *Burns* **1999**, *25*, 345–351. [CrossRef]
44. Freiburg, C.; Igneri, P.; Sartorelli, K.; Rogers, F. Effects of Differences in Percent Total Body Surface Area Estimation on Fluid Resuscitation of Transferred Burn Patients. *J. Burn Care Res.* **2007**, *28*, 42–48. [CrossRef] [PubMed]
45. Irwin, L.R.; Reid, C.A.; McLean, N.R. Burns in Children: Do Casualty Officers Get It Right? *Injury* **1993**, *24*, 187–188. [CrossRef]
46. Klippel, C.H. Surface Area versus Skin Area. *N. Engl. J. Med.* **1979**, *301*, 730. [PubMed]
47. Wallace, A.B. The Exposure Treatment of Burns. *Lancet* **1951**, *257*, 501–504. [CrossRef]
48. Berry, C.C.; Wachtel, T.; Frank, H.A. Differences in Burn Size Estimates Between Community Hospitals and a Burn Center. *J. Burn Care Rehabil.* **1982**, *3*, 176–178. [CrossRef]
49. Giretzlehner, M.; Dirnberger, J.; Owen, R.; Haller, H.L.; Lumenta, D.B.; Kamolz, L.-P. The Determination of Total Burn Surface Area: How Much Difference? *Burn. J. Int. Soc. Burn Inj.* **2013**, *39*, 1–7. [CrossRef]
50. Livingston, E.H.; Lee, S. Percentage of Burned Body Surface Area Determination in Obese and Nonobese Patients. *J. Surg. Res.* **2000**, *91*, 106–110. [CrossRef] [PubMed]
51. Williams, R.Y.; Wohlgemuth, S.D. Does the "Rule of Nines" Apply to Morbidly Obese Burn Victims? *J. Burn Care Res. Off. Publ. Am. Burn Assoc.* **2013**, *34*, 447–452. [CrossRef] [PubMed]
52. Yu, C.-Y.; Lin, C.-H.; Yang, Y.-H. Human Body Surface Area Database and Estimation Formula. *Burn. J. Int. Soc. Burn Inj.* **2010**, *36*, 616–629. [CrossRef] [PubMed]
53. Rossiter, N.D.; Chapman, P.; Haywood, I.A. How Big Is a Hand? *Burn. J. Int. Soc. Burn Inj.* **1996**, *22*, 230–231. [CrossRef]
54. Nagel, T.R.; Schunk, J.E. Using the Hand to Estimate the Surface Area of a Burn in Children. *Pediatric Emerg. Care* **1997**, *13*, 254–255. [CrossRef]
55. Berry, M.G.; Evison, D.; Roberts, A.H. The Influence of Body Mass Index on Burn Surface Area Estimated from the Area of the Hand. *Burn. J. Int. Soc. Burn Inj.* **2001**, *27*, 591–594. [CrossRef]
56. Butz, D.R.; Collier, Z.; O'Connor, A.; Magdziak, M.; Gottlieb, L.J.; Connor, A.O.; Magdziak, M.; Gottlieb, L.J. Is Palmar Surface Area a Reliable Tool to Estimate Burn Surface Areas in Obese Patients? *J. Burn Care Res. Off. Publ. Am. Burn Assoc.* **2015**, *36*, 87–91. [CrossRef] [PubMed]
57. Laing, J.H.; Morgan, B.D.; Sanders, R. Assessment of Burn Injury in the Accident and Emergency Department: A Review of 100 Referrals to a Regional Burns Unit. *Ann. R. Coll. Surg. Engl.* **1991**, *73*, 329–331. [PubMed]
58. Cone, J.B. What's New in General Surgery: Burns and Metabolism. *J. Am. Coll. Surg.* **2005**, *200*, 607–615. [CrossRef]
59. Sheng, W.; Zeng, D.; Wan, Y.; Yao, L.; Tang, H.; Xia, Z. BurnCalc Assessment Study of Computer-Aided Individual Three-Dimensional Burn Area Calculation. *J. Transl. Med.* **2014**, *12*, s12967–s014. [CrossRef]

60. Wachtel, T.L.; Brimm, J.E.; Knight, M.A.; Heisterkamp, S.; Frank, H.A.; Inancsi, W. Research: Computer Assisted Estimation of the Size of Burns. *J. Burn Care Rehabil.* **1983**, *4*, 255–259. [CrossRef]
61. Barnes, J.; Duffy, A.; Hamnett, N.; McPhail, J.; Seaton, C.; Shokrollahi, K.; James, M.I.; McArthur, P.; Pritchard Jones, R. The Mersey Burns App: Evolving a Model of Validation. *Emerg. Med. J.* **2015**, *32*, 637–641. [CrossRef]
62. Morris, R.; Javed, M.; Bodger, O.; Gorse, S.H.; Williams, D. A Comparison of Two Smartphone Applications and the Validation of Smartphone Applications as Tools for Fluid Calculation for Burns Resuscitation. *Burns* **2014**, *40*, 826–834. [CrossRef]
63. Neuwalder, J.M.; Sampson, C.; Breuing, K.H.; Orgill, D.P. A Review of Computer-Aided Body Surface Area Determination: SAGE II and EPRI's 3D Burn Vision. *J. Burn Care Rehabil.* **2002**, *23*, 55–59. [CrossRef]
64. Knaysi, G.A.; Crikelair, G.F.; Cosman, B. The Role of Nines: Its History and Accuracy. *Plast. Reconstr. Surg.* **1968**, *41*, 560–563. [CrossRef] [PubMed]
65. Lee, R.C.; Kieska, G.; Mankani, M.H. A Three-Dimensional Computerized Burn Chart: Stage I: Development of Three-Dimensional Renderings. *J. Burn Care Rehabil.* **1994**, *15*, 80–83. [CrossRef]
66. Mankani, M.H.; Kicska, G.; Lee, R.C. A Three-Dimensional Computerized Burn Chart: Stage II: Assessment of Accuracy. *J. Burn Care Rehabil.* **1994**, *15*, 191–192. [CrossRef]
67. Parvizi, D.; Giretzlehner, M.; Wurzer, P.; Klein, L.D.; Shoham, Y.; Bohanon, F.J.; Haller, H.L.; Tuca, A.; Branski, L.K.; Lumenta, D.B.; et al. BurnCase 3D Software Validation Study: Burn Size Measurement Accuracy and Inter-Rater Reliability. *Burns* **2016**, *42*, 329–335. [CrossRef]
68. Yu, C.-Y.; Lo, Y.-H.; Chiou, W.-K. The 3D Scanner for Measuring Body Surface Area: A Simplified Calculation in the Chinese Adult. *Appl. Ergon.* **2003**, *34*, 273–278. [CrossRef]
69. Stockton, K.A.; McMillan, C.M.; Storey, K.J.; David, M.C.; Kimble, R.M. 3D Photography Is as Accurate as Digital Planimetry Tracing in Determining Burn Wound Area. *Burns* **2015**, *41*, 80–84. [CrossRef] [PubMed]
70. Wurzer, P.; Giretzlehner, M.; Kamolz, L.-P. 3D Photography Is an Accurate Technique for Measuring Small Wound Areas. *Burns* **2015**, *41*, 196–197. [CrossRef]
71. Yu, C.-Y.; Hsu, Y.-W.; Chen, C.-Y. Determination of Hand Surface Area as a Percentage of Body Surface Area by 3D Anthropometry. *Burn. J. Int. Soc. Burn Inj.* **2008**, *34*, 1183–1189. [CrossRef]
72. Goldberg, H.; Klaff, J.; Spjut, A.; Milner, S. A Mobile App for Measuring the Surface Area of a Burn in Three Dimensions: Comparison to the Lund and Browder Assessment. *J. Burn Care Res.* **2014**, *35*, 480–483. [CrossRef]
73. Thumfart, S.; Giretzlehner, M.; Wurzer, P.; Höller, J.; Ehrenmüller, M.; Pfurtscheller, K.; Haller, H.L.; Kamolz, L.-P.; Schmitt, K.; Furthner, D. Burn Size Measurement Using Proportionally Correct 3D Models of Pediatric Patients. In Proceedings of the Supplement to Journal of Burn Care & Research, Las Vegas, NV, USA, 3–6 May 2016; Volume 37, p. 80.
74. Siegel, J.B.; Wachtel, T.L.; Brimm, J.E. Automated Documentation and Analysis of Burn Size. *J. Trauma Inj. Infect. Crit. Care* **1986**, *26*, 44–46. [CrossRef] [PubMed]
75. Kinnunen, U.-M.; Saranto, K.; Ensio, A.; Iivanainen, A.; Dykes, P. Developing the Standardized Wound Care Documentation Model: A Delphi Study to Improve the Quality of Patient Care Documentation. *J. Wound Ostomy Cont. Nurs.* **2012**, *39*, 397–407. [CrossRef]
76. Panfil, E.; Linde, E. *Kriterien Zur Wunddokumentation–Literaturanalyse*; Hessisches Institut Für Pflegeforschung: Frankfurt, Germany, 2006.
77. Giretzlehner, M.; Haller, H.L.; Faucher, L.D.; Pressman, M.A.; Salinas, J.; Jeng, J.C. One Burn, One Standard. *J. Burn Care Res.* **2014**, *35*, e372. [CrossRef]
78. Törnvall, E.; Wahren, L.K.; Wilhelmsson, S. Advancing Nursing Documentation–an Intervention Study Using Patients with Leg Ulcer as an Example. *Int. J. Med. Inf.* **2009**, *78*, 605–617. [CrossRef]
79. Hübner, U.; Flemming, D.; Schultz-Gödker, A. Software Zur Digitalen Wunddokumentation: Marktübersicht und Bewertungskriterien. *Wundmanagement* **2009**, *3*, 16–25.
80. Ingenerf, J. Computergestützte Strukturierte Befundung Am Beispiel der Wunddokumentation. *Wundmanagement* **2009**, *3*, 104–108.
81. Parvizi, D.; Giretzlehner, M.; Dirnberger, J.; Owen, R.; Haller, H.L.; Schintler, M.V.; Wurzer, P.; Lumenta, D.B.; Kamolz, L.P. The Use of Teleemedicine in Burn Care: Development of a Mobile System for Tbsa Documentation and Remote Assessment. *Ann. Burn. Fire Disasters* **2014**, *7*, 94.

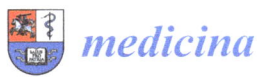

Review

Historical Evolution of Skin Grafting—A Journey through Time

Michael Kohlhauser [1,2,*], Hanna Luze [1,2], Sebastian Philipp Nischwitz [1,2] and Lars Peter Kamolz [1,2]

1. COREMED—Cooperative Centre for Regenerative Medicine, Joanneum Research Forschungsgesellschaft mbH, 8010 Graz, Austria; hanna.luze@joanneum.at (H.L.); sebastian.nischwitz@joanneum.at (S.P.N.); lars.kamolz@medunigraz.at (L.P.K.)
2. Division of Plastic, Aesthetic and Reconstructive Surgery, Department of Surgery, Medical University of Graz, 8036 Graz, Austria
* Correspondence: michael.kohlhauser@joanneum.at; Tel.: +43-316-876-6003

Abstract: Autologous skin grafting was developed more than 3500 years ago. Several approaches and techniques have been discovered and established in burn care since then. Great achievements were made during the 19th and 20th century. Many of these techniques are still part of the surgical burn care. Today, autologous skin grafting is still considered to be the gold standard for burn wound coverage. The present paper gives an overview about the evolution of skin grafting and its usage in burn care nowadays.

Keywords: skin grafting; skin transplantation; skin substitutes; history; burns

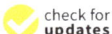

Citation: Kohlhauser, M.; Luze, H.; Nischwitz, S.P.; Kamolz, L.P. Historical Evolution of Skin Grafting—A Journey through Time. *Medicina* 2021, 57, 348. https://doi.org/10.3390/medicina57040348

Academic Editors: Rytis Rimdeika and Gadi Borkow

Received: 4 March 2021
Accepted: 2 April 2021
Published: 5 April 2021

Publisher's Note: MDPI stays neutral with regard to jurisdictional claims in published maps and institutional affiliations.

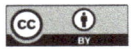

Copyright: © 2021 by the authors. Licensee MDPI, Basel, Switzerland. This article is an open access article distributed under the terms and conditions of the Creative Commons Attribution (CC BY) license (https://creativecommons.org/licenses/by/4.0/).

1. Introduction

The skin is not only the largest organ of the human body but also the first line of defense against harmful influences such as mechanical forces, microorganisms, or radiation. It maintains thermoregulation and fluid balance as well as acts as a sensory organ that is able to register pressure, temperature, and pain, due to specific receptors. The integrity of human skin plays an essential role in maintaining physiological homeostasis of the body. A large skin loss caused by e.g., burns, can cause a disturbance of this integrity [1,2]. To date, autologous skin grafting is commonly considered as the gold standard for the coverage of large skin defects. While the usage of meshed split thickness skin grafting is the best option for the treatment of extensive burns, unmeshed sheet grafting is used for small burns and in aesthetically important regions. Full-thickness skin grafting achieves the best aesthetic and functional results in burn injury reconstruction [3–5].

The origin of skin grafting can be traced back for more than 3500 years. Many techniques and adjustments have been established over time. This article gives an overview about the historical evolution of skin grafting, including the development of common techniques, and further explains their usage in burn care nowadays. In addition, the development and the usage of further established techniques are presented. Finally, the split-thickness skin graft associated donor site problems are analyzed, and solutions are discussed.

2. The Origin of Skin Grafting

Skin grafting was already practiced in the Egyptian Empire. This ancient skin graft technique was already taking place 1500 before Christ (BC) and was documented in an old papyrus role called "Ebert papyrus" [6]. According to the "Sushruta Samhita", one of the early texts of Ayurveda, skin grafting was also performed by the ancient Hindu more than 3000 years ago. Members of the Koomas Caste used subcutaneous fat and skin from the gluteal region as free skin graft [6–8]. In the 1st and 2nd century, Celsus and Galen used skin grafts to treat facial defects. Furthermore, Celsus developed a method to reconstruct the foreskin of Jewish men in historical Roman Empire [7]. During a long period, most of the knowledge was forgotten. For example, the earlier known techniques of free skin grafting got lost in the Middle Ages. The method seemed to be forgotten until the early 19th century. In 1804, Giuseppe Baroni demonstrated successful transplantations of free skin grafts in ram. Seventeen years later, the first verified successful nasal reconstruction by usage of free skin autografting was performed by Professor Bünger, which was inspired by the ancient Indian method [8–10].

In 1869, Jaques-Louis Reverdin, a Swiss surgeon, presented a successful experiment of free skin grafting [6,7,9,11]. By using the tip of a lancet, Reverdin harvested epidermal small bits from the arm of the patient and fixed them into the middle of wound with a diachylon bandage. Although the procedure is known as "Pinch Graft" today, Reverdin called his technique "Epidermic Grafting" [6,7]. In May 1870, Georg David Pollock was the first surgeon who performed a successful pinch graft in a burn victim case. His patient was an 8-year-old girl who suffered a large defect of her right thigh by severe burns [6,7,12,13]. Pollock transplanted two small pieces from the abdomen to the middle of the lower part of the defect. Three weeks later, a second series was transplanted into the wound. After 6 weeks, all grafts grew well and divided the defect into two parts. Two further pinch grafts, harvested from the abdomen, were successfully transplanted. Pollock also performed the first known allografts to a burned patient in combination with autologous pinch grafts. However, the allogeneic grafts did not grow and were gradually destroyed, but they seemed to stimulate the spontaneous healing of the autologous pinch grafts [12,13].

3. The Split-Thickness Skin Graft

The history of split-thickness skin grafting dates back to the late 19th century. The earliest known split-thickness skin grafting method was developed by Ollier in 1872. His results revealed not only a faster healing but also less scar formation and therefore less scar contractures by covering the whole wound surface with skin grafts. Since these grafts included epidermis as well parts of the dermis, Ollier called his technique "dermo-epidermic grafting" [6]. Prof. Carl Thiersch, chairman of the surgery department in Leipzig, presented his technique at the 15th Congress of German Surgical Association in 1886 [6,14]. His technique advised to cut the skin with a razor blade as thin as possible via sharp horizontal incisions to produce thin strips of epidermis, only including small parts of dermis [6,7,15]. Thiersch's technique obtained national publicity, which is known as "Thiersch Graft" [6]. Caused by the similarity of both discoveries, the method is also known as "Ollier–Thiersch graft". In 1929, Blair and Brown presented their method of "split skin grafts" of intermediate thickness. These grafts differ from "Ollier–Thiersch graft" in regard of the thickness due to included layers of dermis. While Ollier and Thiersch advised to include only little more than the epithelial layer, the split skin grafts of intermediate thickness also included an appreciable amount of the dermal layer. The idea was to preserve the advantages of both, the "Ollier–Thiersch graft", as well those of the full-thickness skin graft [16]. In 1941, Earl C. Padgett, an American surgeon, developed a new method of split-thickness skin grafting by using a manual dermatome. The "three-quarter"-thickness skin graft demonstrated good graft take, and the dermatome enabled the possibility of new skin donor sites, which were not available by free hand skin grafting methods [17].

The current STSG classification is based according to their thickness into thin STSGs (0.15 to 0.3 mm), intermediate STSGs (0.3 to 0.45 mm), and thick STSGs (0.45 to 0.6 mm) [18]. The different thickness layers are displayed in Figure 1.

In 1970, Janzekovic demonstrated her concept of early excision and wound coverage with autologous split-thickness skin grafts [19]. This method is considered as the current gold standard in surgical burn treatment, even today [4,5]. A major advantage of split-thickness skin grafting is the possibility of using the same donor site repeatedly after healing, which typically occurs within 7–14 days [20,21]. Further benefits are less morbidity and less scar formation in donor sites, which increase the contemplable donor sites, compared with full-thickness skin grafts [22]. Commonly used donor sites are thighs, legs, abdomen, back, arms, forearms, and chest [22,23]. In extensive burns, with a lack of eligible skin, the scalp or even scrotum can be used as last resort donor sites [24–27]. A distinction must be made between unmeshed STSGs (sheet grafts) and STSGs extended by specifically expanding methods. Sheet grafts are commonly used for small burns, while meshed split-thickness skin grafting depicts the best alternative for the coverage of large burns [23,28,29].

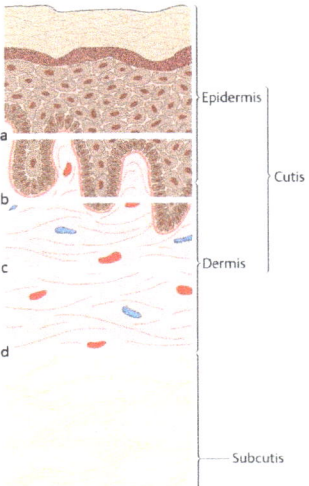

Figure 1. The classification of split thickness skin grafts (**a**–**c**) and full thickness skin graft (**d**) according to the thickness of the layer. a = 0.15–0.3 mm; b = 0.3–0.45 mm; c = 0.5–0.6 mm; d > 0.6 mm.

3.1. Sheet Graft

Sheet grafting is considered to be the gold standard for the treatment of small burns and to cover sensitive areas [5,28,30]. Sheet grafts accelerate the end of the inflammatory phase and offer a better vascularization and re-innervation. Further benefits are the lower tendency for scar formation and contractures, a better aesthetic outcome, and no permanent mesh pattern in contrast to meshed skin grafts. Therefore, sheet grafts are appropriate to cover visible and functionally important areas [28,30]. Sheet grafts can as well be used to cover aesthetic and functional important areas in severe burns, in order to save donor sites instead of initial coverage with full-thickness skin grafts [31]. The disadvantages of sheet grafting are the need of larger donor sites, the risk of hematoma formation, the danger of losing the graft because of its impermeability, and the inability to cover severe burns, which is caused by a lack of donor sites [28].

3.2. Mesh Graft

Professor Otto Lanz was dissatisfied with the fact that the donor site of a Thiersch graft was still an open wound, while the initial defect already healed. He investigated various methods, but none of the experiments led to a satisfactory result. Due to a childhood game, which was used to build a paper accordion, he was encouraged to use the same method for skin grafting. Lanz developed an accordion-like expansion of a Thiersch graft in 1908, which not only served the purpose of covering the defect but also the newly formed wound of the donor site [32].

In 1964, James C. Tanner, a plastic surgeon at the Long Memorial Hospital, Atlanta developed a new method to produce expanded STSGs by usage of a new device named "Tanner–Vandeput mesh dermatome". By rolling split-thickness skin grafts through the novel dermatome, the machine cuts the skin grafts into a mesh with ribbons of skin 0.050-inches wide. Tanner's mesh grafting enabled skin grafts expanding up to a ratio 1:3, reducing the area of the donor site and offering the possibility of covering more wound area [33]. Nowadays, ratios up to 1:6 or even 1:9 are possible by using special devices [23]. Complete wound coverage can be achieved in approximately 10 days through rapid epithelialization in the absence of infection. Furthermore, a drainage of exudate and hemorrhage, as well regaining of areas lost by shrink is possible, due to the mesh-like structures. These properties are ideal for the treatment of burn injuries and large defects with limited donor sites [34,35]. The advantage of fluid drainage and a similar cosmetic outcome as with sheet grafts is achievable with a meshing ratio of 1:1 [28]. Additionally, mesh grafting shows a high percentage of graft take and enables covering large wound areas. Further benefits are the decrease of operating time and the reduction of the required number of necessary surgeries to achieve full rehabilitation.

Due to the advantages described above, the mesh skin graft method is well established and is considered as the standard method to surface large areas in severe burn treatment, even today [4,5,23,36].

3.3. Meek Technique

In 1958 Cicero Parker Meek, a general practitioner at the Aiken Country Hospital in South Carolina known for his great interest in burn care, published an article called "Successful microdermagrafing using the Meek–Wall microdermatome". The Meek–Wall microdermatome consisted of 13 blades driven by an electronic engine. Flat cork plates served as carriers for the skin grafts [37,38]. The functions were described by a case report of a 14-year-old burn victim with 25% total body surface area. Meek cut conventional split-thickness skin grafts (0.0125 inches) into units 1/16 inches square (40 mm^2). Subsequently, the microdermagrafts were saturated in plasma and evenly distributed to prefold parachute silk bandages, which were placed directly on the wound. After ten days, the grafted areas could be left exposed [37]. Meek's microdermal grafting enabled the possibility of covering large denuded areas after severe burns successfully by widely expanded stamp autografts [39]. In 1965, Meek published another article to describe his method step by step in detail and reported about the experience he made with the Meek–Wall dermatome [40]. The Meek technique was slowly forgotten after the development of the mesh grafting technique by Tanner in 1964. In the early 1990s, Meek's technology was rediscovered and improved by Dutch surgeons at the burn unit of the Red Cross Hospital in Beverwijk. The Meek technique was used successfully in the treatment of severe burns, when insufficient suitable donor sites were available for wound coverage with mesh grafts only. The clinical results of this modified Meek technique were first published by Kreis et al. in 1993 [41]. Thenceforth, the Meek technique returned in the clinical setting. The usage of the Meek technique offers many advantages, especially in the treatment of severe burns, which are often affected by the lack of donor sites. The Meek technique enabled an expansion of surface area coverage from 1:3 up to 1:9. The micro grafts allow a shorter duration and more uniform epithelialization than other techniques. Another benefit is the easy application compared to the difficult handling of higher expanded mesh grafts (1:6 or 1:9) [42–46]. In shortage of donor sites, Meek enabled the expansion of smaller grafts, as well the usage of donor sites, which cannot be grabbed by other grafting techniques [46,47]. Furthermore, the re-epithelialization time seems to be shorter with the Meek technique compared to mesh grafts [43]. Some graft takes failed by contamination, but these were mostly restricted to a partial area without affecting nearby skin islands [42,48], while the observed total take rate with Meek grafts was described by several authors between 82.3% and 90% [42,44,45,48–50]. Major disadvantages of Meek's method are the protracted procedure as well the necessity of more staff in the operating theater [42,45].

4. The Full-Thickness Skin Graft

If the skin graft includes the entire thickness of the dermis, the appropriate term is full-thickness skin graft (FTSG) [51,52]. Full-thickness skin grafts are not widely used for emergency burn care but are ideal for the reconstruction after initial treatment and for scar corrections [31,53].

The first known full-thickness skin graft technique was presented by John Reissberg Wolfe in 1875. Wolfe described the correction of an ectropium by using a full-thickness skin graft after cutting accurately to the shape of the defect. A similar technique was described by Georg Lawson in 1870 and 1871, even though his name is not associated with the development of the full-thickness skin graft [7,54,55]. Fedor Krause, a German surgeon based in Hamburg, established the usage of full-thickness skin grafts. At the XXIII Congress of the German Surgical Association in 1893, Krause advised the usage of the Wolfe graft for all cases, where the Thiersch graft showed unsatisfactory outcomes and reported 21 cases in which full-thickness skin grafts were successfully transplanted. Krause's knowledge was well received not only nationally but also internationally, and the full-thickness graft achieved great popularity [6].

Nowadays, FTSGs are considered to achieve best results in burn deformity reconstructions due to less scar formation, good plasticity, elasticity, mobility, and aesthetic outcome, as well due to providing improved texture and color matching. After a long-term period, full-thickness skin grafts are almost similar to intact skin. Especially facial and palmar burns are one of the most challenging problems in burn injury treatment, but they are also a burden to the individual's psychological sentiment by functional disorders, structural defects, scars formation, scar contractures, as well soft tissue or hard tissue defects [56,57]. Hand burns often affect children in particular, leading to scar contracture and resulting in functional implications and disturbed evolution of the child's hand [22]. Full-thickness skin grafts are able to achieve excellent results in reconstruction, are aesthetically as well functionally superior to those obtained from sheet grafts, and therefore are the ideal choice for treatment of facial and palmar defects and scars suffered by burns [53,56–58]. Despite this occurrence of excellent results, various influencing factors must be observed by the performing surgeon at the selection of the eligible donor site: skin quality, skin color, texture, damage due to ultraviolet radiation, skin thickness, convenience, size, possibility of contractility, and scar formation after graft taking, as well the fact that donor sites can only be harvested once [53]. Summarizing, the usage of FTSGs achieves better aesthetic and functional results compared with STSGs. However, FTSGs have various limitations; thus, their usage should be reserved for the reconstruction of late deformities, especially in sensitive areas.

5. Allogeneic and Xenogeneic Transplants

The earliest proposals using foreign human skin or animal skin for burn injuries date back to the 19th century, but these failed [12,13,59–61]. Nevertheless, the first successes occurred not until the middle of the 20th century [31,62]. Even these days, allografts, usually taken by cadaver and xenografts, mostly from porcine skin, are used as temporary skin substitutes ahead to final coverage with autologous skin grafting, which provides a temporary coverage for up to 14 days, followed by the immunoreaction and rejection [5,63]. Currently, two common types of foreign skin are available, cryo-preserved or glycerol-preserved allografts [64]. Both preservation procedures have shown different benefits. While cryo-preserved allografts demonstrated a better tissue viability, the glycerol preservation is cost-efficient, can reduce the antigenicity, and leads to longer storage periods [65–68].

The usage of porcine skin as a temporary wound dressing became popular in the 1960s, and it is still the most commonly used xenograft [62]. The major advantages of porcine skin include its easy availability and histopathological similarity to human skin [69,70]. Novel approaches are the usage of fish skin as a temporary biological dressing [71–73]. Alam and Jeffery demonstrated complete re-epithelialization in the absence of infection or adverse reaction in a case series of 10 patients with partial thickness burns treated with fish skin [72]. Bruno et al. presented Nile Tilapia fish skin as an easily available and cost-effective option as a xenograft [73]. A phase II randomized controlled trial showed that patients treated with Nile Tilapia fish skin had a statistically significant reduction of the mean time for re-epithelialization, significant pain reduction, and lower requirement of dressing changes compared with patients under silver sulfadiazine treatment [71]. According to these findings, fish skin seems to be a promising candidate as an effective and low-cost biological dressing for burn treatment, especially in middle- to low-income countries. However, for the introduction into the hospital setting, further investigations need to be done.

Sandwich Technique

Another option for the treatment of extensive loss of skin is the combined application of autologous STSGs and allografts. In 1981, Alexander et al. first publicized the successful usage of widely meshed autologous split-thickness skin grafts (1:6), which were overlayed by meshed allogeneic skin grafts (ratio 1:2) [74]. Although the usage of widely expanded mesh grafts has shown a bad outcome, the dressing with allografts enabled this method for the treatment of extensive burns, despite the lack of donor sites [74–76]. Good clinical results and a high rate of re-epithelization were achieved with the sandwich technique [74,77].

6. A Brief History of Skin Substitutes and Their Use Today

Despite the great achievements of the expansion methods of Tanner and Meek, the treatment of extensive burns still presents crucial problems. Due to insufficient amounts of healthy native skin during the acute phase, an initial coverage with autologous skin is sometimes not possible. Therefore, several methods were developed over the past years to handle the absence of donor sites.

6.1. Cell Cultures

The first published formation of epidermis-like tissue by in vitro cultivation of human epidermal keratinocytes was performed by Rheinwald and Green in 1975 [78]. Ten years later, the first usage of human cultured epidermal autografts (CEAs) in a clinical case series were performed in 1980 by Connor et al [79]. Nowadays, the usage of CEAs is reserved for extensive burn injuries as a last resort opportunity when significantly less donor sites are remaining and other alternatives are not applicable. However, the application of CEAs is extremely time-consuming; these grafts are very fragile and susceptible to shear forces, and they additionally have a higher rate of blistering and re-grafting requirement [80,81]. A novel approach in the wound closure of extensive burned patients is the conjunction of CEAs with split-thickness skin grafting using high expansion techniques [82–84]. These methods enable the coverage of fragile body parts susceptible to pressure or shear forces with autologous STSGs, while insensitive areas can be covered with CEAs [82]. Another benefit is the reduction of donor sites [82,84]. Since 2007, cell therapies such as CEAs are considered as "Advanced Therapy Medicinal Products" (ATMP) by European Directives along with associated Regulations by the European Parliament. The aim of this adaption was to improve the safety and efficiency of cell therapy by standardization. Due to these new regulations, cell cultures need to be accomplished in an approved laboratory, along with new quality inspection measures and complex pathways, which the medical practitioner has to assess before deciding if a technique should be introduced [85]. Furthermore, the compliance of Good Manufacturing Practice requirements, as well the marketing authorization, for cell therapy production in hospital settings leads to higher costs [86]. Although it is important to ensure the safety for burn patients, these changes present a major challenge for clinical research not only in burn care but also in other cell research facilities in the hospital settings [85]. Gardien et al. showed the possibility of conducting a multicenter clinical trial that follows all requirements consistent with the ATMP guidelines [87].

6.2. Dermal Substitutes

In the last decades, burn care research has shifted from pure survival to a better quality of survival by focusing on improvement of the scars outcome and contractures prevention. Better functional and aesthetical results can be achieved through the use of dermal substitutes during the acute phase of burns [88]. Therefore the gain in importance of alloplastic or mixed synthetic–biological carriers with different alloplastic materials as dermal substitutes were observed in recent decades.

The first dermal analoga called "Integra®" was developed in the 1980s by Yannas and Burke as an alternative burn injury treatment [89,90]. Integra® consists of a dermal layer of bovine collagen and chondroitin-6-sulfate glycos-aminoglycan (GAG), as well an epidermal layer of silicone, and it was designed for the treatment of fresh excised full-thickness burns. The silicone layer has to be removed and replaced by a split-thickness skin graft after 2 or 3 weeks [91,92]. Aesthetic and functional results similar to healthy skin can be achieved in burned hands treated with Integra® and STSGs [93,94]. Currently, Integra® represents the most accepted artificial skin substitute due to favorable long-term use and outcomes [88,91,92]. Recently, a single layer version of Integra® was developed. The aim of this single layer version was to enable a one-step procedure with the simultaneous application of autologous STSGs [95]. However, further studies are necessary to establish an Integra® single layer in burn care.

Another option is the treatment with Matriderm®, a single layer dermal substitute, which consists of a collagen-based matrix and allows a one-step procedure in combination with an autologous split-thickness skin graft as an alternative for the missing epidermal layer [96,97]. The use of Matriderm® in the treatments of burns in aesthetic and functional important areas achieved good results. Two studies by Ryssel et al. demonstrated an improved skin quality and range of motion in full-thickness burns of the hand's dorsum treated with STSGs and Matriderm® compared with ones treated by STSGs alone [98,99]. Furthermore, Matriderm® is useful for the treatment of facial burns [96,100]. According to Jackson and Roman, the combination of Matriderm® with split-thickness skin grafts is a safe and effective method to achieve better aesthetic and functional results in full-thickness facial burns [96].

Hyaluronic acid-based wound dressings were also introduced as an alternative for the dermal layer. Hyaluronic acid has a supportive role in the healing process, such as the stimulation of epidermal cell proliferation and migration, as well the promotion of fibroblast differentiation into myofibroblasts. Furthermore, hyaluronic acid improves the re-epithelization and granulation [101,102]. Hyalomatrix® was designed as a temporary dressing in cases of deep burns and full-thickness wounds for wound bed preparation prior to definitive coverage with STSGs [103–105]. Faga et al. demonstrated that the application of STSGs followed by Hyalomatrix® supports the dermis regeneration. The long-term biopsies showed that the regenerative skin was similar to healthy skin [106]. Gravante et al. even described that the aesthetic long-term result of patients treated with Hyalomatrix® were similar to those treated with the combination of STSGs and Hyalomatrix® [103].

In conclusion, the introduction of dermal substitutes led to burn care innovations, which enabled better functional and aesthetic outcomes. A major disadvantage is the dependence of the application of native skin. Future perspectives include the development of skin substitutes that are able to replace the dermal and the epidermal layer.

6.3. Cell Suspension

In 1895, Mangold described the first successful clinical application of scraped epithelial cells, which are known as a precursor of keratinocyte suspensions in modern burn care nowadays [107]. However, the technology was not able to be implemented due to the lack of an eligible carrier substance. Hunyadi et al. performed the first successful suspension of uncultured keratinocytes fixed on a fibrin carrier to treat chronic wounds in 1987 [108]. Nowadays, ReCell® is a common method for the preparation of non-cultured autologous cells by the isolation of cells from a small donor site and immediate autologous replantation by spraying to promote the healing process. ReCell® shows similar aesthetic results as STSGs and achieves an expansion ratio up to 1:80 [109–111]. The major benefit is the reduction of required donor sites for the treatment of high skin losses in severe burns [109–111]. However, the procedure is very time-consuming, which leads to greater surgical stress for the patients and additional surgery costs [110].

7. The Curse of Donor Site Morbidity

Donor site morbidity is a considerable problem in surgery burn care that has attracted attention in recent years. Despite the advantages of split-thickness skin grafting, the harvesting of donor sites creates secondary injuries. These injuries need wound care and can be associated with donor site morbidities such as pain, pruritus, wound infection, and hyperpigmentation as well unaesthetic and unpleasant hypertrophic scars [112,113]. While morbidities such as pain and scars are common, the infection rate seems to be low [113]. Almost no findings are available on the prevalence of hypertrophic scars associated with donor site [114,115]. According to retrospective analyses, 34% of reviewed patients were affected by persistent hypertrophic scarring [114]. Karlsson et al. demonstrated that 28% of the patients in a randomized longitudinal clinical trial had donor site hypertrophic scars [115]. However, scar formation seems to be a major problem for affected patients. In a cohort study, Legemate et al. evaluated the long-term scar quality of donor sites as stated by burn patients. Patients assessed the scar quality at 12 months after burn by using the Patient and Observer Scar Assessment Scale (POSAS) version 2.0. The patients' overall opinion of the donor site scars was conspicuously high. The overall PSOAS score was 3.2 (1–10), even 1 year after surgery [116].

The usage of techniques, such as regrafting of the donor site or minced skin grafting, is described to reduce donor-site morbidity. Regrafting of the donor site is based on taking a larger amount of skin to cover not only the initial defect but also the donor site [117–119]. Several studies described an acceleration in re-epithelization, an improved scar quality, less pain, and a better aesthetic outcome by regrafting the donor site [117–119]. According to Bradow et al., all remaining pieces of a split-thickness skin graft should be placed back to the donor site. They also supposed that patients with poor healing potential could benefit from additional skin harvesting just for regrafting [117]. However, not all patients seem to benefit from the regrafting procedure. Legemate et al. demonstrated a worse result of the regrafted part compared with a non-grafted part in a follow up control of a 26-year-old woman 12 months after regrafting. While the non-grafted part was only a little erythematous, the regrafted part showed an irregular surface and a mix of hypo- and hyperpigmentation [120].

The technique of minced skin grafting is based on the use of the exceeded split skin, remaining after the application at the regular recipient area. These leftovers are prepared with tissue scissors until they get pasty enough to be dispensed onto the donor site [121,122]. Several studies showed a better quality of healing in terms of re-epithelialization and pigmentation, as well in a reduction of hypertrophic scarring and pruritus [121–123].

In conclusion, the application of STSG leftovers seems to be a promising way for the donor site treatment to reduce unpleasant morbidities. Especially, patients expected to develop a donor site morbidity could benefit from such procedures. Overall, a risk–benefit analysis could be useful to decide which patients could benefit by such procedures and who might not. Another technique to reduce donor site morbidity is dermal grafting, which is described below [124,125].

8. The Dermis Graft—A Novel Approach

Dermis grafting is a method to obtain a de-epithelialized split-thickness skin graft [124]. The technique of dermis grafting is based on the simultaneous harvesting of a purely dermal split-thickness graft from the same donor site after taking the standard split-thickness skin graft [124,125]. In this procedure, two grafts are obtained, and the dermis graft is always transferred to the recipient site, while the ordinary split-thickness skin graft can serve as an additional graft [125], or it can be used for donor site coverage [124]. Lindeford et al. observed no difference in the healing duration between the dermal grafts and standard split-thickness skin grafts [125]. According to Han et al., the dermis grafting is superior to the regular STSG technique not only due to the accelerated and improved healing of the donor site but also in terms of pigmentation, height, and vascularity at the recipient sites [124]. Altogether, dermal grafting is an interesting method, which enables obtaining two grafts from a single donor site to minimize the need of available skin in extended burns and to reduce donor site-associated morbidity.

9. Conclusions

Great achievements in the development of skin grafting were made, especially over the past 200 years. Many of them are still part of the current burn injury treatment. Nowadays, autologous split-thickness skin grafting is considered as the gold standard for the treatment of major traumatic loss of skin caused by burns. The development of expansion methods enables the coverage of large wound surfaces and increases the survival of severely burned patients. Additionally, to the survival of severe burns, the quality of survival, by preventing scars formation and contractures, is one of the main goals in burn injuries management. A more cosmetic and functional result can be obtained by the usage of full-thickness skin grafts in reconstruction. However, autologous skin grafting is limited by available donor sites, especially in the initial treatment of severely burned patients. Historically, various attempts were already made to reproduce the properties of healthy skin to fill this gap. Significant progresses were made in the development of skin substitutes, which are a great discovery and fulfill their purpose in the burn injuries treatment. However, commonly used skin substitutes are not able to achieve the properties of native skin. Almost all products are only able to replace one: the epidermal or dermal skin layers. As a current challenge, donor site morbidity, such as wound infection, hyperpigmentation, and hypertrophic scarring attract attention. Several approaches were already made to solve this problem. However, further investigations are needed. The long-term objective is the development of novel methods or combined techniques allowing covering large burn surfaces without the necessity of high amounts of donor sites. In summary, the desired result has not been achieved, and despite several drawbacks, autologous skin grafting remains the method of choice for burn coverage, even more than 3000 years after its discovery.

Limitations: This review has some inherent limitations. Many of the original articles are not written in the English language or are not available through the online database, which is caused by the fact that they are even older than the internet. Therefore, the content of this review is reliant on reprints and biographical literature. Finally, our review is limited to articles retrieved from PubMed and Google Scholar only with the possibility of missed publications.

Author Contributions: Conceptualization, Methodology, and Data Acquisition, M.K.; Writing—Original Draft Preparation, M.K.; Review and Editing, H.L. and S.P.N.; Supervision, L.P.K. All authors have read and agreed to the published version of the manuscript.

Funding: This research received no external funding.

Institutional Review Board Statement: Ethical review and approval were waived caused by exclusive use of data from the literature.

Informed Consent Statement: Patient consent was not necessary due to exclusive use of data from the literature.

Data Availability Statement: No new data were created or analyzed due to this study. Data sharing is not applicable to this article.

Conflicts of Interest: All authors declare no conflict of interest.

References

1. Church, D.; Elsayed, S.; Reid, O.; Winston, B.; Lindsay, R. Burn Wound Infections. *Clin. Microbiol. Rev.* **2006**, *19*, 403–434. [CrossRef]
2. Sorg, H.; Tilkorn, D.J.; Hager, S.; Hauser, J.; Mirastschijski, U. Skin Wound Healing: An Update on the Current Knowledge and Concepts. *Eur. Surg. Res.* **2017**, *58*, 81–94. [CrossRef]
3. Brusselaers, N.; Pirayesh, A.; Hoeksema, H.; Richters, C.D.; Verbelen, J.; Beele, H.; Blot, S.I.; Monstrey, S. Skin Replacement in Burn Wounds. *J. Trauma Inj. Infect. Crit. Care* **2010**, *68*, 490–501. [CrossRef] [PubMed]

4. Jeschke, M.G.; Shahrokhi, S.; Finnerty, C.C.; Branski, L.K.; Dibildox, M. Wound Coverage Technologies in Burn Care: Established Techniques. *J. Burn. Care Res.* **2018**, *39*, 313–318. [CrossRef] [PubMed]
5. Jeschke, M.G.; Van Baar, M.E.; Choudhry, M.A.; Chung, K.K.; Gibran, N.S.; Logsetty, S. Burn injury. *Nat. Rev. Dis. Prim.* **2020**, *6*, 11. [CrossRef] [PubMed]
6. Ehrenfried, A. Reverdin and Other Methods of Skin-Grafting: Historical. *Boston Med Surg. J.* **1909**, *161*, 911–917. [CrossRef]
7. Ang, G.C. History of skin transplantation. *Clin. Dermatol.* **2005**, *23*, 320–324. [CrossRef]
8. Hauben, D.J.; Baruchin, A.; Mahler, A. On the History of the Free Skin Graft. *Ann. Plast. Surg.* **1982**, *9*, 242–245. [CrossRef]
9. Hattery, E.; Nguyen, T.; Baker, A.; Palmieri, T. Burn Care in the 1800s. *J. Burn. Care Res.* **2015**, *36*, 236–239. [CrossRef]
10. McDowell, F. Successful attempt of reconstruction of a nose from a completely separated piece of skin from the leg, by Prof. Dr. Bünger, Marburg, Germany. (Journal der Chirurgie and Augenheilkunde, 4: 569, 1822). Translated from the German by Dr. Hans May. *Plast. Reconstr. Surg.* **1969**, *44*, 486–490.
11. Fariña-Pérez, L.A. Jaques-Louis Reverdin (1842–1929): The surgeon and the needle. *Arch. Esp. Urol.* **2010**, *63*, 269–274. [CrossRef]
12. Freshwater, M.F.; Krizek, T.J. Skin grafting of burns: A centennial. A tribute to George David Pollock. *J. Trauma* **1971**, *11*, 862–865. [CrossRef]
13. Freshwater, M.F.; Krizek, T.J. George David Pollock and the Development of Skin Grafting. *Ann. Plast. Surg.* **1978**, *1*, 96–102. [CrossRef]
14. Rogers, B.O. Historical Development of Free Skin Grafting. *Surg. Clin. N. Am.* **1959**, *39*, 289–311. [CrossRef]
15. McDowell, F. Carl Thiersch, microscopy, and skin grafting. *Plast. Reconstr. Surg.* **1968**, *41*, 369–370. [PubMed]
16. Blair, V.P.; Brown, J.B. The use and uses of large split skin grafts of intermediate thickness. *Plast. Reconstr. Surg.* **1968**, *42*, 65–75. [CrossRef]
17. Padgett, E.C. Skin grafting and the "three-quarter"-thickness skin graft for prevention and correction of cicatricial, formation. *Ann. Surg.* **1941**, *113*, 1034–1049. [CrossRef] [PubMed]
18. Braza, M.E.; Fahrenkopf, M.P. *Split-Thickness Skin Grafts*; StatPearls Publishing: Treasure Island, FL, USA, 2021. [PubMed]
19. Janzekovic, Z. A new concept in the early excision and immediate grafting of burns. *J. Trauma* **1970**, *10*, 1103–1108. [CrossRef] [PubMed]
20. Barret, J.P.; Dziewulski, P.; Wolf, S.E.; Desai, M.H.; Nichols, R.J.; Herndon, D.N. Effect of topical and subcutaneous epinephrine in combination with topical thrombin in blood loss during immediate near-total burn wound excision in pediatric burned patients. *Burns* **1999**, *25*, 509–513. [CrossRef]
21. Masella, D.P.C.; Balent, E.M.; Carlson, D.T.L.; Lee, B.K.W.; Pierce, D.L.M. Evaluation of Six Split-thickness Skin Graft Donor-site Dressing Materials in a Swine Model. *Plast. Reconstr. Surg.* **2013**, *1*, 1–11. [CrossRef]
22. Chan, Q.E.; Barzi, F.; Harvey, J.G.; Holland, A.J.A. Functional and Cosmetic Outcome of Full- Versus Split-Thickness Skin Grafts in Pediatric Palmar Surface Burns: A prospective, independent evaluation. *J. Burn. Care Res.* **2013**, *34*, 232–236. [CrossRef]
23. Pripotnev, S.; Papp, A. Split thickness skin graft meshing ratio indications and common practices. *Burns* **2017**, *43*, 1775–1781. [CrossRef] [PubMed]
24. Van Niekerk, G.; Adams, S.; Rode, H. Scalp as a donor site in children: Is it really the best option? *Burns* **2018**, *44*, 1259–1268. [CrossRef] [PubMed]
25. Mimoun, M.; Chaouat, M.; Picovski, D.; Serroussi, D.; Smarrito, S. The Scalp Is an Advantageous Donor Site for Thin-Skin Grafts: A Report on 945 Harvested Samples. *Plast. Reconstr. Surg.* **2006**, *118*, 369–373. [CrossRef] [PubMed]
26. Desai, M.H.; Herndon, D.N.; Rutan, R.L.; Parker, J. An Unusual Donor Site, a Lifesaver in Extensive Burns. *J. Burn Care Rehabil.* **1988**, *9*, 637–639. [CrossRef]
27. Wyrzykowski, D.; Chrzanowska, B.; Czauderna, P. Ten years later—Scalp still a primary donor site in children. *Burns* **2015**, *41*, 359–363. [CrossRef]
28. Nikkhah, D.; Booth, S.; Tay, S.; Gilbert, P.; Dheansa, B. Comparing outcomes of sheet grafting with 1:1 mesh grafting in patients with thermal burns: A randomized trial. *Burns* **2015**, *41*, 257–264. [CrossRef]
29. Greenhalgh, D.G. Management of burns. *N. Engl. J. Med.* **2019**, *380*, 2349–2359. [CrossRef]
30. Archer, S.B.; Henke, A.; Greenhalgh, D.G.; Warden, G.D. The Use of Sheet Autografts to Cover Extensive Burns in Patients. *J. Burn. Care Rehabil.* **1998**, *19*, 33–38. [CrossRef]
31. Brown, J.B.; McDowell, F. Massive repairs of burns with thick split-skin grafts: Emergency dressings with homografts. *Ann. Surg.* **1942**, *115*, 658–674. [CrossRef]
32. Clodius, L. The classic reprint. Die Transplantation Betreffend by Prof. Otto Lanz. *Plast. Reconstr. Surg.* **1972**, *50*, 395–397. [PubMed]
33. Tanner, J.C.; Vandeput, J.; Olley, J.F. The mesh skin graft. *Plast. Reconstr. Surg.* **1964**, *34*, 287–292.
34. Tanner, J.C.; Vandeput, J.J.; Bradley, W.H. Mesh skin grafting: Report of a typical case. *J. Occup. Med.* **1965**, *7*, 175–176. [CrossRef] [PubMed]
35. Salisbury, R.B. Use of the Mesh Skin Graft in Treatment of Massive Casualty Wounds. *Plast. Reconstr. Surg.* **1967**, *40*, 161–162. [CrossRef] [PubMed]
36. Macmillan, B.G. The Use of Mesh Grafting in Treating Burns. *Surg. Clin. N. Am.* **1970**, *50*, 1347–1359. [CrossRef]
37. Meek, C.P. Successful microdermagrafting using the Meek-Wall microdermatome. *Am. J. Surg.* **1958**, *96*, 557–558. [CrossRef]
38. Ottomann, C.; Hartmann, B.; Branski, L.; Krohn, C. A tribute to Cicero Parker Meek. *Burns* **2015**, *41*, 1660–1663. [CrossRef]
39. Meek, C.P. Medical Debridement and Microdermagrafting of Burns. *South. Med J.* **1963**, *56*, 1074–1076. [CrossRef]

40. Meek, C.P. Microdermagrafting: The Meek technic. *Hosp. Top.* **1965**, *43*, 114–116. [CrossRef]
41. Kreis, R.; Mackie, D.; Vloemans, A.; Hermans, R.; Hoekstra, M. Widely expanded postage stamp skin grafts using a modified Meek technique in combination with an allograft overlay. *Burns* **1993**, *19*, 142–145. [CrossRef]
42. Lumenta, D.B.; Kamolz, L.-P.; Frey, M. Adult Burn Patients With More Than 60% TBSA Involved–Meek and Other Techniques to Overcome Restricted Skin Harvest Availability–The Viennese Concept. *J. Burn. Care Res.* **2009**, *30*, 231–242. [CrossRef] [PubMed]
43. Dahmardehei, M.; Vaghardoost, R.; Saboury, M.; Zarei, H.; Saboury, S.; Molaei, M.; Seyyedi, J.; Maleknejad, A.; Hospital, I.F. Comparison of Modified Meek Technique with Standard Mesh Method in Patients with Third Degree Burns. *World J. Plast. Surg.* **2020**, *9*, 267–273. [CrossRef] [PubMed]
44. Lee, S.Z.; Halim, A.S.; Sulaiman, W.A.W.; Saad, A.Z.M. Outcome of the Modified Meek Technique in the Management of Major Pediatric Burns. *Ann. Plast. Surg.* **2018**, *81*, 295–301. [CrossRef] [PubMed]
45. Lari, A.R.; Gang, R.K. Expansion technique for skin grafts (Meek technique) in the treatment of severely burned patients. *Burns* **2001**, *27*, 61–66. [CrossRef]
46. Wanjala, N.F.; Paul, O.J.; Sephania, O.R. Meek Micro-grafting Technique in Reduction of Mortality and Hospital Stay in Patients with Extensive Burns in a Resource Constrained Setting. *J. Surg.* **2018**, *6*, 154. [CrossRef]
47. Sánchez-García, A.; Vanaclocha, N.; García-Vilariño, E.; Salmerón-González, E.; Vicente-Pardo, A.; Pérez-Del Caz, M.D. Use of the Meek Micrografting Technique for Coverage of Extensive Burns: A Case Report. *Plast. Surg. Nurs.* **2019**, *39*, 44–47. [CrossRef]
48. Houschyar, K.S.; Tapking, C.; Nietzschmann, I.; Rein, S.; Weissenberg, K.; Chelliah, M.P.; Duscher, D.; Maan, Z.N.; Philipps, H.M.; Sheckter, C.C.; et al. Five Years Experience With Meek Grafting in the Management of Extensive Burns in an Adult Burn Center. *Plast. Surg.* **2018**, *27*, 44–48. [CrossRef]
49. Lee, S.Z.; Halim, A.S. Superior long term functional and scar outcome of Meek micrografting compared to conventional split thickness skin grafting in the management of burns. *Burns* **2019**, *45*, 1386–1400. [CrossRef]
50. Munasinghe, N.; Wasiak, J.; Ives, A.; Cleland, H.; Lo, C.H. Retrospective review of a tertiary adult burn centre's experience with modified Meek grafting. *Burn. Trauma* **2016**, *4*, 6. [CrossRef]
51. Kilner, T.P. The Full-Thickness Skin Graft. *Postgrad. Med J.* **1935**, *11*, 279–282. [CrossRef]
52. Padgett, E.C. Indications for determination of the thickness of split skin grafts. *Am. J. Surg.* **1946**, *72*, 683–693. [CrossRef]
53. Çeliköz, B.; Deveci, M.; Duman, H.; Nişanci, M. Recontruction of facial defects and burn scars using large size freehand full-thickness skin graft from lateral thoracic region. *Burns* **2001**, *27*, 174–178. [CrossRef]
54. Somma, A.M.; Somma, L.M. John Reissberg Wolfe (1823–1904): A plastic surgeon in Garibaldi's Army. *J. Med Biogr.* **2010**, *18*, 77–80. [CrossRef] [PubMed]
55. Sykes, P.J. Wolfe's Part in the Italian Risorgimento and His Skin Graft. *Ann. Plast. Surg.* **2012**, *69*, 228–231. [CrossRef] [PubMed]
56. Bogdanov, S.B.; Gilevich, I.V.; Melkonyan, K.I.; Sotnichenko, A.S.; Alekseenko, S.N.; Porhanov, V.A. Total full-thickness skin grafting for treating patients with extensive facial burn injury: A 10-year experience. *Burns* **2020**. [CrossRef]
57. Weeks, D.; Kasdan, M.L.; Wilhelmi, B.J. Forty-Year Follow-up of Full-Thickness Skin Graft After Thermal Burn Injury to the Volar Hand. *Eplasty* **2016**, *16*, e21.
58. Merrell, S.W.; Saffle, J.R.; Schnebly, W.A.; Kravitz, M.; Warden, G.D. Full-Thickness Skin Grafting for Contact Burns of the Palm in Children. *J. Burn. Care Rehabil.* **1986**, *7*, 501–507. [CrossRef]
59. Seghers, M.J.; Longacre, J.J. Paul Bert and his animal grafts. *Plast. Reconstr. Surg.* **1964**, *33*, 178–186. [CrossRef]
60. Cooper, D.K.; Ekser, B.; Tector, A.J. A brief history of clinical xenotransplantation. *Int. J. Surg.* **2015**, *23 Pt B*, 205–210. [CrossRef]
61. Bromberg, B.E.; Song, I.C.; Mohn, M.P. The use of pig skin as a temporary biological dressing. *Plast. Reconstr. Surg.* **1965**, *36*, 80–90. [CrossRef]
62. Yamamoto, T.; Iwase, H.; King, T.W.; Hara, H.; Cooper, D.K. Skin xenotransplantation: Historical review and clinical potential. *Burns* **2018**, *44*, 1738–1749. [CrossRef]
63. Rowan, M.P.; Cancio, L.C.; Elster, E.A.; Burmeister, D.M.; Rose, L.F.; Natesan, S.; Chan, R.K.; Christy, R.J.; Chung, K.K. Burn wound healing and treatment: Review and advancements. *Crit. Care* **2015**, *19*, 1–12. [CrossRef] [PubMed]
64. Wang, C.; Zhang, F.; Lineaweaver, W.C. Clinical Applications of Allograft Skin in Burn Care. *Ann. Plast. Surg.* **2020**, *84*, S158–S160. [CrossRef] [PubMed]
65. Blome-Eberwein, S.; Jester, A.; Kuentscher, M.; Raff, T.; Germann, G.; Pelzer, M. Clinical practice of glycerol preserved allograft skin coverage. *Burns* **2002**, *28*, 10–12. [CrossRef]
66. Hoekstra, M.J.; Kreis, R.W.; du Pont, J.S. History of the Euro Skin Bank: The innovation of preservation technologies. *Burns* **1994**, *20*, S43–S47. [CrossRef]
67. Hermans, M.H. Preservation methods of allografts and their (lack of) influence on clinical results in partial thickness burns. *Burns* **2011**, *37*, 873–881. [CrossRef]
68. Kua, E.H.J.; Goh, C.Q.; Ting, Y.; Chua, A.; Song, C. Comparing the use of glycerol preserved and cryopreserved allogenic skin for the treatment of severe burns: Differences in clinical outcomes and in vitro tissue viability. *Cell Tissue Bank.* **2012**, *13*, 269–279. [CrossRef] [PubMed]
69. Debeer, S.; Le Luduec, J.-B.; Kaiserlian, D.; Laurent, P.; Nicolas, J.-F.; Dubois, B.; Kanitakis, J. Comparative histology and immunohistochemistry of porcine versus human skin. *Eur. J. Dermatol.* **2013**, *23*, 456–466. [CrossRef]

70. Sykes, D.S. Transplanting organs from pigs to humans Megan. *Physiol. Behav.* **2016**, *176*, 100–106. [CrossRef]
71. Júnior, E.M.L.; Filho, M.O.D.M.; Costa, B.A.; Rohleder, A.V.P.; Rocha, M.B.S.; Fechine, F.V.; Forte, A.J.; Alves, A.P.N.N.; Júnior, F.R.S.; Martins, C.B.; et al. Innovative Burn Treatment Using Tilapia Skin as a Xenograft: A Phase II Randomized Controlled Trial. *J. Burn. Care Res.* **2020**, *41*, 585–592. [CrossRef]
72. Alam, K.; Jeffery, S.L. Acellular Fish Skin Grafts for Management of Split Thickness Donor Sites and Partial Thickness Burns: A Case Series. *Mil. Med.* **2019**, *184*, 16–20. [CrossRef]
73. Costa, B.A.; Júnior, E.M.L. Use of Tilapia Skin as a Xenograft for Pediatric Burn Treatment: A Case Report. *J. Burn Care Res.* **2020**, *40*, 714–717. [CrossRef] [PubMed]
74. Alexander, J.W.; Macmillan, B.G.; Law, E.; Kittur, D.S. Treatment of severe burns with widely meshed skin autograft and meshed skin allograft overlay. *J. Trauma* **1981**, *21*, 433–438. [PubMed]
75. Phipps, A.R.; Clarke, J.A. The use of intermingled autograft and parental allograft skin in the treatment of major burns in children. *Br. J. Plast. Surg.* **1991**, *44*, 608–611. [CrossRef]
76. Qaryoute, S.; Mirdad, I.; Hamail, A. Usage of autograft and allograft skin in treatment of burns in children. *Burns* **2001**, *27*, 599–602. [CrossRef]
77. Horch, R.E.; Stark, G.; Kopp, J.; Spilker, G. Cologne Burn Centre experiences with glycerol-preserved allogeneic skin: Part I: Clinical experiences and histological findings (overgraft and sandwich technique). *Burns* **1994**, *20*, S23–S26. [CrossRef]
78. Rheinwatd, J.G.; Green, H. Serial cultivation of strains of human epidermal keratinocytes: The formation of keratinizing colonies from single cells. *Cell* **1975**, *6*, 331–343. [CrossRef]
79. O'Connor, N.; Mulliken, J.; Banks-Schlegel, S.; Kehinde, O.; Green, H. Grafting of burns with cultured epithelium prepared from autologous epidermal cells. *Lancet* **1981**, *317*, 75–78. [CrossRef]
80. Barret, J.P.; Wolf, S.E.; Desai, M.H.; Herndon, D.N. Cost-Efficacy of Cultured Epidermal Autografts in Massive Pediatric Burns. *Ann. Surg.* **2000**, *231*, 869–876. [CrossRef]
81. Matsumura, H.; Matsushima, A.; Ueyama, M.; Kumagai, N. Application of the cultured epidermal autograft "JACE®" for treatment of severe burns: Results of a 6-year multicenter surveillance in Japan. *Burns* **2016**, *42*, 769–776. [CrossRef] [PubMed]
82. Ottomann, C.; Küntscher, M.V.; Hartmann, B. The Combination of Cultured Epidermal Autograft (CEA) and Split Thickness Skin Graft Technique (Meek) in Therapy for Severe Burns. *Osteosynth. Trauma Care* **2007**, *15*, 29–33. [CrossRef]
83. Menon, S.; Li, Z.; Harvey, J.G.; Holland, A.J. The use of the Meek technique in conjunction with cultured epithelial autograft in the management of major paediatric burns. *Burns* **2013**, *39*, 674–679. [CrossRef] [PubMed]
84. Akita, S.; Hayashida, K.; Yoshimoto, H.; Fujioka, M.; Senju, C.; Morooka, S.; Nishimura, G.; Mukae, N.; Kobayashi, K.; Anraku, K.; et al. Novel Application of Cultured Epithelial Autografts (CEA) with Expanded Mesh Skin Grafting Over an Artificial Dermis or Dermal Wound Bed Preparation. *Int. J. Mol. Sci.* **2018**, *19*, 57. [CrossRef] [PubMed]
85. Dimitropoulos, G.; Jafari, P.; de Buys Roessingh, A.; Hirt-Burri, N.; Raffoul, W.; Applegate, L.A. Burn patient care lost in good manufacturing practices? *Ann. Burn. Fire Disasters* **2016**, *29*, 111–115.
86. Abdel-Sayed, P.; Michetti, M.; Scaletta, C.; Flahaut, M.; Hirt-Burri, N.; Roessingh, A.D.B.; Raffoul, W.; Applegate, L.A. Cell therapies for skin regeneration: An overview of 40 years of experience in burn units. *Swiss Med Wkly.* **2019**, *149*, w20079. [CrossRef]
87. Gardien, K.L.M.; Marck, R.E.; Bloemen, M.C.T.; Waaijman, T.; Gibbs, S.; Ulrich, M.M.W.; Middelkoop, E. Outcome of Burns Treated with Autologous Cultured Proliferating Epidermal Cells: A Prospective Randomized Multicenter Intrapatient Comparative Trial. *Cell Transplant.* **2016**, *25*, 437–448. [CrossRef]
88. Arno, A.I.; Jeschke, M.G. The Use of Dermal Substitutes in Burn Surgery: Acute Phase. *Dermal Replace. Gen. Burn Plast. Surg. Tissue Eng. Clin. Pr.* **2014**, *9783709115*, 193–210. [CrossRef]
89. Yannas, I.V.; Burke, J.F. Design of an artificial skin. I. Basic design principles. *J. Biomed. Mater. Res.* **1980**, *14*, 65–81. [CrossRef]
90. Yannas, I.V.; Burke, J.F.; Gordon, P.L.; Huang, C.; Rubenstein, R.H. Design of an artificial skin. II. Control of chemical composition. *J. Biomed. Mater. Res.* **1980**, *14*, 107–132. [CrossRef]
91. Heimbach, D.M.; Warden, G.D.; Luterman, A.; Jordan, M.H.; Ozobia, N.; Ryan, C.M.; Voigt, D.W.; Hickerson, W.L.; Saffle, J.R.; Declement, F.A.; et al. Multicenter Postapproval Clinical Trial of Integra® Dermal Regeneration Template for Burn Treatment. *J. Burn. Care Rehabil.* **2003**, *24*, 42–48. [CrossRef]
92. Branski, L.K.; Herndon, D.N.; Pereira, C.; Mlcak, R.P.; Celis, M.M.; Lee, J.O.; Sanford, A.P.; Norbury, W.B.; Zhang, X.-J.; Jeschke, M.G. Longitudinal assessment of Integra in primary burn management: A randomized pediatric clinical trial. *Crit. Care Med.* **2007**, *35*, 2615–2623. [CrossRef] [PubMed]
93. Danin, A.; Georgesco, G.; Le Touze, A.; Penaud, A.; Quignon, R.; Zakine, G. Assessment of burned hands reconstructed with Integra® by ultrasonography and elastometry. *Burns* **2012**, *38*, 998–1004. [CrossRef]
94. Cuadra, Á.; Correa, G.; Roa, R.; Piñeros, J.L.; Norambuena, H.; Searle, S.; Heras, R.L.; Calderon, W. Functional results of burned hands treated with Integra®. *J. Plast. Reconstr. Aesthetic Surg.* **2012**, *65*, 228–234. [CrossRef]
95. Koenen, W.; Felcht, M.; Vockenroth, K.; Sassmann, G.; Goerdt, S.; Faulhaber, J. One-stage reconstruction of deep facial defects with a single layer dermal regeneration template. *J. Eur. Acad. Dermatol. Venereol.* **2010**, *25*, 788–793. [CrossRef] [PubMed]
96. Jackson, S.R.; Roman, S. Matriderm and Split Skin Grafting for Full-Thickness Pediatric Facial Burns. *J. Burn Care Res.* **2019**, *40*, 251–254. [CrossRef]

97. Phillips, G.S.A.; Nizamoglu, M.; Wakure, A.; Barnes, D.; Dziewulski, P. The use of dermal regeneration templates for primary burns surgery in a UK regional burns centre. *Ann. Burn. Fire Disasters* **2020**, *XXXIII*, 245–252.
98. Ryssel, H.; Gazyakan, E.; Germann, G.; Öhlbauer, M. The use of MatriDerm® in early excision and simultaneous autologous skin grafting in burns—A pilot study. *Burns* **2008**, *34*, 93–97. [CrossRef]
99. Ryssel, H.; Germann, G.; Kloeters, O.; Gazyakan, E.; Radu, C. Dermal substitution with Matriderm® in burns on the dorsum of the hand. *Burns* **2010**, *36*, 1248–1253. [CrossRef]
100. Greenhalgh, D.G.; Hinchcliff, K.; Sen, S.; Palmieri, T.L. A Ten-Year Experience with Pediatric Face Grafts. *J. Burn. Care Res.* **2010**, *34*, 576–584. [CrossRef] [PubMed]
101. Graça, M.F.; Miguel, S.P.; Cabral, C.S.; Correia, I.J. Hyaluronic acid—Based wound dressings: A review. *Carbohydr. Polym.* **2020**, *241*, 116364. [CrossRef]
102. Longinotti, C. The use of hyaluronic acid based dressings to treat burns: A review. *Burn. Trauma* **2014**, *2*, 162–168. [CrossRef] [PubMed]
103. Gravante, G.; Sorge, R.; Merone, A.; Tamisani, A.M.; Di Lonardo, A.; Scalise, A.; Doneddu, G.; Melandri, D.; Stracuzzi, G.; Onesti, M.G.; et al. Hyalomatrix PA in Burn Care Practice: Results from a national retrospective survey, 2005 to 2006. *Ann. Plast. Surg.* **2010**, *64*, 69–79. [CrossRef]
104. Erbatur, S.; Coban, Y.K.; Aydın, E.N. Comparision of clinical and histopathological results of hyalomatrix usage in adult patients. *Int. J. Burn. Trauma* **2012**, *2*, 118–125.
105. Gravante, G.; Delogu, D.; Giordan, N.; Morano, G.; Montone, A.; Esposito, G. The Use of Hyalomatrix PA in the Treatment of Deep Partial-Thickness Burns. *J. Burn. Care Res.* **2007**, *28*, 269–274. [CrossRef] [PubMed]
106. Faga, A.; Nicoletti, G.; Brenta, F.; Scevola, S.; Abatangelo, G.; Brun, P. Hyaluronic acid three-dimensional scaffold for surgical revision of retracting scars: A human experimental study. *Int. Wound J.* **2013**, *10*, 329–335. [CrossRef] [PubMed]
107. Mangoldt, F. Die Epithelsaat zum Verschlußeiner großen Wundfläche. *Med. Wochenscher* **1895**, *21*, 798–903. [CrossRef]
108. Hunyadi, J.; Farkas, B.; Bertényi, C.; Oláh, J.; Dobozy, A. Keratinocyte Grafting: Covering of Skin Defects by Separated Autologous Keratinocytes in a Fibrin Net. *J. Investig. Dermatol.* **1987**, *89*, 119–120. [CrossRef] [PubMed]
109. Holmes, J.; Molnar, J.; Shupp, J.; Hickerson, W.; King, B.T.; Foster, K.; Cairns, B.; Carter, J. Demonstration of the safety and effectiveness of the RECELL® System combined with split-thickness meshed autografts for the reduction of donor skin to treat mixed-depth burn injuries. *Burns* **2019**, *45*, 772–782. [CrossRef] [PubMed]
110. Gravante, G.; Di Fede, M.; Araco, A.; Grimaldi, M.; De Angelis, B.; Arpino, A.; Cervelli, V.; Montone, A. A randomized trial comparing ReCell® system of epidermal cells delivery versus classic skin grafts for the treatment of deep partial thickness burns. *Burns* **2007**, *33*, 966–972. [CrossRef]
111. Iv, J.H.H.; Molnar, J.; Carter, J.; Hwang, J.; Cairns, B.; King, B.T.; Smith, D.J.; Cruse, C.W.; Foster, K.N.; Peck, M.D.; et al. A Comparative Study of the ReCell® Device and Autologous Split-Thickness Meshed Skin Graft in the Treatment of Acute Burn Injuries. *J. Burn. Care Res.* **2018**, *39*, 694–702. [CrossRef]
112. Otene, C.; Olaitan, P.B.; Ogbonnaya, I.S.; Nnabuko, R. Donor site morbidity following harvest of split-thickness skin grafts in south eastern nigeria. *J. West Afr. Coll. Surg.* **2016**, *1*, 86–96.
113. Asuku, M.; Yan, Q.; Yu, T.-C.; Boing, E.; Hahn, H.; Hovland, S.; Donelan, M.B. 522 Skin Graft Donor-site Morbidity: A Systematic Literature Review. *J. Burn. Care Res.* **2020**, *41*, S98–S99. [CrossRef]
114. Rotatori, R.M.; Starr, B.; Peake, M.; Fowler, L.; James, L.; Nelson, J.; Dale, E.L. Prevalence and Risk Factors for Hypertrophic Scarring of Split Thickness Autograft Donor Sites in a Pediatric Burn Population. *Burns* **2019**, *45*, 1066–1074. [CrossRef] [PubMed]
115. Karlsson, M.; Elmasry, M.; Steinvall, I.; Sjöberg, F.; Olofsson, P.; Thorfinn, J. Scarring At Donor Sites After Split-Thickness Skin Graft: A Prospective, Longitudinal, Randomized Trial. *Adv. Ski. Wound Care* **2018**, *31*, 183–188. [CrossRef]
116. Legemate, C.M.; Ooms, P.J.; Trommel, N.; Middelkoop, E.; van Baar, M.E.; Goei, H.; van der Vlies, C.H. Patient-reported scar quality of donor-sites following split-skin grafting in burn patients: Long-term results of a prospective cohort study. *Burns* **2021**, *47*, 315–321. [CrossRef] [PubMed]
117. Bradow, B.P.; Hallock, G.G.; Wilcock, S.P. Immediate Regrafting of the Split Thickness Skin Graft Donor Site Assists Healing. *Plast. Reconstr. Surg. Glob. Open* **2017**, *5*, e1339. [CrossRef]
118. Goverman, J.; Kraft, C.T.; Fagan, S.; Levi, B. Back Grafting the Split-Thickness Skin Graft Donor Site. *J. Burn. Care Res.* **2017**, *38*, e443–e449. [CrossRef]
119. Bian, Y.; Sun, C.; Zhang, X.; Li, Y.; Li, W.; Lv, X.; Li, J.; Jiang, L.; Li, J.; Feng, J.; et al. Wound-healing improvement by resurfacing split-thickness skin donor sites with thin split-thickness grafting. *Burns* **2016**, *42*, 123–130. [CrossRef]
120. Legemate, C.M.; Lucas, Y.; Oen, I.M.M.H.; Van Der Vlies, C.H. Regrafting of the Split-Thickness Skin Graft Donor-Site: Is It Beneficial? *J. Burn. Care Res.* **2020**, *41*, 211–214. [CrossRef]
121. Miyanaga, T.; Kishibe, M.; Yamashita, M.; Kaneko, T.; Kinoshita, F.; Shimada, K. Minced Skin Grafting for Promoting Wound Healing and Improving Donor-Site Appearance after Split-Thickness Skin Grafting: A Prospective Half-Side Comparative Trial. *Plast. Reconstr. Surg.* **2019**, *144*, 475–483. [CrossRef]
122. Kumar, P.; Ajai, K.S.; Sharma, R.K. The role of recruited minced skin grafting in improving the quality of healing at the donor site of split-thickness skin graft—A comparative study. *Burns* **2019**, *45*, 923–928. [CrossRef]
123. Miyanaga, T.; Haseda, Y.; Sakagami, A. Minced skin grafting for promoting epithelization of the donor site after split-thickness skin grafting. *Burns* **2017**, *43*, 819–823. [CrossRef] [PubMed]

124. Han, S.-K.; Yoon, T.-H.; Kim, J.-B.; Kim, W.-K. Dermis Graft for Wound Coverage. *Plast. Reconstr. Surg.* **2007**, *120*, 166–172. [CrossRef] [PubMed]
125. Lindford, A.J.; Kaartinen, I.S.; Virolainen, S.; Kuokkanen, H.O.; Vuola, J. The dermis graft: Another autologous option for acute burn wound coverage. *Burns* **2012**, *38*, 274–282. [CrossRef] [PubMed]

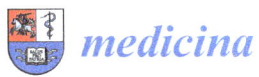

Review

A Narrative Review of the History of Skin Grafting in Burn Care

Deepak K. Ozhathil *, Michael W. Tay, Steven E. Wolf and Ludwik K. Branski

Department of Surgery, University of Texas Medical Branch at Galveston, Galveston, TX 77550, USA; mitay@utmb.edu (M.W.T.); swolf@utmb.edu (S.E.W.); lubransk@utmb.edu (L.K.B.)
* Correspondence: deepak.ozhathil@gmail.com; Tel.: +1-508-654-8246

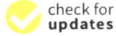

Citation: Ozhathil, D.K.; Tay, M.W.; Wolf, S.E.; Branski, L.K. A Narrative Review of the History of Skin Grafting in Burn Care. *Medicina* **2021**, *57*, 380. https://doi.org/10.3390/medicina57040380

Academic Editor: Lars P. Kamolz

Received: 4 March 2021
Accepted: 7 April 2021
Published: 15 April 2021

Publisher's Note: MDPI stays neutral with regard to jurisdictional claims in published maps and institutional affiliations.

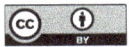

Copyright: © 2021 by the authors. Licensee MDPI, Basel, Switzerland. This article is an open access article distributed under the terms and conditions of the Creative Commons Attribution (CC BY) license (https://creativecommons.org/licenses/by/4.0/).

Abstract: Thermal injuries have been a phenomenon intertwined with the human condition since the dawn of our species. Autologous skin translocation, also known as skin grafting, has played an important role in burn wound management and has a rich history of its own. In fact, some of the oldest known medical texts describe ancient methods of skin translocation. In this article, we examine how skin grafting has evolved from its origins of necessity in the ancient world to the well-calibrated tool utilized in modern medicine. The popularity of skin grafting has ebbed and flowed multiple times throughout history, often suppressed for cultural, religious, pseudo-scientific, or anecdotal reasons. It was not until the 1800s, that skin grafting was widely accepted as a safe and effective treatment for wound management, and shortly thereafter for burn injuries. In the nineteenth and twentieth centuries skin grafting advanced considerably, accelerated by exponential medical progress and the occurrence of man-made disasters and global warfare. The introduction of surgical instruments specifically designed for skin grafting gave surgeons more control over the depth and consistency of harvested tissues, vastly improving outcomes. The invention of powered surgical instruments, such as the electric dermatome, reduced technical barriers for many surgeons, allowing the practice of skin grafting to be extended ubiquitously from a small group of technically gifted reconstructive surgeons to nearly all interested sub-specialists. The subsequent development of biologic and synthetic skin substitutes have been spurred onward by the clinical challenges unique to burn care: recurrent graft failure, microbial wound colonization, and limited donor site availability. These improvements have laid the framework for more advanced forms of tissue engineering including micrografts, cultured skin grafts, aerosolized skin cell application, and stem-cell impregnated dermal matrices. In this article, we will explore the convoluted journey that modern skin grafting has taken and potential future directions the procedure may yet go.

Keywords: skin graft; history; autograft; burn; dermatome; mesh; split-thickness; xenograft; CEA; CSS; Spray-on-Skin; ReCell

1. Introduction

"(A Spaniard) upon a time walked in the field, and fell at words with a soldier, and began to draw (his sword); the soldier seeing that, struck him with the left hand, and cut off his nose, and there it fell down in the sand. I then happened to stand by, and took it up, and pissed thereon to wash away the sand, and dressed it with our balsama artificiato, and bound it up, and so left it to remain 8 or 10 days, thinking that it would have come to matter; nevertheless when I did unbind it I found it fast conglutinated, and then I dressed it only once more, and he was perfectly whole."—Leonardo Fioravanti [1].

The above is an excerpt from the sixteenth century works of Leonardo Fioravanti (1517–1588), a charismatic Italian surgeon, who was controversial in his time for his vocal rejection of Galenic doctrine and credited with performing the first splenectomy on Italian soil [1]. Fioravanti was also the first in the western world to document the successful reattachment of a severed body part, in this case a nose. The excerpt describes a 29-year-old gentleman named Signor Andreas Gutiero living in Africa, who, much to his own misfortune, chose to engage in a heated argument with a soldier stationed there. As described above, this interaction did not go well and left Gutiero breathless and detached from his nose. Leonardo Fioravanti happened upon this encounter and was able to achieve an outcome that would be considered remarkable for any time period, and certainly in his. Though this anecdotal story is not a true description of a skin grafting per se, the practice of tissue restitution lays the foundation for the development of modern skin grafting. Following Fioravanti's report, numerous similar descriptions of nasal restitution subsequently appear throughout the literature as criminal punishment with nasal disfigurement was a common practice in those days. Arguably, auto-transplantation of tissue to its own donor site is the precursor to cutaneous autografting.

Burn injuries and their treatments are intertwined with human history dating back to the origins of mankind's relationship with fire. In fact, the rich history of burn wound treatments predates civilization. Archeologists have found cave paintings depicting Neanderthal-man having treated burn wounds with plant-based extracts [2,3]. Numerous concoctions over the ages have been utilized to treat burn wounds. In the ancient world, the Ebers Papyrus (1500 BC) describes Egyptian physicians making salves derived from animal, plant, and mineral byproducts and combining their application with religious ceremonies to the Goddess Isis. Burn wounds were then dressed with bandages moistened with the milk derived from the mothers of male infants [4]. The Romans had a pharmacopeia of products to treat burn wounds, ranging from mixtures of honey and bran to cork and ashes [3]. For millennia, physicians have attempted to treat burn wounds with all manner of products and combinations therein, but were met with middling success due to the lack of scientific understanding about burn wound pathophysiology. Independent of burn injuries, the history of skin grafting followed a similar trajectory with limited success for several centuries due to a combination of inefficient tissue collection methods, inappropriately thick grafts, and a lack of understanding of the physiology behind skin grafting. It would not be until the nineteenth century on the wave of numerous medical advances in burn care that the Swiss surgeon Jacques-Louis Reverdin (1842–1929) and the English surgeon George Pollock (1897–1917) would first apply skin grafting techniques to the treatment of burn wounds [5].

Modern burn care is the result of numerous advances in wound care, understanding of burn sepsis pathophysiology, operative technology, and surgical technique. The single most significant advancement credited for heralding the modern age of burn care is the utilization of skin grafting after early wound excision first introduced in the 1940s [6]. Today, autografting of full thickness burn wounds is the standard of care, having a direct effect on time-till-wound-closure, and a substantial impact on morbidity and mortality for burn victims. In this historical review, we will trace the evolution of surgical techniques, the development of operative instruments and the advancement in physiologic knowledge about skin grafting through the ages. We hope to integrate a common thread of the lessons hard-learned by numerous exceptional surgeons in our timeline to best appreciate how the state of modern burn care came to be. Furthermore, the author hopes to explore techniques and cutting-edge technologies that are anticipated to play a significant role in the burn care of tomorrow.

2. Skin Grafts in Antiquity: 3000 BC–476 AD

Facial mutilation was a common punishment in the ancient world and practiced in much of Asia and Europe. It was often performed by cutting off the nose or ear of victims as a punishment for crimes committed, but also served as a warning to other would-be wrong-doers. The silver lining of centuries of this painful and humiliating practice was that it inspired the development of skin grafting [7]. One of the oldest descriptions of nasal mutilation comes from an ancient Indian Sanskrit epic from 1500 BC, the Ramayana, in which Lady Surpunakha (Meenakshi), angry after being scorned by Prince Rama, attacks his wife Princess Sita. As punishment, her nose is amputated by Rama's brother, Prince Lakshmana. The cultural significance of this act is that the nose is synonymous with respect. As a consequence, King Ravana orders her nose be reconstructed [7]. Although this legend leaves many details to the imagination, it highlights how commonplace such practices were. For example, in 1769 the Ghoorka King of India captured the city of Kirtipoor in modern day Nepal. He ordered the nasal mutilation of all 865 male inhabitants and changed the name to Naskatapoor, which translates to "city without noses" [8]. The cultural influence of more than three millennia of this practice is undeniable, exemplified by idiomatic expressions such "loosing face" which alludes to a loss of dignity and wonton embarrassment. In Urdu and Punjabi there is a colloquial expression "mera noc kart gaya" meaning "you have hurt my feelings", but literally translated as "you have cut off my nose" [7]. It is therefore no surprise that nasal reconstruction is the oldest form of facial surgery.

The first operative description of tissue translocation was performed by the Indian surgeon Sushruta (approximately 750–800 BC), considered by many historians to be the "Father of Indian Surgery". Indian surgeons (referred to as Hindoo surgeons in early texts) underwent an extensive period of training on anatomy and hand dexterity. He described the instruments and surgical techniques he used in Sanskritt hymns called Vedas. The best known of these is the Sushruta Samitá and serves both as an educational and religious text [5]. Sushruta outlined the progenitor for the modern pedicle flap by rotating and advancing tissues from the cheek [9]. This method, now called the "Indian cheek flap", is the oldest documented method of skin translocation and is sometimes referred to as the "Indian Method" of nasal restitution. Sushruta also documented more than 15 methods to repair mutilated ears and lips. Our modern understanding of skin grafting originates directly from the Indian Method as it would be distributed and discovered several times over the years. The Indian Method by way of migrating surgeons would make it is way to Egypt, Greece, Arabia (the Middle East), and ultimately Italy over the centuries. Knowledge of the procedure would be discovered and credit misappropriated several times. The "French Method" for example, is considered to be a recapitulation of Sushruta's techniques several centuries later. The Indian cheek flap, in our modern nomenclature, would be considered an advancement of sliding flap [10].

In the time of Buddha (562–472 BC), progress in Indian surgery came to a standstill because of social and religious pressures. Although great respect to the field of medicine was afforded by the Buddhists, animal experimentation and direct contact with bodily fluids and diseased tissues was considered to be spiritually defiling [10]. Therefore, surgical responsibilities fell by default to the second lowest cast in the Hindu system, the Shudras. Called by various names (Koomás), and described later by Europeans based on their profession (potters, bricklayers, and tile-makers), the Shudras were considered unclean and therefore not at risk of being further defiled by the handling of blood and pus, necessary in the practice of surgery. Being generally uneducated compared to the surgeons of Sushruta's day, much fundamental surgical wisdom would be lost for an age.

The origin of the techniques practiced by the Shudra is controversial and discrepant by several millennia, depending on the source, due to the entanglement of surgical folklore and oral traditions—3000 BC, 600 BC, 1000 AD, and 1440 AD have all been reported. [5,11,12]. Their techniques, now more commonly referred to as the "Ancient Indian Method", actually referred to two different procedures. The first procedure would be described as a median forehead pedicle flap. The patients were operated upon awake and in an upright position to minimize blood-loss and protect their airway. In addition, a handkerchief around the neck would reportedly be used to induce transient venous congestion. This procedure was first described in 1794 by the British Army surgeon Cully Lyon Lucas, who was stationed in Madras (Chennai, India). At the time, Tipú Sultán, the ruler of Mysore (Karnataka, India) waged a guerilla war against the British Crown by placing a bounty on the noses of any Indian's who helped transport grain for the British. Lucas described in detail a median forehead flap for nasal restitution performed on one such victim named Cowasjee, who had his nose and one hand mutilated. He would publish his observation in the Gentleman's

Magazine (London, UK) [13]. The reconstructed "Hindoostan noses" were subsequently observed by others, who commented on their likeness to native nasal tissue and sturdiness to tolerate sneezing and nose-blowing [5].

The second procedure would be considered a free full-thickness skin graft. In this technique, a wooden sandal would be used to percuss the gluteal region until it had been contused and inflamed sufficiently to generate local edema. Then, the skin and underlying subcutaneous fat would be harvested and applied immediately to the nasal wound, along with a proprietary surgical cement that was described to have healing properties [12]. These procedures, as well as the equipment and products used at the time (topical hemostasis, cotton sutures, intranasal splints, various leaves, and ant-heads as skin staples), were closely guarded secrets passed down from father to son within families [5].

Stories of these methods slowly made their way to ancient Egypt and Rome, carried by "students and itinerant surgeons" [12]. In 1600 BC, the Edwin Smith Papyrus is a record of a number of ancient Egyptian treatments for those who have suffered mutilations to the face, though none would be considered reconstructive. In the first century, the Roman encyclopedist Aurelius Cornelius Celsus (25 BC–50 AD) wrote De Medicina, which depicted a multitude of skin flaps used to repair ears, noses, and lips [14,15]. Celsus even described how to reconstruct foreskin to enable circumcised Jewish men to be more accepted by the Romans [5]. In the second century, the famous Roman surgeon Claudius Galen (129–210 AD) described a number of procedures to reconstruct facial injuries with local tissue advancement flaps. The works and theories of Galen would form the Galenic doctrine, which would make up the mainstay of medical education and practice for the next thousand years [16].

3. Skin Grafts in the Middle Ages and Renaissance: 476–1789 AD

The majority of early medical knowledge in Europe during the Middle Ages rested with the Catholic Church and was preserved in monastic texts. In 1215 AD, however, Pope Innocent III banned any priest, deacon, or sub-deacon from performing any surgical procedure due to the religious misgivings that bloodshed was "incompatible with the divine mission" [10]. Following the Pope's decree, and quite similar to the impediments that befell surgical practice in ancient India, academic progress in Europe came to a standstill and ultimately much surgical wisdom was lost for several centuries [10].

In the eighth century, the Sushruta Samhitá was translated into Arabic and along the silk road made its way to Italy. The first European surgeon to practice the cheek-flap technique was Gustavo (Branca) de'Branca in Catania (Sicily) in the fifteenth century. His son, Antonio Branca further developed the procedure into a six-stage rhinoplasty that utilized a myocutaneous flap from the arm. This method remained a closely held secret within the Branca family for nearly a century. Though first documented in 1460 by Heinrich von Pfolspeundt, a knight of the Teutonic Order, it would not be until 1493 that a detailed description of the procedure would be make available to the public by Alessandro Benedetti (1450–1512) a professor at Padua University (Italy). More than a hundred years later, the famous Italian surgeon Gaspare Tagliacozzi (1545–1599), while practicing at the Hospital of Death would cite Benedetti and build upon the Branca technique in his own work De Curtorum Chirurgia per Insitionem (published in 1597). For his contributions, Tagliacozzi is considered a pioneer in reconstructive and plastic surgery and credited for the "(Ancient) Italian Method" of tissue translocation [17].

Not surprising for the time, Tagliacozzi incurred the antagonism of the Catholic Church, which viewed reconstructive surgery as a form of sacrilege that meddled with God's creations [2]. His writings were, therefore, declared heretical and burned by decree. The Church even went so far as to exhume Tagliacozzi's body in order to rebury in unconsecrated ground [7]. As a few copies of his writings survived the purge, a number of Tagliacozzi's followers attempted to reproduce his techniques. Unfortunately, they could not replicate his results. After numerous failed attempts and the slow passage of time, Tagliacozzi's reputation would slowly slide into mockery and denigration. For nearly

200 years, little progress would be achieved. In fact, by the end of the eighteenth century the Paris Academy of Surgery would declare Tagliacozzi's (Italian) Method impossible. Once again, we see history repeat itself as short-lived advances in skin translocation are prematurely abandoned due to social and religious pressures of the age.

In the sixteenth century the French Barber–Surgeon Ambroise Paré (1510–1590 AD), who served in the royal courts of Kings Henry II, Francis II, Charles IX, and Henry III, wrote voluminously on the importance of procedural interventions to reduce pain and suffering. His efforts are thought to have laid the foundation for empiricism and the modern concept of evidence-based practice. In addition, Paré helped prompt the transition of Barber–Surgeons to their contemporary status as physicians [18]. Barber–Surgeons were entrusted with performing operations under the supervision of physicians due to their familiarity with handling blades. Galenic doctrine had been the mainstay of western medical education for more than a thousand years and it emphasized theory over empirical knowledge [18]. For example, the recommended treatment for burn wounds from gunpowder was to 'detoxify' the patient by cauterizing the wounds with boiling oils. The method was so common that it was referred to in Shakespeare's *King John*, where Cardinal Pandulph says to King Philip:

> "And falsehood falsehood cures; as fire cools fire within the scorched veins of one new-burned." King John (Act 3, Scene 1).

Paré was trained at the renowned Hôtel Dieu and was appointed as a surgeon in the military directly out of his training. Perhaps fortunately for Paré, the beginning half of the sixteenth century was a time of great turmoil in Europe. The ambitious French king, François I, seeking to increase his domains and influence waged multiple wars against the industrious Emperor of Germany, Charles V. One such battle took place in 1535 when Anne de Montmorenci, commanding the armies of France, pursued the retreating imperial army from Provence to the Pas de Suze (the Suza Pass). It was on this campaign through the Alps that Paré first gained experience caring for burn injuries. At the time, Paré served under the inferior title of "surgeon" as he had not yet been confirmed into the ranks of Barber–Surgeons, having been sent to the Italian front prior to completing his certifying examinations. Ironically, however, it was as a surgeon that Paré made many of the observations for which he is credited for today [19].

During the battle of Pas de Suze, Paré ran out of boiling oil, the recommended treatment for burn wounds. He, therefore, improvised and created a soothing balm made from egg yolks, rose oil, and turpentine. The following morning, he found that the patients treated with the balm were resting comfortably, while those treated in the traditional manner remained ill and febrile [20]. This simple observation would change the fundamental practice of medicine and the treatment of burn injuries from theory-based to evidence-based practice. Paré, upon seeing the dramatic difference in his patient groups, broke from his Galenic teachings. He would go on to characterize various degrees of burn wounds and contractures, and even pioneer the practice of burn wound excision [21]. Although Paré did write about skin grafting, he viewed its benefits with considerable skepticism [10]. This is not surprising for two important reasons. First, knowledge of burn wound pathophysiology remained fundamental and severely injured patients failed to receive appropriate resuscitation that would be considered acceptable by modern standards. Second, access to surgical interventions was limited, especially for those who would benefit from it the most. As general anesthesia and the technique of transfusing blood had not yet been invented, surgical excision of large burns was not considered possible. Therefore, Paré's perspective was influenced by a selection bias — that is to say patients who survived long enough to be considered for surgery would likely continue to survive independent of the treatment they then received. Nonetheless, his efforts to promote evidence-based wound care would play an incredibly important role in the development of modern skin grafting.

4. Skin Grafts in the Early Modern Era—Age of Revolution: 1789–1849 AD

The nineteenth century was unique in that it marked the dawn of the Contemporary Age. Important notable advancements in medicine during this time included the discovery of anesthesia and the dawn of microbiology. The introduction of general anesthesia is credited to the Boston dentist William Thomas Green Morton (1819–1868), who on 16th October 1846 performed his famous demonstration with diethyl ether at Massachusetts General Hospital on Mr. Edward Gilbert Abbott during the excision of a cervical mass. The introduction of anesthesia made it possible to perform more invasive procedures including larger surface area skin grafting, with improved safety and tolerance to the patient.

Another momentous achievement came through Louis Pasteur and Joseph Lister's work on microbiology. Their research on antiseptic techniques revolutionized anti-microbial wound care and improved post-operative outcomes [10]. Riding on the coattails of scientific breakthroughs in multiple fields including microbiology, anatomy and physiology, medicine itself was dramatically changing in response to evidenced-based practices. Both the Indian and Italian methods would see their revivals during this period. The English surgeon Joseph Carpue (1746–1840) recapitulated the Ancient Indian Method (median forehead flap), as originally documented by Lucas in 1816, effectively reviving it in Europe [5]. Similarly, the German surgeon Karl Ferdinand von Gräfe (1787–1840) would successfully revive the Italian Method in 1817 [2].

The Indian and the Italian Methods of nasal reconstruction, though important in the origin of the (free) skin graft, were nonetheless technically not skin grafts themselves, but pedicle flaps. The transition from the pedicle flap to the skin graft is not, however, as linear a narrative as one would imagine. Although potentially first performed by the Shudras of India (Ancient Indian Method), credit or even proof of their achievements cannot be well validated as there is no specific documentation of their surgical technique or outcomes from prior to the nineteenth century. In 1941, the American surgeon Sumner L. Koch (1888–1976) wrote [22]:

Although it has been said that in India the restoration of the nose with the free grafts of skin and subcutaneous tissue was successfully accomplished. I have been unable to find any definite record of it and if it was actually carried out it remains an achievement that the surgeon of today has not been able to equal. Sumner L. Koch [22].

It would not be until the latter half of the nineteenth century that surgeons like Jacques-Louis Reverdin, George Pollock, and John Reissberg Wolfe would successfully perform and proselytization the proper technique for (free) skin grafting. To this affect, in 1874 Wolfe wrote the following:

This pedicle (flap) has, in my opinion, been a source of great embarrassment to surgeons, and tended rather to retard the progress of plastic surgery. (. . .) I have long held it demonstrated, that in most cases the pedicle is not essential, if indeed it (does) contribute anything, to the vitality of (the) flap. John R. Wolfe [22].

Wolfe's beliefs, however forward thinking for his day, were built upon the works of pioneers in the first half of the nineteenth century. The British surgeon Sir Astley Paston Cooper (1768–1841), for example, transferred a full-thickness skin graft from a severed thumb in order to cover the amputation stump in 1817 [23]. The German surgeon Johann Friedrich Dieffenbach (1792–1847) wrote voluminously on tissue transplant techniques to reconstruct various body parts mutilated by a number of etiologies including burns [11]. Dieffenbach is also recognized for his numerous animal experiments. In his book Surgical Observations on the Restoration of the Nose and on the Removal of Polyps and other Tumors from the Nostrils (London, 1833), Dieffenbach writes about his failed attempts to re-attach severed bodily appendages of different mammalian species: tails from cats and dogs, ears from dogs and rabbits, and even human fingers. Dieffenbach also dabbled in xenografting—transplanting pigskin to pigeons for example [24]. Despite a handful on controversial exceptions, the vast majority of Dieffenbach's experiments were met with failure.

The separate history of zoologic experimentation and skin xenografts is worth mentioning here as it is likely nearly as influential, if not more so, than nasal restitution in the origin or (free) skin grafts. Unfortunately, as many early zoological experiments resulted in failure, the literature is sparsely populated with confirmed experiments. In 1663, Robert Hooke (1635–1703), a British scientist for the Royal Society of London, performed a handful of successful skin transplants on chickens and dogs [25]. In the nineteenth century, a number of surgeons experimented with live xenografts (inter-species pedicle flaps) between various animals (cats, dogs, rats, rabbits, sheep, birds, and frogs) and human subjects. In these experiments, the donor animal was typically immobilized and affixed to the patient for several days in an effort to promote vascularization of the xenografted tissue [26,27]. Despite some disputed claims of success, the majority of these experiments are also believed to have failed.

It would not be until the early nineteenth century when the Italian physician Giuseppe Baronio (1759–1811) would successfully and reproducibly perform a series of (free) skin grafts on sheep [28]. Baronio was an interesting individual with eclectic interests, underappreciated in his time, who failed to achieve promotion and died unmarried at a young age. His interest in autologous skin translocation derived directly from the nasal reconstruction techniques of the Branca family and Tagliacozzi mentioned earlier. In 1804, Baronio describes in his book, *Degli Innesti Animali* (On Grafting in Animals), the three experiments he performed at the estate farm of Count Anguissola of Albignano (Milan, Italy). In the first experiment, Baronio harvested skin from the back of a ram and immediately grafted it to a new site on the back of the same sheep. The graft was secured with adhesive dressings rather than sutures. In the second experiment, a similar procedure was performed on the same unfortunate animal, but with an 18 min delay between graft collection and placement. In the third experiment, this delay was extended to one hour. Not surprisingly, the first graft took perfectly, the second incurred some inflammation and likely superficial necrosis. The third graft failed altogether. The surviving grafts were cut into 10–12 days after transplantation and were noted to be well vascularized [29,30]. Baronio went on to perform similar experiments on 27 animals (sheep, goats, dogs, a horse, and a cow) in total. Unfortunately, his accomplishment went unnoticed, and he died in relative obscurity, but his findings mark the first scientifically documented reports of successful autologous skin grafts performed in mammals.

The German surgeon Christian Bünger (1782–1842) was the first to theorize that free tissue transfers may also be viable in humans. In 1823, Bünger performed a rhinoplasty on a 33-year-old woman named Wilhelmina in Marburg, Germany. The patient was considered to be quite beautiful at one time, but suffered from a skin condition resulting in severe disfigurement to her face. The lack of usable adjacent tissue on the face obviated the use of an advancement flap. Using a variation of the Ancient Indian Method (full-thickness skin graft), Bünger transferred tissue from her buttock to reconstruct the patient's nasal defect. This was done with a much thinner graft free of any subcutaneous tissue and likely without the preparatory tissue percussion recommended in the original technique. This operation was applauded by many as the first verified (free) skin graft performed in Europe. However, controversy surrounded Bünger's achievement as some stated that the surgery had only been partially successful. Furthermore, Bünger's contemporaries would not successfully replicate his results for more than a decade [12,31].

In the United States, Jonathan Mason Warren (1811–1867) was a Harvard trained surgeon who is best remembered for being the first surgeon to administer anesthesia to a pediatric patient. In 1834, he also became the first surgeon in North America to reconstruct a nose using a median forehead pedicle flap, and in 1840 he became the first surgeon to successfully use a (free) skin graft to reconstruct a nose. Warren was a fruitful writer, who recorded his use of full-thickness skin grafts to repair eyelids and noses. In 1844, Joseph Pancoast (1805–1882) from Philadelphia, a contemporary of Warren's, described the reconstruction of an earlobe with a (free) skin graft in his Treatise of Operative Surgery [30].

5. Skin Grafts in the Late Modern Era—Preceding World War II: 1850–1938 AD

On 8th December 1869 Swiss surgeon Jacques-Louis Reverdin (1842–1929) reported the successful use of [free] skin grafts on granulating wounds to the Société Impériale de Chirurgie in Paris, France. He described taking extremely small and very thin pieces of skin, which he called "epidermic grafts" and placing them on the granulating wound bed to act as centers of epithelization [32]. His first case involved a man who had injured his thumb. Reverdin placed two 1 mm pieces of skin onto the wound. Then, two weeks later, he observed that each graft formed a small island of epithelization and with the same amount of epidermal proliferation. Therefore, he attempted to increase the surface area treated by increasing the number of (small) grafts applied [5]. Because Reverdin's technique involved picking up skin with forceps and excising a small piece with scissors, it became known as "pinch grafts". Reverdin's accomplishment were paradigm changing and gained him the reputation of Father of Skin Grafting. Nonetheless, his technique had some significant shortcomings. Due to the small size of the grafts, large wounds would suffer significant contracture. Due to the friability and the prolonged time till wound closure, it was less effective around joints. Lastly, it was not an aesthetically pleasing graft, forming bumps and pits at both the donor and graft sites [12]. Some historians also attribute credit to Reverdin for the use of skin grafting in burn wounds because he is reputed to have used skin from his own arm as allograft to treat the burn wounds on a patient's back. Many historians, however, question the validity of this story.

Credit for treating burn wounds with skin grafts lies with George Davis Pollock (1876–1950), who presented his work titled "Cases of Skin Grafting and Skin Transplantation" before the Clinical Society of London in 1870. In his paper, Pollock described a series of 16 cases where he applied thin skin grafts to open wounds, of which 8 were successful. Pollock credited Reverdin in his work, but his very first case, an eight-year-old girl named Anne, is the first documented successful report of the use of skin grafts for the treatment of burn wounds. Anne suffered significant burn injuries to her lower extremities after her dress caught on fire. After two years of insufficient wound care, she presented to Pollock with a large persistent ulcerations on the right thigh. Pollock applied two small pieces of skin from the patient's abdomen to the ulcer and noticed six weeks later that the ulcer had healed considerably with the small skin grafts acting as a node for secondary epithelialization (secondary intention). By 1872, despite their description as epidermic grafts, Reverdin and Pollock had both admitted that their grafts contained a portion of dermis.

Around the same time (1870), the British surgeon George Lawson (1831–1903) presented to the Clinical Society of London his experience using a full-thickness skin graft from the upper arm to repair a complete ectropion of the upper eyelid. Lawson's method described meticulous dissection of all subcutaneous tissues from the dermis. Due to its size of only 32 mm, his grafts were affectionately referred to as "Fourpenny Grafts" [33]. Despite his accomplishment, however, Lawson is largely overlooked by historians. It would not be until 1875 that Polish-born John Reissberg Wolfe (1824–1904), an ophthalmologist from Glasgow (United Kingdom), would describe his experiences in the *British Medical Journal* that the medical community would take notice. Wolfe used even larger grafts (2.5 cm × 5 cm) from the forearm to reconstruct lower eyelid ectropions in a manner much like Lawson's. Then, 20 years later (1896), Fedor Krause (1857–1937), a neurosurgeon in Hamburg (Germany), emulated the same practice as Wolfe in a larger series. In 1893, he recommended the use of Wolfe's techniques to the 23rd *Kongress der Deutschen Gesellschaft für Chirurgie* (Congress of the German Surgical Association) and highlighted the specific instances where predecessors had failed. He also pointed out the benefits of full-thickness skin grafts over thinner grafts: resistance to scar contracture, improved joint range of motion, and more favorable aesthetic results. For his efforts Krause is credited with popularizing full-thickness skin grafting [12]. Although neither Wolfe nor Krause can reasonably be credited for discovering full-thickness skin grafts, their contributions to popularizing the technique, which is ubiquitously used today, is why the dermo-epidermal graft is still remembered under the eponym "Wolfe–Krause graft" [34].

The evolution of the split-thickness skin grafting technique follows a parallel timeline. Certainly, Reverdin's pinch grafts were historic in the origin of skin graft of all degrees of thickness. In his initial description of the grafts, Reverdin suggested that they were composed almost entirely of epidermis. It was not until later that he would admit to some dermal inclusion. In 1872, the French surgeon Leopold Louis Xavier Édouard Léopold Ollier (1830–1900) of Lyon (France) published his experiences with thin skin grafts ranging from 4 to 8 cm^2 in size, substantially larger than previously performed by Reverdin or Pollock [5]. Ollier's grafts, though described in the same nomenclature as full-thickness skin grafts at the time, were considered intermediate thickness as they included the entire epidermis and only a thin portion of dermis. Today, we would consider Ollier's grafts to be split-thick skin grafts (STSG). Due to the technologic limitations at the time, the collection of such grafts required remarkable technical dexterity [5,12]. Ollier's grafts were, however, more advantageous over full thickness grafts in two remarkable ways. The first is that the grafts experienced less shrinkage and curling at the time of collection due to the decreased amount of dermal elements. The second is that the donor site required far less time to heal [14].

Carl Thiersch (1822–1895), a German surgeon who trained under Dieffenbach, believed himself to have perfected skin grafting with his technique, which involved minimal dermal inclusion in the graft. He demonstrated his method to the 15th Kongress der Deutschen Gesellschaft für Chirurgie in 1886, and for a time his grafts were referred to as "razorgrafts" [22]. Critics attest that Thiersch's conclusion that the "ideal skin graft" should be excised as superficially as possible reinforced the incorrect notion that there could only be one optimal graft thickness, and that such idealism delayed the development of modern full-thickness skin grafting techniques. Thiersch emphasized his opinion in a number of his own publications and was broadly influential within the medical community due to his reputation as a brilliant surgeon [35]. Today, we recognize that there is no ideal thickness for skin grafts. Rather, grafts of different thicknesses can be used in a diverse variety of applications. Furthermore, despite not ascribing any credit in his writings to Ollier, who published similar findings 14 years earlier, both are credited by historians for their advancement of surgical knowledge and technique. The Ollier–Thiersch graft is now synonymous with STSG. Despite Thiersch's emphasis on meticulous technique, grafts performed by his contemporaries would, progressively over time, get thicker. Eventually, inclusion of nearly half the dermis was still considered an Ollier–Thiersch graft. This distinction would be obviated with advances in surgical technology in the twentieth century.

Thiersch was in many ways was obsessed with the microscope, taught lectures on microscopic anatomy and was even described as a "dexterous microscopist" in his obituary, for his integration of his passions for cellular physiology and surgery. Thiersch is reported to have rigorously studied the microvascular anastomosis between skin grafts and wound beds. He described layers in the granulation tissue that formed, distinguishable by the orientation of the vasculature. Through his study, he discovered that superficial granulation tissue actually hinders skin graft implantation.

> "The only alternative, therefore, is elimination of the superficial portion of the granulation (layer) and implantation of the skin (graft) directly upon the tense underlying tissue. This substratum is exposed by sharp, horizontal incision, hemorrhage is permitted to run its course completely, and then skin graft is placed upon this greyish wound surface, whose vessels and tissues are in excellent condition for immediate inflammatory adhesion."—Carl Thiersch [22].

Thus, through the efforts of countless surgeons, the basic tenants of skin grafting from epidermal to full-thickness grafts, as well as the optimal preparation of the wound bed were established by the end of the nineteenth century.

6. Skin Grafts in the Contemporary Era—World War II and After: 1939–2020 AD
6.1. Burn Wound Management

The use of skin grafting in acute burn wound treatment did not occur until the utility of early wound excision in full thickness burn wounds was understood. Although the importance of early burn wound excision was first described by Paré in the sixteenth century. Wilhelm Fabricius Hildanus (1560–1634) is considered the "Father of German Surgery" and the first to write a book dedicated to the management of burn wounds, De Combustionibus (On Burns) in 1607. In his book, Hildanus advocated for the surgical removal of burn eschar to facilitate improved medication penetration. Although certainly ahead of his time in a surgical regard, Hildanus was ignorant of the teaching of Paré nearly 70 years prior, as many of the medications he utilized were of medieval origin [32]. In the eighteenth century, Dieffenbach would describe the use of skin grafts to reconstruct wounds caused by burn injuries and in the late nineteenth century both Reverdin and Pollock would be credited with the successful use of skin grafts in chronic burn wounds. However, it would not be until the 1940 that skin grafting following tangential excision of acute burn wounds wound be connected in a therapeutic sequence.

The 1940s was a period of significant advancement in the understanding of burn shock management, not in any small part due to the immense loss of life precipitated by multiple man-made disasters. In 1921, Frank Pell Underhill (1877–1932) a surgeon at Yale University, treated more than 20 victims of the infamous Rialto Theater fire in New Haven, Connecticut. Underhill noted similarities in the serous fluid within skin blisters and plasma, and went on to suggested that acute shock in burn victims was primarily a hypovolemic process due to fluid losses from injured skin [36]. Then, 20 years later, Oliver Cope (1902–1994) and Francis D. Moore (1913–2001) from Massachusetts General Hospital would treat nearly 40 victims of the Coconut Grove Nightclub in Boston, Massachusetts. Their work would connect the amount of body surface injured to the volume of resuscitation fluid needed to stave off the precipitating shock [37]. In 1942, Forrest Young of the University of Rochester correlated that victims of burn injuries suffered from sepsis and shock as a result of fluid losses and bacterial colonization of their wounds. He also surmised that full-thickness burn injuries would only heal by secondary intention. Therefore, he advocated for early excision and skin grafting to improve mortality by removing the source of sepsis [38]. During this era, however, many believed it inopportune to operate during the acute period of shock, so the term "early surgical intervention" referred to a period of 10–21 days after the injury [39,40].

In 1960, Douglas MacGilchrist Jackson (1916–2002) and colleagues from Birmingham, England described in detail a series of cases where early excision down to fascia was performed on the day of injury for full thickness burn wounds and hemodynamic management with aggressive hemoglobin monitoring and transfusions as needed. They determined that 20–30% total body surface area (TBSA) burns could be operated on the day of injury without any increased risk of death, while achieving much earlier rates of graft take and wound closure [41]. Other surgeons would advocate for similar time frames for early excision of burn wounds, but there was little momentum in the surgical community because like Jackson, they could not demonstrate a mortality improvement over the method that delayed excision by 2–3 weeks. This would change in the early 1970s when an unknown Eastern European surgeon, Zora Janžekovič (1918–2015) from the Slovenian city of Maribor, published her findings after performing tangential excisions on deep-second and third-degree burn wounds on 2615 patients [42,43]. Janžekovič described the austere post-war conditions in which she found herself practicing in isolation. Later in her life, Janžekovič wrote:

> "The daily changing of dressings of the burn patient, piles of dressings full of pus, the terrible stench, but above all the horrible suffering of the patients—mostly children who were scared to death and emaciated, was a cry for help and a challenge for our personal engagement. Their suffering became our suffering. The feeling of our own helplessness and the incompetence of the then medical

science were destroying us ... Confronted with this terrible situation, I was forced to search for any kind of solution."—Zora Janžekovič [44].

She went on to abandon delaying wound excision until the wound had fully demarcated through the sequela of infection out of necessity. She believed that she could circumvent pathologic process by shaving the wound down to healthy tissue before infection had set in. Janžekovič found that tangential excision needed to be performed down to bleeding tissue, otherwise any applied graft would desiccate and fail. Beginning with small wounds and gaining confidence with larger injuries, Janžekovič is credited with formalizing the technique of tangential excision with immediate skin graft placement within 5 days of injury. Her results showed that patients with up to a 20% TBSA could be healed within 10 days, which was unheard-of at other more prestigious burn centers [44]. Janžekovič would go on to be the first woman to receive the Evens Medal from the American Burn Association and the Zora Janžekovič (Golden Razor) Award from the European Club for Paediatric Burns. It should be noted that Janžekovič technique was primarily for deep second-degree burns that were small enough to be addressed with a single operative intervention. In the decades that followed her publication, more than 200 surgeons from around the world would come to learn her technique first-hand and go on to further build upon her accomplishments. John Francis Burke (1922–2011) and his colleagues from Harvard University showed that the combination of tangential excision for smaller burns and full-fascial excision for larger burns followed by immediate autograft placement markedly reduced mortality and allowed the successful treatment of children up to 80% TBSA [45]. In the decades since, numerous surgeons continue to validate and build upon Janžekovič's technique. Today tangential excision of all non-viable tissues within 72 h of injury followed by immediate skin graft placement for full-thickness wounds is considered the standard of care.

6.2. Operative Equipment

Prior to the nineteenth century, skin grafts were collected using scalpels and knives adapted for surgical procedures, such as the Catlin knife (also called the Catling knife, Amputation knife, and Interosseous knife), which was a double-bladed instrument that was typically 17 cm long and 1.5 cm wide with a simple handle at one end, as seen in Figure 1a [12]. As a basic single-piece instrument, it lacked any mechanism by which to control depth of excision. It was also used surgically for a number of different tasks [12]. Although commonly used as far back as the seventeenth century, the Catling knife is still used by many surgeons today when performing extremity amputations. As one might imagine, the fine task of harvesting skin grafts with such a blunt instrument was challenging even in the most experienced hands and generally resulted in inconsistent graft thickness.

In 1920, the Thiersch's skin grafting knife was introduced and was a rectangular stainless steel single-bladed instruments weighted toward the handle. This rectangular design, as seen in Figure 1b, has persisted with nearly all subsequent hand-held skin grafting instruments. Vilary Papin Blair (1871–1975) an American surgeon at Washington University in St. Louis, who is best remembered as a pioneer for helping to distinguish plastic surgery from general surgery. Much of his reconstructive experience came from his time as a surgeon in the United States Army during World War I. He introduced the Blair knife in 1930, which was used in conjunction with a suction apparatus that put the skin under tension during harvest. This markedly improved the consistency of the grafts and allowed surgeons to harvest skin free-hand [12]. The Hofmann and Finochietto knives were introduced shortly thereafter, both of which were equipped with rudimentary guards that could be adjusted with lateral screws to allow the surgeon to calibrate the depth of dissection.

Improving upon this design, Thomas Graham Humby (1909–1970) a British plastic surgeon training at the Great Ormonde Street Hospital for Sick Children (London, UK) under the famous Sir Heneage Ogilvie introduced the Humby knife in 1934, as seen in Figure 2a [46]. Humby added a guard with a roller mechanism to his knife that allowed detailed calibration of the depth of tissue excised. In addition, the Humby knife had a rectangular metal frame equipped with 1/8th inch hooks at either end and a ratchet mechanism that enabled the surgeon to keep the donor tissue under tension while sliding the knife within the construct of the frame. Its use revolutionized skin grafting, enabling surgeons to single handedly and consistently excise rectangular strips of skin of consistent depth. The framework of the Humby knife was later abandoned as it could not reasonably be used for a number of potential donor sites. Subsequent variations of the Humby knife design include the Modified Humby (1936, fixed blade for rigidity), Bodenham (1949, partially supported replaceable blade that must be dismantled to change blades), Braithwaite (1955, leaf-type fully supportive replaceable blade that can be changed without disassembly) [47–49]. All of these knives shared two design flaws. First, the mechanism for depth adjustment is dependent on two separate knurled collars mounted on either end of the back of the handle allowing room for asymmetry and user error. Second, the roller guard and the handle are fixed while the blade must have some slack in the end-bearings in order for it to slide freely from side-to-side during use. As a result, grafts would often curl around the guard, become irregular and at times became gradually thicker across a harvest.

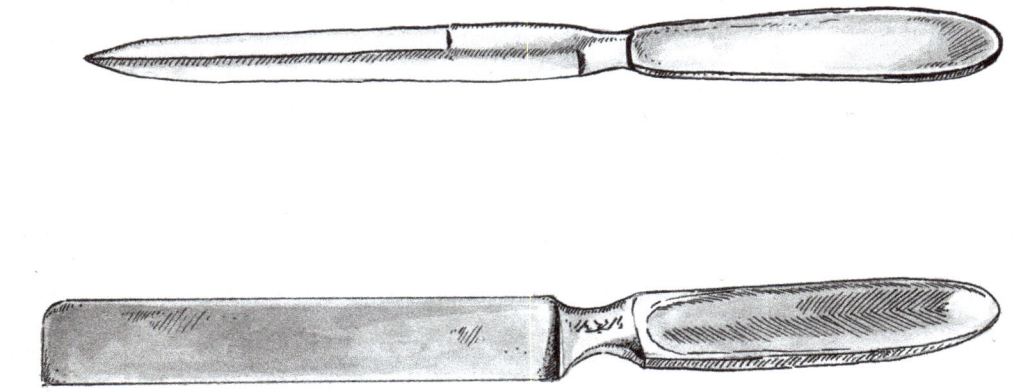

Figure 1. Early skin grafting knives: (**a**) The Catlin knife from the 19th century and earlier; (**b**) Thiersch's knife in 1920.

John Watson (1914–2009), who served as a pilot in the Royal Air Force during World War II, went on to become a plastic surgeon at the Queen Victoria Hospital in East Grinstead, United Kingdom, after the war. There, he would operate on many former aircrew who had sustained disfiguring burn injuries during the war. Inspired by a potato peeler and wanting to create a user-friendly instrument that emulated the renowned dexterity of his mentor Sir Archibald McIndoe (1900–1960). So inspiring was McIndoe's work that he was knighted for his contributions in reconstructing injured veterans of World War II. Watson introduced his knife in the year of McIndoe's passing, 1960. The Watson knife, as seen in Figure 2b, is unique in its simple design with a single more ridged knurled control knob for depth adjustment and precision-fit end-bearings that do not slide [50,51]. The result was a knife that is easier to operate and maintain, and for this reason the Watson knife is still used at many burn centers today.

In 1937, a remarkable advancement in surgical technology occurred with the introduction of the Padgett–Hood dermatome. Earl Calvin Padgett (1893–1946), an American physician from Kansas City who trained under Blair during residency. Padgett in collaboration with his colleague George J. Hood from the Department of Engineering designed a simple to use dermatome that allowed calibrated collection of skin grafts and presented their invention at the Western Surgical Association in 1938. Unlike many of its predecessors, the Padgett–Hood dermatome earned instant recognition. One of the founding members of the American Board of Plastic Surgery, George Warren Pierce, called it "the greatest contribution in many decades to the technique of skin grafting" [52].

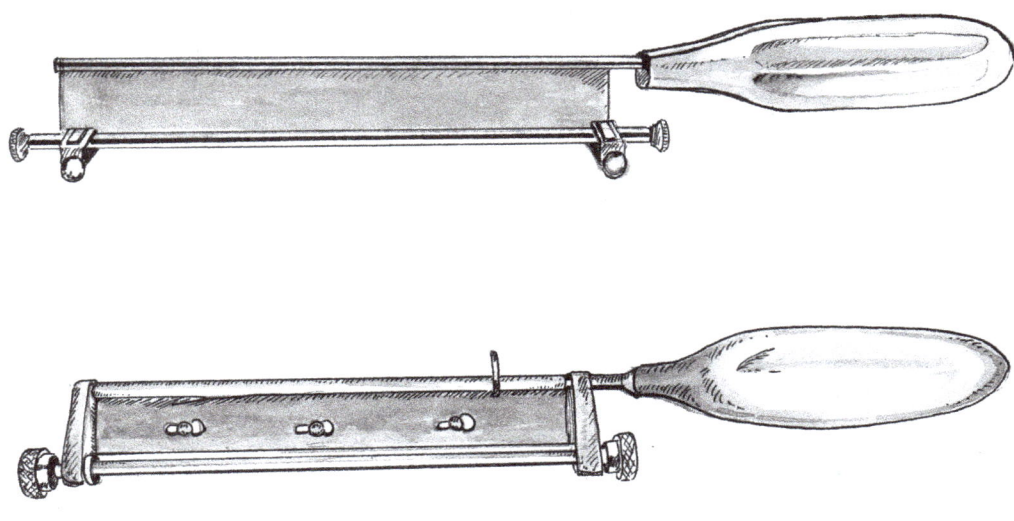

Figure 2. Skin grafting knives with modifiable depth: (**a**) The Humby knife in 1934; (**b**) The Watson knife in 1960.

The Padgett–Hood dermatome consisted of an aluminum drum that utilizes a traction-adhesion principle to feed donor tissue into a rotating blade, as seen in Figure 3a. The distance between the blade and the rotary drum can be calibrated down to a thousandth of an inch. The Padgett–Hood dermatome had several advantages compared to previous free hand tools. It vastly improved the quality and consistency of harvested graft, even when utilized on uneven donor surfaces. This not only increased the body surface that could be considered for donor harvest, but also increased the pool of surgeons that could perform skin grafting. No longer were skin grafts an art restricted to the most dexterous and experienced plastic surgeons, rather, now they could be performed by nearly any surgeon in training. Padgett's fortunate timing just prior to the onset of World War II cannot be understated [29]. Blair Rogers claims the Padgett–Hood dermatome "probably did more than any other single achievement in our specialty to bring the advantages of rapid, free skin transplantation to the innumerable casualties of that conflict" [31].

Following the war, John Davies Reese (1893–1958) would improve upon the Padgett–Hood dermatome in 1946. In contrast to the cast-aluminum of its predecessor, the Reese dermatome was a heavily machined, more precise and more reliable instrument. Notable disadvantages of the Reese dermatome were its considerable weight and inability for depth to be adjusted during a graft harvest [53]. The Reese dermatome would be overshadowed by the introduction of the first electric dermatome by the American surgeon Harry M. Brown (1914–1948) in 1948, as seen in Figure 3b [12]. Brown's dermatome was hand-held and relatively easy to operate, which allowed the harvest of large amounts of skin graft rather quickly with minimal effort. Brown actually thought of this new instrument while being held prisoner by the Japanese during World War II, but unfortunately was killed in a tragic accident shortly after his invention was introduced. A number of contemporary electric dermatomes including the Stryker, Padgett, and the Zimmer are based directly on the design of the Brown electric dermatome [12].

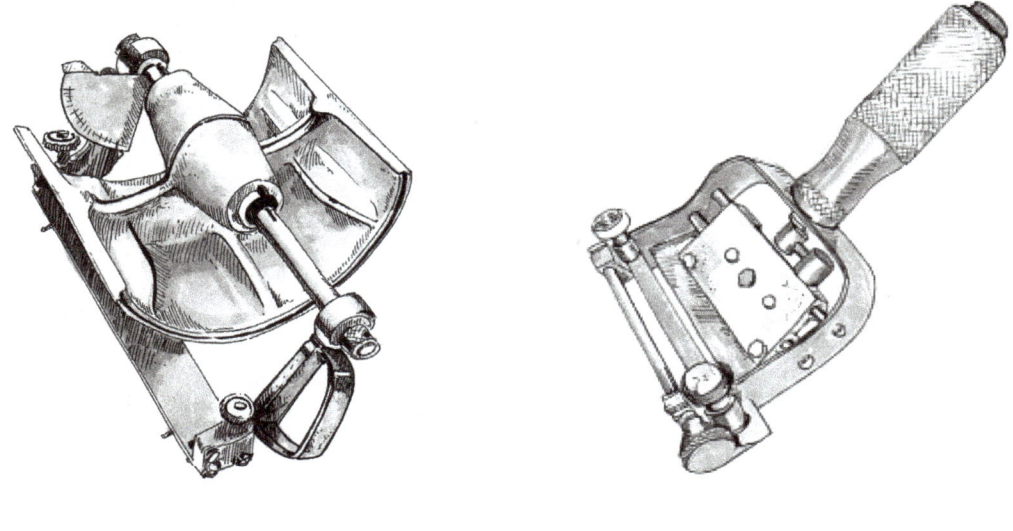

(a) (b)

Figure 3. Early dermatome designs: (**a**) The Padgett–Hood dermatome in 1937; (**b**) The Brown electric dermatome in 1948.

6.3. Skin Graft Expansion

Split thickness skin grafts first became popular in the 1930s after Blair and James Barrett Brown (1899–1971) first articulated the differences between full-thickness, intermediate-thickness and epidermal skin grafts. Their work showed that donor sites for STSG healed through epithelialization from local hair follicles and the underlying basal layer. The preservation of donor tissue so that it could potentially be re-harvested made STSG an attractive option over full thickness grafts, particularly in the treatment of large surface area wounds. The invention of the dermatome made the collection of STSG common practice to any interested surgeon. Building upon these advancements, Cicero Parker Meek (1914–1979) from South Carolina introduced a novel micrografting technique in 1958 that enabled a graft to be utilized over a wound ranging from six to nine-fold greater in size [54]. Meek built upon the early wisdom of Reverdin's pinch grafts and Lawson's Fourpenny grafts by recognizing that epithelialization occurred from the graft edge. He hypothesized that by maximizing the epithelialization boarder he could expedite wound healing. Therefore, Meek would cut each square inch of harvested graft in a 16 by 16 grid pattern (generating 256 micrografts each $1/16^{th}$ of a square inch) using the Meek–Wall microdermatome. The result increased the epithelialization boarder 16-fold from 4 inches to 64 inches. The micrografts would then be placed onto bandages and applied to the wound [55]. In addition to the expansion of applicable surface area for harvested donor tissue, the Meek's technique allowed serosanguineous fluids to drain freely around the micrografts. Although the Meek–Wall microdermatome is still utilized at many specialized burn centers today, its routine use did not gain momentum as it was expensive to acquire and cumbersome to operate.

Although the concept of micrografting would not be forgotten, at this time in history the Meek's technique served as the bridge to skin meshing, which also allowed for wound fluid drainage and expansion of donor tissue over a larger wound surface area. Credit for the first prototype skin mesher belongs to the Swiss surgeon Otto Lanz (1865–1935) in Amsterdam (Netherlands), who trained under the Emil Theodor Kocher (1841–1917) the first surgeon to be awarded the Nobel Prize. Lanz invented a tool in 1907 he called the Hautschlitzapparat, which made 19 parallel cuts into a harvested skin graft, allowing it to expand in a manner that he described as a skin-net [56]. The Hautschlitzapparat and the accompanying tissue pattern are depicted in Figure 4a. Lanz described that the meshed skin graft would allow it to cover twice the surface area as the original donor tissue, a principle called the concertina effect. Lanz would apply one-half of the graft over the wound of interest and the other half would be used to re-cover the donor wound. Lanz's idea was based on the children's activity where a strip of paper is cut in alternating intervals to make an accordion-toy. He did this because it bothered him that when using Thiersch grafts often the wound would heal prior to the donor site. In 1930 Beverly Douglas (1891–1975) described the "sieve graft", which was a skin graft where he punched out holes. The removed "holes" were then re-applied on the donor site, while the graft was applied to the wound. The intention of the sieve graft was to facilitate drainage of wound fluids, which if undrained can dissociate the graft from the underlying wound bed and compromise viability. In 1937, multiple surgeons like Lester Reynolds Dragstedt (1893–1975) and František (Francis) Burian (1881–1965) continued to adapt and modify the sieve graft by manually making staggered incisions in the graft instead of hole-punches. As a result, fluid drainage was still achieved while the graft could now expand to cover larger surface areas. Although at that time, this technique was used primarily on full-thickness skin grafts, today it has been adapted for STSG and is commonly referred to as "pie-crusting".

In 1964 James Carlton Tanner Jr. (1921–1996) and his chief resident Jacques J. Vandeput from Grady Memorial Hospital in Atlanta, Georgia created a simple device called the Tanner–Vandeput mesh-dermatome that could expand STSG by a ratio of 1:3. The Tanner–Vandeput mesh-dermatome and its accompanying tissue pattern are depicted in Figure 4b. In their landmark paper titled "The Mesh Skin Graft" they introduced the term "meshed graft" [57]. The Tanner–Vandeput mesher consisted of two four-inch rollers, one knurled to grip the skin and the other with multiple parallel staggered cutting blades to cause the meshing pattern. Harvested skin grafts were placed between the two rollers and then rotated to incise a meshed pattern into the graft [58]. As mentioned, however, micrografting would not be forgotten. In 1966, Vandeput combined the concepts of the Meek–Wall dermatome and the Tanner–Vandeput mesher to create "ultra-postage skin grafts" that were 1/20th of an inch squared [59].

The Tanner–Vandeput mesher was originally sold under the commercial name Mesh-Dermatome I by the Zimmer Company (Dover, OH, USA) in 1964 and utilized a plastic feeding tray called a dermacarrier. A number of iterations have since been made over the years to improve upon the design. The Mesh-Dermatome II (Zimmer Company) introduced in 1970 changed the blade angles relative to the dermacarrier and the meshing pattern (hexagon) to allow variability in the meshing ratio from 1:1 up to 9:1. In 1991, the Zimmer Skingraft Mesher (Zimmer Company) utilized a ratchet and cog-wheel mechanism to pull the dermacarrier through the cutting mechanism. This model also allowed interchangeable bladed rollers to allow for rapid variation in ratio (ranging from 1:1 to 4:1). The two companies did away with the dermacarrier and introduced a double-cutting-roller design—Collin (Arcueil, France) in 1986 and Brennen Med (St. Paul, MN, USA) in 1988. The primary benefit of the double-roller model is that it did not require sharpening as it did not relay on blades piercing the skin graft in order to form interstices. Rather, the two rollers, one of which is notched, performed a scissor-like pinching action. The Brennen Skingraft Mesher (Brennen Med) which was modified in 1993 from the original design to be more user-friendly offers a number of meshing patterns, but, unlike its Zimmer counterpart, a different instrument is needed for each meshing ratio (ranging from 1:1 to 8:1) [60]. Meshed grafts are the mainstay of modern burn wound care and use nearly universally by all burn centers. They have several key advantages over unmeshed (sheet) grafts beyond surface area expansion, fluid drainage, and expedited wound closure. Meshed grafts are more versatile as the interstices allow the shape of the donor tissue to be adapted to asymmetric wounds and across irregular body contours [58]. Unmeshed skin grafts in contrast develop more robust vascularization, reduced scar contracture and are more aesthetically pleasing due to the lack of interstices.

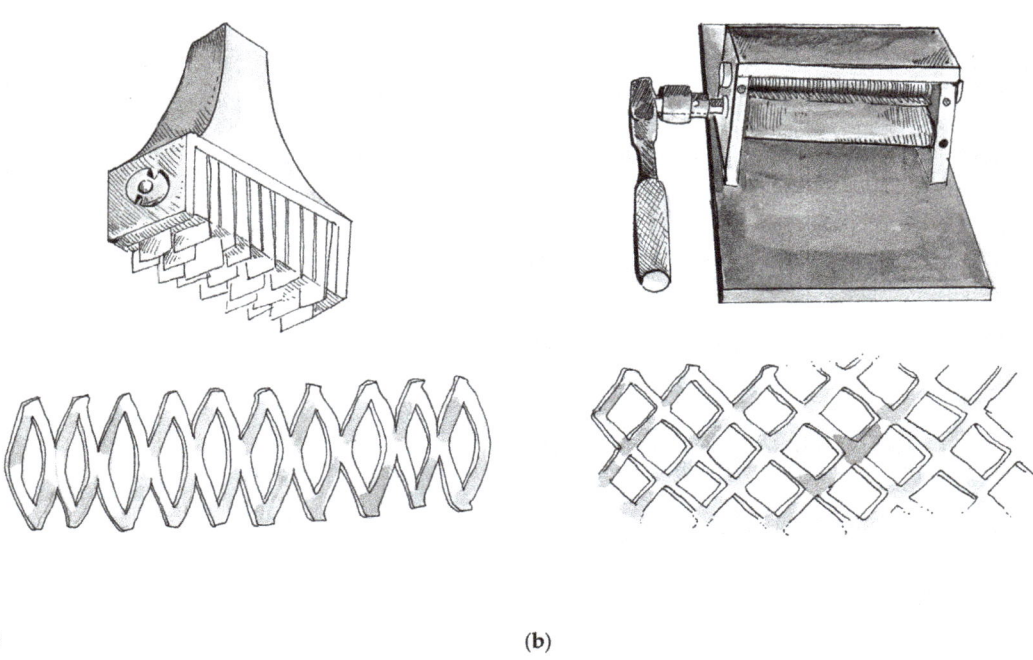

(a) (b)

Figure 4. Instruments for skin graft expansion: (**a**) The Hautschlitzapparat by Lanz in 1907; (**b**) The Tanner–Vandeput mesh-dermatome in 1964.

Severely injured burn victims and limited donor site availability have continued to challenge burn surgeons to push the limits of skin graft expansion. In 2012, Florian Hackl and colleagues from Brigham and Women's Hospital in Boston, Massachusetts described the Xpansion™ technique, which afforded an expansion ratio of 100:1 by mincing skin grafts into 0.8 mm × 0.8 mm micrografts and then spreading them onto the wound bed [61]. Studies have found that mincing grafts leads to over expression of growth factors like tumor necrosis factor alpha, platelet-derived growth factor, and basic fibroblast growth factor, which are thought to promote wound healing [62]. Further, developing Hackl's technique, Denesh Kadam an Indian surgeon from Karnataka, India developed a technique called "Pixel Grafting". Similar to the Xpansion™ technique, skin grafts are minced into digital pixel sized grafts (0.3 mm × 0.3 mm) and are able to achieve expiation ratio of up to 700:1 [63].

6.4. Homografts and Immunologic Discoveries in Skin Grafting

When Reverdin first introduced the concept of skin grafting it gained popularity rapidly due to the remarkable nature of the short-term results. By the 1870s, however, Reverdin's techniques were losing popularity because of their less impressive long-term results. From our modern perspective it is not intuitive why this might be. At the time these shortcomings were attributed to impracticality of the concept of skin grafting itself, but in fact the reason had to do with the unintentional introduction of homografting—the use of skin grafts across members of the same species. Reverdin, along with numerous other surgeons of his age, held the conviction that homografts were for all intents and purposes interchangeable with autografts. In fact, in many publications from that period the authors failed to bother specifying what type of graft was even used. Reverdin's reputation in burn surgery hinges on reports that he used his own skin to treat injured patients. In 1872, he wrote about the care of a burn victim:

> "In my first grafts I used skin from the patient himself, but I soon became convinced that the results was the same when I used skin from another individual. This has been demonstrated with certainty."—Jacques-Louis Reverdin [64].

Although the idea of a surgeon using their own skin seems remarkably philanthropic by our modern cultural norms, during Reverdin's time many surgeons would excise fragments of their own skin to demonstrate to patients who were particularly scared that the procedure was in fact not as painful as the patient might imagine. The modern surgeon might even equate it to a form of informed consent. Surgeons also reported that many patient's relatives were more than willing to donate fragments of their own skin to aid in the healing of a loved one [65]. Going one step further, in the Berlin Military Hospital a skin graft donor could be found for as little as the price of a beer [66]. Donor tissue were also collected in more creative ways—for example from amputated extremities and circumcised foreskin [67,68]. The timing between graft harvest and placement, as well as the temperature that the collected tissue was stored at, was a matter of great debate in those days. Some surgeons arguing that the procedure needed to occur as soon as possible and that the graft must be kept warm, while others reported success with grafts that had been collected four days prior and were stored at 10 °C [69,70]. This dichotomy resulted in a number or remarkable scenarios. One surgeon described placing the soon-to-be amputees in the same operative theater adjacent to the anticipated skin graft recipient. Another surgeon described his method of keeping grafts warm by placing them in his armpit while transporting them from donor to recipient [70,71]. In addition, despite amputations being routinely performed in those days, disease like smallpox, syphilis and tuberculosis were also equally commonplace. Therefore, the sudden appearance of numerous cases of infectious diseases transmitted through homografts in the literature should come as no surprise to the modern reader [64,72,73]. Surgeons also described progressive graft degradation and failure in a time when the mechanism of graft rejection was not understood. Therefore, for a time homografting was abandoned by most practitioners, and considered to be an inherently unsuccessful enterprise.

In the 20th century, however, with advances in critical care and medical technology, there was an unexpected revival of cadaveric homografting with the introduction of the skin bank and cryopreservation. In 1903, the German physician Johann Wentscher (1852–1913), a contemporary of Thiersch, was the first to document the viability of refrigerated skin grafts at 0 °C for 14 days [74]. Long-term cryopreservation was not possible until the 1930s when effective, reproducible, standardized storage methods were established. It was during World War II that serious investment went into skin banking due to the large number or wounded soldiers that were returning from the war. The sheer burden of injury produced by World War II spurred the development of skin banks and trauma-specific research centers, such as the United States Institute of Surgical Research [75]. Researchers found that harvested skin could be preserved in a glycerol-based cryopreservative for up to up to four months at −79 °C [76]. Such skin banks allowed wartime hospitals to have a read supply of homograft skin for severe burn victim with insufficient donor site.

Around the same time, across the Atlantic, the Battle of Britain (1940) raged and a plane crashed in Oxford near the home of British immunologist and Zoologist, Sir Peter Medawar (1915–1987). The physician caring for the horribly burned pilot consulted Medawar for advice. Although Medawar had no experience caring for burn victims, he believed that skin grafting would afford the airman the best chance of survival. Unfortunately, despite Medawar's efforts, the pilot would not survive. The experience, however, would instill in Medawar a life-long curiosity about the immunological intricacies of skin grafting. During the remainder of the war Medawar collaborated with the Scottish Plastic surgeon Thomas Gibson (1915–1993) to perform homografts and autografts on other soldiers [77]. The two observed that homografts, though initially appearing to incorporate, would go on to be rejected within two weeks' time. In contrast, autografts were often successfully engrafted during the same time frame. Medawar also noticed that if a second homograft from the same donor was re-attempted, graft rejection occurred more quickly. This affirmed Medawar's suspicions that the etiology of graft failure was immune-mediated. He reported his findings to the War Wounds Committee of the Medical Research Council in 1944, The Behaviour and Fate of Skin Autografts and Skin Homografts in Rabbits [78].

In 1945, Ray David Owens (1915–2014) introduced the concept of chimerism while studying dizygotic cattle twins. Owens observed the presence of "mixed blood types" that were the result of in utero genetic exposure [79]. Frank Macfarlane Burnet (1899–1985) an Australian Virologist built upon these findings and proposed the theory of immune tolerance, suggesting that immunologic self-awareness could be influenced, particularly during embryogenesis. Medawar tested this theory by crossing allografts between dizygotic cattle twins. He observed that grafts remained intact for several weeks longer than would typically be expected. Medawar took the experiment one step further using a mouse model. He inoculated fetal mice with splenic cells from a donor (second) mouse strain. After eight weeks, he performed allografts using the donor strain of mice and observed that the transplanted skin was tolerated. As a control, skin from a previously unexposed (third) strain was also grafted and was expectantly rejected [80]. This experiment is credited as the foundation for modern transplant immunology and both Medawar and Burnet were awarded the Nobel Prize in Medicine for their discovery of immune tolerance.

Prior to World War II, Colonel James Barrett Brown (1899–1971) had postulated that homograft rejection was due to the genetic disparity between donor and host. In 1937, he performed the first successful "homograft" in which both the donor and recipient of a skin graft were identical twins. During the war as the Chief of plastic surgery at Valley Forge General Hospital (Phoenixville, Pennsylvania), Brown took Joseph E. Murray (1919–2012), then a surgical intern and First Lieutenant, under his wing. This act of charity spared Murray overseas deployment and afforded him experience caring for wartime victims of burn-related trauma. Similar to Medawar, Murray's first-hand exposure to burn victims would inspire an academic career in tissue transplantation. Murray would lay the foundation for our modern understanding of skin's enhanced antigenicity [81,82]. In the decades that followed World War II, a significant amount of research on the immune response to skin grafts was performed. In the 1950s, major histocompatibility complexes (MHC) were discovered. However, Rupert Everett Billingham (1921–2002) demonstrated that both MHC-matched and mismatched donor homografts resulted graft failure [83]. The 1960s saw a wave of animal experiments with immunosuppressants like phenothiazine derivatives, methylhydrazine derivatives, anti-lymphocyte biologics, steroids, anti-metabolites, and even x-ray irradiation—none of which were effective in reducing skin graft rejection rates or were practical for use in human use [84]. In the 1970s, transplanted skin was found to generate a more robust immune response than solid organs due to its higher antigenicity. Although the exact mechanisms for cell-mediate (T-cell) and innate (Natural Killer cell) mediated acute rejection was not better understood till more recent decades, surgeons have come to understand that homograft do not replace the need for autograft, but serves as temporary bridge to autograft application. Of note, Murray replicated the work of him predecessor, Brown, performing the first living donor kidney transplant between identical twins, and was awarded the Nobel Prize in Medicine for his achievement in 1990 [81].

In 1954, Douglas MacGilchrist Jackson (1916–2002), a contemporary of William Heneage Ogilvie, was a British surgeon from the Birmingham Accident Hospital who is remembered for his "alternate strip method," which involved placing half-inch strips of autograft and homograft in an alternating sequence to cover large posterior thoracic burn wounds. Jackson credited the idea to Rainsford Mowlem (1902–1986), a New Zealander who was appointed to presidency of the British Association of Plastic Surgeons. Jackson performed this method on 16 patients and reported successful results with many patients being able to return to their lives without significant functional disability within a year. Jackson also coined the term "creeping substitution", an observation he noted when epithelialization from the autograft strips boarders would grow underneath the homograft strips and eventually connect adjacent autograft strips. Subsequently, the strips of homograft would separate and reveal an epithelialized wound bed underneath [85].

In 1986, Ming-liang Zhang, a Chinese surgeon from Beijing Jishuitan Hospital, and colleagues further developed this technique by slicing autografts into one millimeter micrografts, which they would place onto a larger sheet of homograft. They called this autograft–homograft composite "Microskin". Sheets of Microskin were then applied to the wound bed and much like in the alternate strip method, autograft epithelial cells proliferated via creeping substitution and eventually separated from the homograft. Over multiple publications, Zhang described the successful use of Microskin grafting in 32 burn patients (ranging from 2.5 to 45% TBSA) and reported expansion ratios as high as 15:1 to 18:1 [86]. Despite its advantages, however, Microskin remains technically challenging and requires specialized equipment to apply routinely. J. Wesley Alexander (1934–2018) and colleagues from the Shriners Burns Institute in Cincinnati, Ohio (now called Shriners Children's Ohio) utilized a method in which 6:1 meshed autograft was reinforced with 3:1 meshed homograft. Alexander noted that by layering homograft on top of the more friable autograft the latter would be protected during the critical period of incorporation. In the 14 patients this method was initially described in, there was a 99% graft take of the underlying autograft with no reported loss at follow-up. The overlying homograft, in contrast, had a 95% initial incorporation within the first three days and a subsequent near-total rejection over the subsequent 30-day period [87]. The Alexander method or, as it is more commonly called, the "Sandwich technique" has been modified since being introduced, but is still widely utilized today at almost every large burn center today for its simplicity and efficiency.

6.5. Skin Substitutes

Bioengineered skin substitutes have also emerged as an area of interest. Research into skin substitutes dates back to 1975 when Ioannis V. Yannas of the Massachusetts Institute of Technology (MIT) and John Francis Burke (1922–2011), the Chief of Staff at Shriners Burns Institute in Boston (now called Shriners Hospital for Children©—Boston) and the Massachusetts General Hospital Burn Service, collaborated to develop the first bio-synthetic skin substitute called Integra® (Integra LifeSciences Corp., Plainsboro, NJ, USA). In recognition for their achievement, Yannas and Burke were inducted into the National Inventors Hall of Fame in 2015. Integra® consists of a layer of cross-linked bovin collagen and shark chondroitin (glycosaminoglycan) with a silicon top-layer. The collagen-chondroitin matrix facilitates the recapitulation of a reticular dermis, while the silicone acts as a temporary protective pseudo-epidermis. After the excision of a full-thickness burn, Integra® allows the wound bed to regenerate a layer equivalent to the dermis. After approximately three weeks, when the dermis has regenerated, the silicon layer is physically removed and replaced with a standard autograft [88]. Products like Integra® are acellular skin substitutes. In contrast, cellular skin substitutes like Transcyte® (Advanced Tissue

Sciences, La Jolla, CA, USA) consist of a synthetic scaffolding seeded with living human cells (fibroblasts).

Cell-based therapies aim to replace lost tissue with cultured skin cells, which was not considered feasible until 1975, when Howard Green (1925–2015) and his graduate student James G. Rheinwald at MIT successfully cultured human keratinocytes [82]. Green and Rheinwald actually made their discovery by accident while they were trying to replicate a teratoma, an altogether different tumor [89]. Their discovery called Cultured Epithelial Autografts (CEA) involves harvesting stems cells from the patient's skin and growing a culture of these cells into an autograft sheet, which can then be applied to burn wounds and was particularly useful when donor sites are limited. In 1983, the mettle of CEA was put to the test when a five-year-old, Jamie Selby, and his seven-year-old brother, Glen Selby, suffered 97% TBSA third-degree burns after playing with flammables in an abandoned building. Both children from Casper, Wyoming were airlifted to Shriners Hospitals for Children©—Boston where Green and his colleagues performed over 350 grafts grown from small patches of donor tissue. Having only produced CEA on a small scale prior to this occasion, Green restructured his laboratory at Harvard University in order to produce CEA around the clock for the two boys. He later went on to found the company BioSurface Technology Inc. (Cambridge, MA, USA). The survival of the two boys, gained CEA national recognition from the medical community. In 2010, Rajiv Sood and his colleagues from Indiana University in Indianapolis, Indiana described their experience with the use of CEA in 88 victims of major burns, ranging from 28 to 98% TBSA over a period of 18-years. They found an overall graft success of 72.7%, and a survival rate of 91%. Sood wrote that "[such results] gives much optimism for continuing to use CEA in critically burned patients" [90]. Despite its significant benefits, the primary barrier to its routine use in the critically ill burn patient is the two to three weeks of incubation-time needed to produce it.

In 1989, Steven T. Boyce from the Shriners Burns Institute in Cincinnati, Ohio and colleagues from the University of California San Diego Medical Center introduced an alternative product which they expected to replace CEA called Cultured Skin Substitutes (CSS). Consisting of a collagen-glycosaminoglycan sheet inoculated with human dermal fibroblasts on one side and epidermal keratinocytes on the other, CSS could potential to preserve donor sites as it did not rely on autologous cell harvesting [91]. Boyce prodigiously published the benefits of CSS, showing in vitro that it could be modified in various ways to emulate the anatomic features of autografts—"lipid supplements" could enhance the epidermal barrier, pigmentation could be optimized to the patient with the addition of melanocytes, the addition of growth factors could enhance wound healing and the CSS itself could be genetically enhances to expedite wound closure [92–95]. For a time, CSS was used at a number of burn centers, especially within the Shriners system, however, it did not gain sufficient traction from the Food and Drug Administration to be adapted for widespread clinical use.

Around the same time, another emerging technology was gaining attention within the tissue translocation community—cellular suspension. Rupert E. Billingham (1921–2002) and Joyce Reynolds of the University College (London, United Kingdom) first introduced cellular suspension in 1952 using an enzymatic preparation with Trypsin [96]. Although the suspended cells were viable, this early technique was not successful because the cells failed to adhere to the wound bed. In 1988, János Hunyadi and colleagues revisited the technique by trypsinizing keratinocytes and suspending them in a fibrin glue solution, a process which they named Keratinocytes in Fibrin Glue Suspension (KFGS). Hunyadi was able to use KFGS technology to successfully treat venous stasis ulcers, but did not apply it to the treatment of burn wounds [97]. In 1994, Hans-Wilhelm Kaiser and colleagues from the University of Bonn Medical School and Burn Centre in Colonge-Merheim, Germany published the use of fibrin glue suspension techniques with cells derived from CEA in the treatment of burn wounds [98]. Several subsequent studies compared and contrasted aerosolized skin cells with and without fibrin glue, and, in 2003, Lachlan J. Currie and colleagues concluded that there was no observable of histologic difference in outcomes [99].

The merger of autologous epithelial cell culturing and cellular suspension occurred in the early 1990s by the British-born Australian plastic surgeon, Fiona Melanie Wood. As the Burn Director of the Royal Perth Hospital, Wood had experienced first-hand the morbid consequence of awaiting CEA production in a critically injured burn patient. After several deaths, which Wood believed could have been salvaged if the production time of CEA could be decreased, she began experimenting with the production process of cultured epithelial cells. In her early work, Wood discovered that CEA could be applied after culture growth of as little as 10 days. Not only would the sub-confluent cultured graft adhere to the wound, but Wood observed that the wound healed quicker. The mechanism for this observation was unknown, but Wood suspected that it was a result of cellular signaling pathways within the wound bed that promote proliferation or that sub-confluent cells inherently had improved proliferative potential having spent less time in culture medium [100]. Edwin A. Deitch and colleagues also found that burn wounds closed after 21 days, independent of the method, incurred a 70% risk of hypertrophic scar formation, while wounds closed within ten days only afforded a 4% risk [101]. Wood recruited Marie L. Stoner, a cell biologist, to help her reduce cultured graft application time table and the two worked tirelessly—successfully minimizing it to 5 days. In their method, a postage-stamp size piece of uninjured donor epidermis is harvested. Keratinocytes are scrapped off and cultured in a concentrated single-cell suspension for 5 days and collected while in the pre-confluent stage. The cells are then placed in solution and aerosolized onto the burn wound using a standard syringe with spray-nozzle attachment. Wood dubbed this process CellSpray (later referred to as Spray-on-Skin™) and she went on to commercialize the technology in 1993 with the help of the Australian biotechnology company Clinical Cell Culture Pty Ltd. (also referred to as C3) [102]. Over the next decade the global burn community would regard Spray-on-Skin™ with skepticism, as Wood did not publish any trials demonstrating its comparative efficacy. Wood continued to use the method routinely in her own practice and insisted that the results spoke for themselves. The lack of scientific evidence and Wood's financial relationship with C3 would raise concerns among her peers and negatively affect global interest in the technology. Therefore, for a time, C3 proved a service, albeit on a humble scale, to burn centers in Australia, New Zealand, and the United Kingdom.

On 12th October 2002, however, Spray-on-Skin™ would return to the international limelight when militant terrorist bombed the tourist-rich Kuta district of Bali, Indonesia. The Royal Australian Air Force transported over a hundred patients to hospitals throughout Australia, of which 28 were brought to Wood's burn unit. In preparation for such an event, Wood had coordinated with Woodside Petroleum, a local energy company, to trial a burn catastrophe response plan the year prior. As part of the plan, the production of Spray-on-Skin™ would be upregulated proportionally to meet the acute needs of the patients. By exercising this plan, Wood and her colleagues were able to save all but three of the patients they had received that day [102]. Naturally, international interest in Spray-on-Skin™ increased. In 2005, Wood introduced another technological achievement in skin transplantation technology—aerosolization of non-cultured epidermal cells. Wood called her novel system ReCell®; in 2008, C3 would be restructured under a new name, Avita Medical, Inc. (Valencia, California), and ReCell® would be their primary product. John Harvey, the president of the Australian and New Zealand Burn Association described Wood's work as "ground-breaking" [103]. In 2005, for her significant contributions to the field of burn care, Wood would be named Australian of the Year.

The ReCell® system is available as a single-use kit that combines the extraction and application of cells into a single process. Cells are harvested from the dermal-epidermal junction of a STSG taken at 6–8/1000th of-an-inch thickness. The tissues are then enzymatically (trypsin) and mechanically disrupted. Keratinocytes, melanocytes, fibroblasts, and Langerhans cells are the suspended in a lactate solution. Each square centimeter of donor STSG generates one milliliter of suspension, which in turn can be applied to approximately 80 cm^2 of wound area (80:1 expansion ratio) [104]. Similar to CellSpray, ReCell® was introduced with little comparative evidence of efficacy relative to other routinely used skin grafting techniques. In fact, it would be Sood and colleagues who would publish the first phase 2 trial comparing outcomes between ReCell® and meshed STSG in 10 patients [105]. Although under-powered, Sood showed that ReCell® demonstrated similar results and required a small donor site. In 2018, a larger multi-institutional randomized control trial was performed by James Hill Holmes IV, and collaborators comparing ReCell® with meshed STSG in deep partial thickness wounds in 83 patients. At four weeks, patients treated with ReCell® demonstrated similar wound closure (98 vs. 100%), pain and scarring compared to controls. In contrast, control donor sites were approximately 40 times larger, incurred more pain, and expectantly took longer to heal than donor sites in the treatment group. Subsequent follow-up one year after treatment revealed that patient's that received ReCell® were considerably more satisfaction than controls [106]. Based on these trails, ReCell® received approval by the Food and Drug Administration in 2018.

Critics of ReCell® also raised concern over the viability of extracted cells after applications. In 2012, a study using ReCell® found 75.5% of cells were viable at the time of harvest and 69.5% survived aerosolization. Critics also argued that application of non-cultured cells result in delayed epithelialization and thin wound coverage, especially when utilized on full thickness wounds that lack existing dermal elements. Initially, Wood responded to these concerns in 2007 by demonstrating the successful combined use of ReCell® and Integra® on a porcine model. Wood performed a single-stage repair of ten full thickness wounds on a pair of Yorkshire swine and histologically compared results with controls treated with Integra® alone and ReCell® alone. Wood's results showed that simultaneous treatment enhanced reconstruction of full thickness wounds compared to controls, but once again did not provide a comparison of her technique with what would be considered a standard of care practice [107]. More than a decade later, in 2019, Holmes IV and collaborators once again performed a second multi-institutional trial comparing the concurrent use of ReCell® and STSG with in-subject controls receiving STSG alone. The trial was performed on 30 patients for treatment of mixed depth wounds including deep partial thickness and full-thickness burns. The mean TBSA was 21% (+/− 13%) and the average area grafted was 2443 cm^2 (+/− 1675 cm^2). The results for treatment with ReCell® and STSG showed non-inferiority for wound healing (92 vs. 85%) and a statistically significant reduction in donor site area (32%; $p < 0.001$) [104]. These results suggest that ReCell® combined with STSG can be a safe and effective treatment for deep burn wounds and can help minimize the amount of donor surface area utilized. As of December 2020, ReCell® is being used at 83 of the nations 132 burn centers and is considered one of the most promising advance in skin translocation technology [108].

7. The Future of Skin Grafting: The Author's Thoughts

In the past, research has focused on optimizing expansion ratios and improving graft-related outcomes. Some would argue that the use of cultured keratinocytes and aerosolization of non-cultured skin grafts is the epitome of such pursuits. The future of burn care, therefore, will rely on the incorporation of new techniques, such as nanotechnology and 3D printing to push the boundaries of skin grafting as we know them. One of the difficulties with engineering artificial tissue is the inability to produce complex tissue layers in a reproducible manner. Computer-aided design (CAD) are used to design and produce 3D printed models. While the majority of 3D printing is done on a macro scale, CADs can be scaled down to the cellular level with the help of nanotechnology. This means it would be possible to fine-tune the composition of artificial skin substitute in a manner that is both precise and reproducible. Current techniques that are being attempted involve bioprinting cellular components onto a premade matrix and directly printing such a construct onto the burn wound.

Stefanie Michael from Hanover Medical School (Hanover, Germany) has reported promising results regarding the former technique. Utilizing Laser-assisted bioprinting (LaBP) and a mouse model, Stefanie created artificial skin using Matriderm® as a foundation and printed fibroblasts and keratinocytes onto the surface. Using Ki67 as a marker for cellular growth, Michael found that his artificial skin mimics similar patterns of proliferation and differentiation found in natural skin. In the stratum basalis of normal skin, keratinocytes typically proliferate and differentiate as they progress towards the skin surface. A gradient of Ki67 was found in the artificial skin with a higher concentration at the base of the graft, mirroring the arrangement of natural skin. These grafts were only left in the mice for 11 days before being removed for examination. Apart from the proliferation patters, researchers also noted blood vessels growing towards the graft [109]. The lack of rete ridges, however, suggests the possible fragility of the artificial skin. While these findings are rudimentary in their clinical applications, they represent an early success in the possibility of 3D printed skin.

Biomedical engineer Aleksander Skardal demonstrated the latter technique of directly printing the artificial skin onto the wound. Not only did his team utilize 3D printing, but they also attempted to capitalize on the versatility and lack of immunogenicity of stem cells by incorporating them into the artificial tissue. Using a bioprinter of their own design, amniotic fluid-derived stem (AFS) cells and bone marrow-derived mesenchymal stem cells (MSC) in a fibrin-collagen gel were printed onto a wound and compared to a wound treated with a fibrin-collagen only gel in mice. The wounds were then evaluated periodically at 0, 7, and 14 days. Comparing the histology of the wounds, the researchers found greater wound closure, and re-epithelization in the stem cell treated wounds compared to the control. Histological sections revealed the AFS cell treated wound showed the greatest microvascular density and capillary diameter, while the fibrin-collagen control showed the least. Fluorescence tracking of the stem cells suggest their presence was transient and further analysis indicated that it is possible that is it the growth factors released by the stems cells which induced wound healing [110]. The direct printing of artificial skin onto a burn could be further augmented by a "portable handheld electrohydrodynamic multi-needle spray gun" described by Sofokleous making the process more accessible and convenient. Appearing similar to a hot glue gun, this device was found to be able to produce multicomponent structures with sub-micrometer precision [111]. This technology has yet to be tested printing artificial skin, but theoretically has many appealing applications. The technologies discussed here are only two of the many currently being explored in the cause of advancing the treatment of burn wounds. While many are still confined to theory and animal models, early data provide many reasons to be hopeful for their future applications in skin grafting.

In this article, we traced the history of modern skin grafting from its brutal roots in simple tissue translocation in the ancient world to modern expansion techniques with aerosolized skin cells. A timeline of this journey can be seen in Figure 5. The future of skin grafting and burn care will continue to be driven by the challenges presented by the most severely injured patients. While there is much work left to be done, reflecting on the past is liable to provoke a greater appreciation of how far modern skin grafting and burn care has already come.

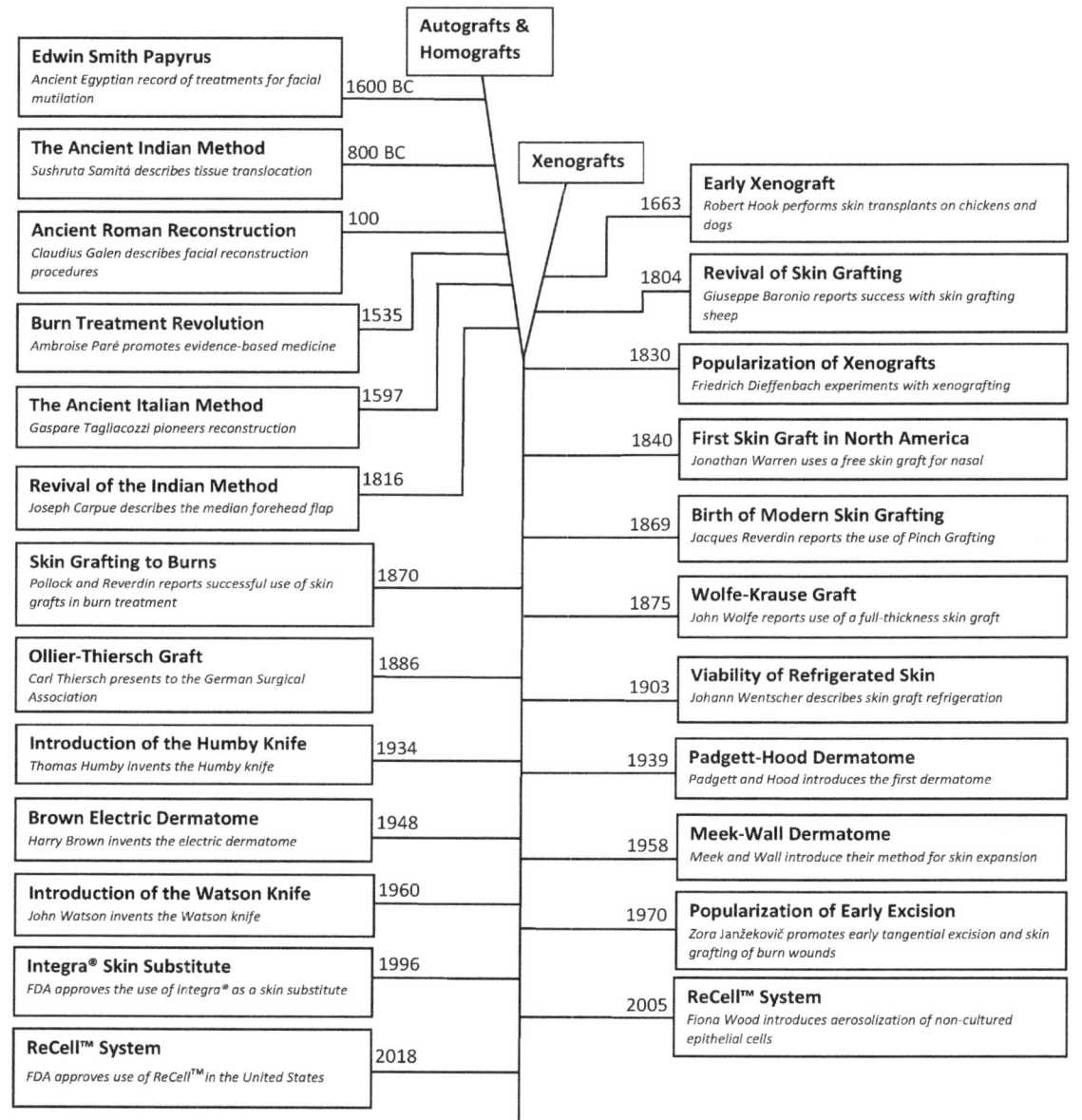

Figure 5. A timeline of the major historic events that preceded modern skin grafting in burn surgery.

Author Contributions: Conceptualization, D.K.O. and L.K.B.; investigation, M.W.T. and D.K.O.; resources, M.W.T.; writing—original draft preparation, M.W.T. and D.K.O.; writing—review and editing, D.K.O., S.E.W., and L.K.B.; visualization, D.K.O.; supervision, S.E.W. and L.K.B.; project administration, D.K.O.; funding acquisition, S.E.W. All authors have read and agreed to the published version of the manuscript.

Funding: The endeavor to compose this manuscript was funded by the British Petroleum Burn Fellowship Program (#C18612), as well as the Remembering the 15 Fund for Burn Research, Education, and Clinical Care (#C19584) provided in part by British Petroleum Products North America Inc.

Institutional Review Board Statement: Not applicable.

Acknowledgments: The authors would like to thank Shephaly Soni for her artistic contributions to this manuscript.

Conflicts of Interest: The authors have no conflicts of interest to declare.

References

1. Hester, J. *Discours of the Excellent Doctour and Knight, Maister Leonardo Phiorauanti Bolognese Uppon Chirurgerie: With a Declaration of Many Thinges, Necessarie to be Knowne, Never Written Before in this Order: Wherunto is Added a Number of Notable Secretes, Found Out by the Saide Author*; Translated out of Italyan into English, by Iohn Hester, Practicioner in the Arte of Distillation; Thomas East: London, UK, 1850; p. 32.
2. Barrow, R.E.; Herndon, D.N. History of treatments of burns. In *Total Burn Care*; Elsevier BV: Amsterdam, The Netherlands, 2007; pp. 1–8.
3. Spitz, L.; Coran, A.G. *Operative Pediatric Surgery*, 6th ed.; Hodder Education Publishers: London, UK, 2006; pp. 957–964.
4. Pećanac, M.; Janjić, Z.; Komarcević, A.; Pajić, M.; Dobanovacki, D.; Misković, S.S. Burns treatment in ancient times. *Med. Pregl.* **2013**, *66*, 263–267. [PubMed]
5. Ang, G.C. History of skin transplantation. *Clin. Dermatol.* **2005**, *23*, 320–324. [CrossRef] [PubMed]
6. Liu, H.-F.; Zhang, F.; Lineaweaver, W.C. History and advancement of burn treatments. *Ann. Plast. Surg.* **2017**, *78*, S2–S8. [CrossRef]
7. Nichter, L.S.; Morgan, R.F.; Nichter, M.A. The impact of Indian methods for total nasal reconstruction. *Clin. Plast. Surg.* **1983**, *10*, 635–647.
8. Keegan, D. *Rhinoplastic Operations*; Tindall & Cox: Baltimore, MD, USA, 1900.
9. Almast, S. History and evolution of the Indian method of rhinoplasty. In *Transactions of the Fourth International Congress of Plastic and Reconstructive Surgery*; Sanvenero-Rosselli, G., Ed.; Exerpta Medica Foundation: Rome, Italy, 1969; p. 49.
10. Davis, J.S. Address of the president: The story of plastic surgery. *Ann. Surg.* **1941**, *113*, 641–656. [CrossRef]
11. Thornton, J.F. Skin grafts and skin substitutes. *Sel. Read. Plast. Surg.* **2004**, *10*, 1–23.
12. Ameer, F.; Singh, A.K.; Kumar, S. Evolution of instruments for harvest of the skin grafts. *Indian J. Plast. Surg.* **2013**, *46*, 28–35. [CrossRef]
13. Letter, B.L. *Gentleman's Magazine*; Nichols: London, UK, 1794; p. 891.
14. Singh, M.; Nuutila, K.; Collins, K.; Huang, A. Evolution of skin grafting for treatment of burns: Reverdin pinch grafting to Tanner mesh grafting and beyond. *Burns* **2017**, *43*, 1149–1154. [CrossRef] [PubMed]
15. Belinfante, L.S. History of Rhinoplasty. *Oral Maxillofac. Surg. Clin. N. Am.* **2012**, *24*, 1–9. [CrossRef] [PubMed]
16. Pasipoularides, A. Galen, father of systematic medicine. An essay on the evolution of modern medicine and cardiology. *Int. J. Cardiol.* **2014**, *172*, 47–58. [CrossRef]
17. Jewett, B.S.; Baker, S.R. History of Nasal Reconstruction. In *Principles of Nasal Reconstruction*, 2nd ed.; Springer: Berlin, Germany, 2010; pp. 3–12.
18. Drucker, C.B. Ambroise Paré and the birth of the gentle art of surgery. *Yale J. Boil. Med.* **2008**, *81*, 199–202.
19. Hernigou, P. Other aspects of Ambroise Paré's life. *Int. Orthop.* **2013**, *37*, 1405–1412. [CrossRef] [PubMed]
20. Ball, J.M. Ambrose Paré, The father of French surgery. 1509–1590. Read before the Des Moines Valley Medical Society, at Ottumwa, Iowa, June 21, 1894. *JAMA* **1894**, *XXIII*, 45. [CrossRef]
21. Artz, C.P. Historical aspects of burn management. *Surg. Clin. N. Am.* **1970**, *50*, 1193–1200. [CrossRef]
22. Koch, S.L. The transplantation of skin and subcutaneous tissue to the hand. *Surg. Gynec. Obst.* **1941**, *72*, 157–177.
23. Brock, R.C. *The Life and Work of Astley Cooper*; Livingstone: Edinburgh, UK, 1952; p. 47.
24. Goldwyn, R.M. Johann Friedrich Dieffenbach (1794–1847). *Plast. Reconstr. Surg.* **1968**, *42*, 19–28. [CrossRef]
25. Cohen, J. Earliest attempt at free skin grafting. *Ann. Plast. Surg.* **1995**, *34*, 552–553. [CrossRef] [PubMed]
26. Gibson, T. Zoografting: A curious chapter in the history of plastic surgery. *Br. J. Plast. Surg.* **1955**, *8*, 234–242. [CrossRef]
27. Cooper, D.K. Xenografting: The early, early years. *Xeno* **1997**, *5*, 21–22.
28. Hauben, D.J.; Baruchin, A.; Mahler, D. On the history of the free skin graft. *Ann. Plast. Surg.* **1982**, *9*, 242–246. [CrossRef]
29. International Society of Aesthetic Plastic Surgery. Available online: https://www.isaps.org/blog/giuseppe-baronio-origins-free-skin-grafting/ (accessed on 8 January 2021).
30. Giuseppe, B. *Degli Innesti Animali*; Tipografia del Genio: Milan, Italy, 1804.
31. Rogers, B.O. Historical development of free skin grafting. *Surg. Clin. N. Am.* **1959**, *39*, 289–311. [CrossRef]
32. Encyclopedia.com. Available online: https://www.encyclopedia.com/science/encyclopedias-almanacs-transcripts-and-maps/ilhelm-fabricius-hildanus (accessed on 25 January 2021).
33. Klasen, H.J. Skin grafting in eyelid surgery. In *History of Free Skin Grafting*; Springer: Berlin/Heidelberg, Germany, 1981; pp. 47–60.

34. Kilner, T.P. The full-thickness skin graft. *Postgrad. Med. J.* **1935**, *11*, 279–282. [CrossRef]
35. McDowell, F. Carl Thiersch, microscopy, and skin grafting. *Plast. Reconstr. Surg.* **1968**, *41*, 369–370.
36. Underhill, F.P. Changes in blood concentration with special reference to the treatment of extensive superficial burns. *Ann. Surg.* **1927**, *86*, 840–849. [CrossRef] [PubMed]
37. Cope, O.; Moore, F.D. THE redistribution of body water and the fluid therapy of the burned patient. *Ann. Surg.* **1947**, *126*, 1010–1046. [CrossRef] [PubMed]
38. Young, F. Immediate skin grafting in the treatment of burns. *Ann. Surg.* **1942**, *116*, 445–451. [CrossRef] [PubMed]
39. Saltonstall, H.; Lee, W.E. Modified technic in skin grafting of extensive deep burns. *Ann. Surg.* **1944**, *119*, 690–693. [CrossRef] [PubMed]
40. McCoekle, H.J.; Silvani, H. Selection of the time for grafting of skin to extensive defects resulting from deep thermal burns. *Ann. Surg.* **1945**, *121*, 285–290. [CrossRef]
41. Jackson, D.; Topley, E.; Cason, J.S.; Lowbury, E.J.L. Primary excision and grafting of large burns. *Ann. Surg.* **1960**, *250*, 167–189. [CrossRef]
42. Janžekovič, Z. A new concept in the early excision and immediate grafting of burns. *J. Trauma Inj. Infect. Crit. Care* **1970**, *10*, 1103–1108. [CrossRef]
43. Janzekovic, Z. Early surgical treatment of the burned surface. *Panminerva Med.* **1972**, *14*, 228–232.
44. Janžekovič, Z. Once upon a time . . . how west discovered east. *J. Plast. Reconstr. Aesthetic Surg.* **2008**, *61*, 240–244. [CrossRef]
45. Burke, J.F.; Bondoc, C.C.; Quinby, W.C. Primary burn excision and immediate grafting. *J. Trauma Inj. Infect. Crit. Care* **1974**, *14*, 389–395. [CrossRef]
46. Humby, G. Apparatus for skin grafting. *Br. Med. J.* **1934**, *1*, 1078.
47. Humby, G. Modified graft cutting razor. *Br. Med. J.* **1936**, *2*, 1086.
48. Bodenham, D.C. A new type of knife for cutting skin grafts, using replaceable blades. *Br. J. Plast. Surg.* **1949**, *2*, 136. [CrossRef]
49. Braithwaite, F. Modification of humby knife. *Lancet* **1955**, *265*, 1004. [CrossRef]
50. Cochrane, T.; Richmond, C. John Watson. *BMJ* **2009**, *338*, b1607. [CrossRef]
51. Watson, J. A skin-grafting knife. *Lancet* **1960**, *276*, 687–688. [CrossRef]
52. Pierce, G.W. Grafting of skin: Advantages of the padgett dermatome. *Calif. West. Med.* **1942**, *57*, 16–18.
53. Stark, R.B. John Davies Reese and the Reese dermatome. *Ann. Plast. Surg.* **1979**, *2*, 80–83. [CrossRef] [PubMed]
54. Kamolz, L.; Schintler, M.; Parvizi, D.; Selig, H.; Lumenta, D. The real expansion rate of meshers and micrografts: Things we should keep in mind. *Ann. Burn. Fire Disasters* **2013**, *26*, 26–29.
55. Meek, C. Successful microdermagrafting using the Meek-Wall microdermatome. *Am. J. Surg.* **1958**, *96*, 557–558. [CrossRef]
56. Haeseker, B. Forerunners of mesh grafting machines. From cupping glasses and scarificators to modern mesh graft instruments. *Br. J. Plast. Surg.* **1988**, *41*, 209–212. [CrossRef]
57. Dragstedt, L.R.; Wilson, H. A modified sieve graft; A full thickness skin graft for covering large defects. *Surg. Gynecol. Obstct.* **1937**, *65*, 104–106.
58. Tanner, J.C., Jr.; Vandeput, J.; Olley, J.F. The mesh skin graft. *Plast. Reconstr. Surg.* **1964**, *34*, 287–292. [PubMed]
59. Vandeput, J.; Tanner, J.C., Jr.; Carlisle, J.D. The ultra postage stamp skin graft. *Plast. Reconstr. Surg.* **1966**, *38*, 252–254. [CrossRef] [PubMed]
60. Vandeput, J.; Nelissen, M.; Tanner, J.; Boswick, J. A review of skin meshers. *Burns* **1995**, *21*, 364–370. [CrossRef]
61. Hackl, F.; Bergmann, J.; Granter, S.R.; Koyama, T.; Kiwanuka, E.; Zuhaili, B.; Pomahac, B.; Caterson, E.J.; Junker, J.P.E.; Eriksson, E. Epidermal regeneration by micrograft transplantation with immediate 100-fold expansion. *Plast. Reconstr. Surg.* **2012**, *129*, 443e–452e. [CrossRef]
62. Pertusi, G.; Tiberio, R.; Graziola, F.; Boggio, P.; Colombo, E.; Bozzo, C. Selective release of cytokines, chemokines, and growth factors by minced skin in vitro supports the effectiveness of autologous minced micrografts technique for chronic ulcer repair. *Wound Repair Regen.* **2012**, *20*, 178–184. [CrossRef]
63. Kadam, D. Novel expansion techniques for skin grafts. *Indian J. Plast. Surg.* **2016**, *49*, 5–15. [CrossRef]
64. Reverdin, J.L. *De la Grelfe Epidermique*; Ancien Interne des Hopitaux de Paris: Paris, France, 1872.
65. Schaper, F. Uebertragung der Pocken durch Implantation waehrend des Prodomalstadiums. *Militairartz* **1872**, 53–57.
66. Bartlett, S.C. Removal of entire scalp; wound healed by skingrafting. *Am. J. Med. Sci.* **1872**, *64*, 573.
67. Om, H.J. Overplantning af Hudstykker (Transplantation of skin) in Norwegian. *Nor. Mag. Laegevidensk* **1871**, *1*, 167–170.
68. Oillier, L. Gretres cutanees ou autoplastiques. *Bull. Acad. Med.* **1872**, *1*, 243–250.
69. Lucas, R. On prepuce grafting. *Lancet* **1884**, *2*, 586–587. [CrossRef]
70. Anger, B. Sur l'heteroplastie. *CR Acad. Sci.* **1874**, *79*, 1210–1212.
71. Jacenko, A. Ueber die Transplantation abgetrennter Hautstiicke. *Med. Jahrb.* **1871**, *3*, 416–424.
72. Martin, G. De la gretre dans le traitement de l'ectropion. *Ann. Ocul.* **1873**, *36*, 110–113.
73. Czerny, V. Ueber die entstehung der tuberculose nach hauttransplantationen. *Verh. Dtsch. Ges. Chir.* **1886**, *1*, 22.
74. Wentscher, J. Ein weiter beitrag zur uberlebensfahigkeit der meschlichen epidermiszellen. *Deutsch Z Chir.* **1903**, *70*, 21–44. [CrossRef]
75. Matthews, D. Storage of skin for autogenous grafts. *Lancet* **1945**, *245*, 775–778. [CrossRef]
76. Billingham, R.; Medawar, P. The freezing, drying, and storage of mammalian skin. *J. Exp. Biol.* **1952**, *19*, 454–468.

77. The Nobel Prize: Peter Medawar—Biographical. Available online: https://www.nobelprize.org/prizes/medicine/1960/medawar/lecture/ (accessed on 26 March 2021).
78. Medawar, P.B. The behaviour and fate of skin autografts and skin homografts in rabbits: A report to the War Wounds Committee of the Medical Research Council. *J. Anat.* **1944**, *78*, 176–199. [PubMed]
79. Owen, R.D. Immunogenetic consequences of vascular anastomoses between bovine twins. *Science* **1945**, *102*, 400–401. [CrossRef] [PubMed]
80. Billingham, R.E.; Brent, L.; Medawar, P.B. 'Actively acquired tolerance' of foreign cells. *Nat. Cell Biol.* **1953**, *172*, 603–606. [CrossRef] [PubMed]
81. The Nobel Prize: Joseph E. Murray—Biographical. Available online: https://www.nobelprize.org/prizes/medicine/1990/murray/facts/ (accessed on 26 March 2021).
82. Murray, J.E. Organ transplantation (skin, kidney, heart) and the plastic surgeon. *Plast. Reconstr. Surg.* **1971**, *47*, 425–431. [CrossRef]
83. Billingham, R.E.; Sabin, A.B. Reactions of graft against their hosts: Transplantation immunity works both ways–hosts destroy grafts and grafts may harm hosts. *Science* **1959**, *130*, 947–953. [CrossRef]
84. Gordon, E.J. Immunological considerations for inducing skin graft tolerance. In *Skin Grafts—Indications, Applications and Current Research*; IntechOpen Limited: London, UK, 2011; pp. 343–368.
85. Jackson, D. A clinical study of the use of skin homografts for burns. *Br. J. Plast. Surg.* **1954**, *7*, 26–43. [CrossRef]
86. Zhang, M.L.; Wang, C.Y.; Chang-Yeh, W.; Cao, D.X.; Han, X.; Ming-Liang, Z.; Zhi-De, C.; Da-Xin, C.; Xun, H. Microskin grafting. II. Clinical report. *Burns* **1986**, *12*, 544–548. [CrossRef]
87. Alexander, J.W.; Macmillan, B.G.; Law, E.; Kittur, D.S. Treatment of severe burns with widely meshed skin autograft and meshed skin allograft overlay. *J. Trauma Inj. Infect. Crit. Care* **1981**, *21*, 433–438.
88. Yannas, I.V.; Orgill, D.P.; Burke, J.F. Template for skin regeneration. *Plast. Reconstr. Surg.* **2011**, *127*, 60S–70S. [CrossRef] [PubMed]
89. Rheinwatd, J.G.; Green, H. Seria cultivation of strains of human epidemal keratinocytes: The formation keratinizin colonies from single cell is. *Cell* **1975**, *6*, 331–343. [CrossRef]
90. Sood, R.; Roggy, D.; Zieger, M.; Balledux, J.; Chaudhari, S.; Koumanis, D.J.; Mir, H.S.; Cohen, A.; Knipe, C.; Gabehart, K.; et al. Cultured epithelial autografts for coverage of large burn wounds in eighty-eight patients: The Indiana university experience. *J. Burn. Care Res.* **2010**, *31*, 559–568. [CrossRef]
91. Hansbrough, J.F.; Boyce, S.T.; Cooper, M.L.; Foreman, T.J. Burn wound closure with cultured autologous keratinocytes and fibroblasts attached to a collagen-glycosaminoglycan substrate. *JAMA* **1989**, *262*, 2125–2130. [CrossRef] [PubMed]
92. Boyce, S.T.; Williams, M.L. Lipid supplemented medium induces lamellar bodies and precursors of barrier lipids in cultured analogues of human skin. *J. Investig. Dermatol.* **1993**, *101*, 180–184. [CrossRef]
93. Boyce, S.T.; Medrano, E.E.; Abdel-Malek, Z.; Supp, A.P.; Dodick, J.M.; Nordlund, J.J.; Warden, G.D. Pigmentation and inhibition of wound contraction by cultured skin substitutes with adult melanocytes after transplantation to athymic mice. *J. Investig. Dermatol.* **1993**, *100*, 360–365. [CrossRef] [PubMed]
94. Le Poole, I.C.; Boyce, S.T. Keratinocytes suppress transforming growth factor-β1 expression by fibroblasts in cultured skin substitutes. *Br. J. Dermatol.* **1999**, *140*, 409–416. [CrossRef]
95. Supp, D.M.; Supp, A.P.; Boyce, S.T.; Bell, S.M. Enhanced vascularization of cultured skin substitutes genetically modified to over-express vascular endothelial growth Factor11The authors declared in writing to have no conflict of interest. *J. Investig. Dermatol.* **2000**, *114*, 5–13. [CrossRef]
96. Billingham, R.; Reynolds, J. Transplantation studies on sheets of pure epidermal epithelium and on epidermal cell suspensions. *Br. J. Plast. Surg.* **1952**, *5*, 25–36. [CrossRef]
97. Hunyadi, J.; Farkas, B.; Bertényi, C.; Oláh, J.; Dobozy, A. Keratinocyte grafting: A new means of transplantation for full-thickness wounds. *J. Dermatol. Surg. Oncol.* **1988**, *14*, 75–78. [CrossRef] [PubMed]
98. Kaiser, H.; Stark, G.; Kopp, J.; Balcerkiewicz, A.; Spilker, G.; Kreysel, H. Cultured autologous keratinocytes in fibrin glue suspension, exclusively and combined with STS-allograft (preliminary clinical and histological report of a new technique). *Burns* **1994**, *20*, 23–29. [CrossRef]
99. Currie, L.J.; Martin, R.; Sharpe, J.R.; James, S.E. A comparison of keratinocyte cell sprays with and without fibrin glue. *Burns* **2003**, *29*, 677–685. [CrossRef]
100. Wood, F.M.; Giles, N.; Stevenson, A.; Rea, S.; Fear, M. Characterisation of the cell suspension harvested from the dermal epidermal junction using a ReCell® kit. *Burns* **2012**, *38*, 44–51. [CrossRef] [PubMed]
101. Deitch, E.A.; Wheelahan, T.M.; Rose, M.P.; Clothier, J.; Cotter, J. Hypertrophic burn scars: Analysis of variables. *J. Trauma: Inj. Infect. Crit. Care* **1983**, *23*, 895–898. [CrossRef]
102. Dennis, C. Hard graft. *Nat. Cell Biol.* **2005**, *436*, 166–167. [CrossRef]
103. The Age. Available online: https://www.theage.com.au/national/jury-still-out-over-spray-on-skin-20050129-gdzgj5.html (accessed on 26 February 2021).
104. Holmes, J.; Molnar, J.; Shupp, J.; Hickerson, W.; King, B.T.; Foster, K.; Cairns, B.; Carter, J. Demonstration of the safety and effectiveness of the RECELL® System combined with split-thickness meshed autografts for the reduction of donor skin to treat mixed-depth burn injuries. *Burns* **2019**, *45*, 772–782. [CrossRef]
105. Sood, R.; Roggy, D.E.; Zieger, M.J.; Nazim, M.; Hartman, B.C.; Gibbs, J.T. A comparative study of spray keratinocytes and autologous meshed split-thickness skin graft in the treatment of acute burn injuries. *Wounds* **2015**, *27*, 31–40.

106. Iv, J.H.H.; A Molnar, J.; E Carter, J.; Hwang, J.; Cairns, B.A.; King, B.T.; Smith, D.J.; Cruse, C.W.; Foster, K.N.; Peck, M.D.; et al. A comparative study of the ReCell® Device and autologous split-thickness meshed skin graft in the treatment of acute burn injuries. *J. Burn. Care Res.* **2018**, *39*, 694–702. [CrossRef]
107. Wood, F.M.; Stoner, M.L.; Fowler, B.V.; Fear, M.W. The use of a non-cultured autologous cell suspension and Integra®dermal regeneration template to repair full-thickness skin wounds in a porcine model: A one-step process. *Burns* **2007**, *33*, 693–700. [CrossRef] [PubMed]
108. GlobeNewswire. Available online: https://www.globenewswire.com/news-release/2020/12/15/2145327/0/en/RECELL-System-Data-Presented-at-American-Burn-Association-Fall-Regional-Burn-Conferences.html (accessed on 26 February 2021).
109. Michael, S.; Sorg, H.; Peck, C.-T.; Koch, L.; Deiwick, A.; Chichkov, B.; Vogt, P.M.; Reimers, K. Tissue engineered skin substitutes created by laser-assisted bioprinting form skin-like structures in the dorsal skin fold chamber in mice. *PLoS ONE* **2013**, *8*, e57741. [CrossRef] [PubMed]
110. Skardal, A.; Mack, D.; Kapetanovic, E.; Atala, A.; Jackson, J.D.; Yoo, J.; Soker, S. Bioprinted Amniotic fluid-derived stem cells accelerate healing of large skin wounds. *Stem Cells Transl. Med.* **2012**, *1*, 792–802. [CrossRef] [PubMed]
111. Sofokleous, P.; Stride, E.; Bonfield, W.; Edirisinghe, M. Design, construction and performance of a portable handheld electrohydrodynamic multi-needle spray gun for biomedical applications. *Mater. Sci. Eng. C* **2013**, *33*, 213–223. [CrossRef] [PubMed]

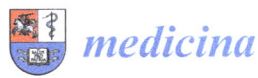

Review

A Short History of Skin Grafting in Burns: From the Gold Standard of Autologous Skin Grafting to the Possibilities of Allogeneic Skin Grafting with Immunomodulatory Approaches

Frederik Schlottmann *, Vesna Bucan, Peter M. Vogt and Nicco Krezdorn

Department of Plastic, Aesthetic, Hand- and Reconstructive Surgery, Hannover Medical School, Carl-Neuberg-Strasse 1, 30625 Hannover, Germany; bucan.vesna@mh-hannover.de (V.B.); vogt.peter@mh-hannover.de (P.M.V.); krezdorn.nicco@mh-hannover.de (N.K.)
* Correspondence: schlottmann.frederik@mh-hannover.de; Tel.: +49-511-532-0

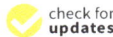

Citation: Schlottmann, F.; Bucan, V.; Vogt, P.M.; Krezdorn, N. A Short History of Skin Grafting in Burns: From the Gold Standard of Autologous Skin Grafting to the Possibilities of Allogeneic Skin Grafting with Immunomodulatory Approaches. *Medicina* **2021**, *57*, 225. https://doi.org/10.3390/medicina57030225

Academic Editor: Lars P. Kamolz

Received: 30 December 2020
Accepted: 22 February 2021
Published: 2 March 2021

Publisher's Note: MDPI stays neutral with regard to jurisdictional claims in published maps and institutional affiliations.

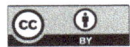

Copyright: © 2021 by the authors. Licensee MDPI, Basel, Switzerland. This article is an open access article distributed under the terms and conditions of the Creative Commons Attribution (CC BY) license (https://creativecommons.org/licenses/by/4.0/).

Abstract: Due to groundbreaking and pioneering developments in the last century, significant improvements in the care of burn patients have been achieved. In addition to the still valid therapeutic standard of autologous split-thickness skin grafting, various commercially available skin substitutes are currently available. Significant progress in the field of tissue engineering has led to the development of promising therapeutic approaches. However, scientific advances in the field of allografting and transplant immunology are of great importance. The achievement of various milestones over the past decades has provided thought-provoking impulses in the field of skin allotransplantation. Thus, biologically viable skin allotransplantation is still not a part of the clinical routine. The purpose of this article is to review the achievements in burn surgery with regards to skin allotransplantation in recent years.

Keywords: burn care; allotransplantation; skin transplantation; skin graft; skin substitute; immunocompatible skin grafts

1. Introduction

According to recent surveys by the German Society for Burn Medicine, a total of 4350 people were affected by burn injuries in Germany in 2016 [1]. In Germany, burn patients, especially those with severe burns, are treated in highly specialized burn centers that have comprehensive technical equipment and specialized personnel and can thus ensure optimal care [2]. In initial care, the focus is on immediate treatment and, in particular, adequate volume replacement therapy within the first 24 h, sufficient ventilation, and timely surgical treatment of burn wounds [3]. Due to the enormous progress in the intensive medical care of severely burned patients and the expansion of the network of burn centers, a significant increase in survival rates has been recorded [4,5]. In addition to the above-mentioned intensive care treatment, the interdisciplinary and multimodal treatment concept of burn injuries primarily includes surgical debridement to establish aseptic wound conditions in order to allow sufficient defect coverage and thus adequate wound healing [6–8]. Despite intensive research efforts, autologous skin grafting still represents the surgical gold standard in the treatment of burn injuries, as no skin substitute has yet succeeded in sufficiently replacing the function of the patient's original skin [9]. The gold standard in burn surgery is still autologous tissue transfer, such as autologous split-thickness skin grafting. Skin grafting has developed significantly during the past decades. Thus, in addition to the optimization of autologous skin grafting, the use of allogeneic skin grafts in particular was investigated, but showed limited success. The purpose of this review is to provide an overview of the historical development of allogeneic skin grafting. In addition to the developments of allogeneic skin grafting, the treatment concepts of autologous skin grafting, the status of allogeneic and xenogeneic skin grafts, and the use of synthetic skin substitutes are discussed. Finally, forward-looking perspectives of immunomodulation of allogeneic skin grafts are highlighted, offering a promising approach for future research projects and clinical applications.

1.1. Concepts of Autologous Split-Thickness Skin Grafting as the Gold Standard in Burn Surgery

Skin grafting has been practiced by European surgeons for little more than 200 years and can be considered as a standardized procedure nowadays [10]. The history of autologous skin grafting dates back to the first experiments of Giuseppe Baronio in 1804. He investigated skin transplantations in a ram by excising a piece of skin from the dorsum and grafting it immediately on the opposite side. Five out of six skin grafts grew in without problems. In another experiment, Baronio performed transplantation of skin pieces between a cow and a horse. However, without knowing the basic principles of immunology and graft rejection, these attempts of xenogeneic transplantations were not crowned with success [11]. Over the following years, other surgeons such as Johann Friedrich Dieffenbach and Alfred Armand Velpeau focused their research on autologous skin grafting and tried to reproduce the results of Baronio, but hat limited success. It took until 1869 to perform the first successful autologous skin graft on a human by the Swiss-born surgeon Jacques Louis Reverdin [12]. In the following decades, developments and discoveries in the field of allogeneic skin grafting increased rapidly so thatsplit-thickness skin grafting is now clinically well established after many years of experience [13]. Despite intensive scientific efforts, autologous skin grafting, particularly split-thickness skin grafting, represents the workhorse for the reconstructive surgeon in the management of burn injuries. However, donor site limitations and morbidity are major constraints to the use of autologous skin grafts especially in patients with extended skin injuries [14]. In addition, any skin grafting is associated with a donor site defect and aesthetic impairment [3,13]. In particular, permanent wound closure with a satisfactory aesthetic result continues to be a challenge in the treatment of extensive burn wounds. Considering socioeconomic costs for the care of chronic wounds as well as the expected increase in costs due to demographic change, a complete and as early as possible wound closure should be aimed for [15,16].

Since the first successful in vitro cultivation of keratinocytes by Rheinwald and Green in 1975, keratinocytes have increasingly become the focus of research as a promising approach for the production of an artificial skin substitute [17,18]. In the course, various research approaches focused in on the transplantation of autologous keratinocytes [19,20]. For example, autologous keratinocytes are currently commercially available as a cell sheet (EpiCel™, (Vericel Corporation, Cambridge, MA, USA)) [21] or as a spray suspension (ReCell™ (Valencia, CA, USA) or the autologous keratinocyte spray suspension of Deutsches Institut für Zell- und Gewebeersatz gGmbH, Berlin, Germany) [22,23] and are part of the clinical care of burn patients. However, the application remains very limited due to high costs of production and a cultivation time of several weeks [24]. In addition, graft healing rates still vary significantly [25,26]. Both delivery forms also lack the dermal skin component, so that sufficient stability of the grafts, especially in handling during production, but also during transplantation, is not given [3]. The effect on scar formation has also not been conclusively investigated.

1.2. The History of Allogeneic Transplantations

The history of burn wound care and treatment dates back to ancient Greece and Rome [27]. The desire to replace lost limbs and facial parts is as old as mankind's history and many attempts have been made. In reality, ancient allotransplantation attempts all failed and the scientific and surgical success of the first allografts did not occur until about 60 years ago [28]. Due to the severe injuries and burns of war victims in World War II, the foundation for the field of modern transplant biology was laid out of necessity. The young biologist Peter B Medawar was assigned to the service of the British surgeon Dr Thomas Gibson to determine if skin allografts could be used to treat war injuries. In the early 1940s, Medawar began to work on the subject of immune tolerance and transplantation.

He published his first fundamental work in this field together with Thomas Gibson in 1943. They proved that the rejection of organs derived from unrelated donors is based on immunological principles [10]. In the following years, Medawar focused on the immunity of homologous skin grafts and their immunological tolerance [29–32]. For example, he first described the immune privilege of the anterior chamber of the eye using homologous skin grafts [29]. For his fundamental and groundbreaking discoveries, Medawar received a Nobel Prize in 1960 and was knighted [28]. For these discoveries, he is considered the founding father of modern transplantation immunology. However, more than six decades after the first experiments of Medawar, the precise mechanisms of skin allograft rejection are still not fully understood and it has not been possible to achieve reliable clinical tolerance of skin allotransplants [33]. Despite this, human mankind still began to aim for solid organ transplantation. Joseph E Murray, John P Merrill and J Hartwell Harrison in Boston (USA) performed the first solid organ transplant in 1954. They transplanted a human kidney donated between identical twins [34,35]. With advancements in the field of immunology, transplantation and regenerative medicine the transplantation of complex composite tissue allotransplantations became possible. Important milestones in this regard are the discovery and development of immunosuppressive drugs after allotransplantation to prevent rejection making it feasible to transplant facial structures, extremities, larynx, tongue, abdominal wall and external ear and scalp [28]. Along with the growing field of clinical experience in allotransplantation, insights into the pathophysiological and immunological background have been made.

Animal studies have shown that skin grafting between unrelated mouse inbred strains can be expected to occur after ten to 13 days and result in a primary rejection reaction [36,37]. In addition to primary rejection, secondary rejection is also known to occur much more rapidly over the six- to eight-day period and has been observed in repeated transplantation of skin to a recipient animal that had previously rejected a skin graft from the same donor animal [36,37]. The clinical diagnosis of rejection is made based on various parameters, such as clinical symptoms in the form of epidermolysis, hemorrhage, or necrosis, as well as laboratory chemical analyses and histologic evaluation of tissue biopsy. In this context, important rejection features include the infiltrating immune cells and their ratio to each other, structural matching of tissue anatomy, and histological confirmation of damage to local blood vessels [38–40]. As shown later, the compatibility of major histocompatibility complex (MHC) molecules between donor and recipient can significantly improve the transplantation outcome and prevent rejection [41,42]. In recent years, the success of organ transplantation in particular has been significantly improved by matching the MHC profiles between donor and recipient [42,43]. However, even accurate MHC typing of the graft cannot always prevent rejection of the recipient organism. A perfect match is rarely achievable in clinical practice because the donor and recipient must usually be related to have a genetic similarity of MHC molecules. Moreover, because of a mismatch between the supply and demand of donor organs, the selection of an MHC-compatible organ is severely limited [44]. In humans, the genes encoding MHC molecules are located in the human leukocyte antigen (HLA) gene region and has high genomic diversity [45–47]. Due to this, an ideal donor who has an identical genomic MHC profile is usually not available despite an existing relationship [42,44,47]. The reasons for this are, in particular, that despite extensive progress the available methods of HLA typing make accurate typing almost impossible due to polygenetic diversity and the resulting complexity [47]. Moreover, it is known that even MHC-identical transplants, for example in HLA-identical siblings, are rejected with a time delay. The rejection reaction is based on the minor histocompatibility antigens, which are individual-specific antigens that are not part of the MHC proteins [48–50]. Minor histocompatibility antigens will not be discussed in detail here.

Despite various research approaches, it has not yet been possible to inhibit the specific immune response against allografted tissue without compromising the immune response of the entire recipient organism [51]. Therefore, most transplantations often require the use of immunosuppressive drugs that cause general immune compromise [51,52]. Thus, clinical success in solid organ transplantation is largely attributable to advances in the development of immunosuppressive drugs. However, systemic immunomodulation of an organism can be toxic and is associated with impaired immunocompetence and thus an increased risk of infection [51]. The main driver of success of allogeneic tissue or organ transplantation depends on MHC typing of the graft, the use of effective immunosuppression, and the operative skills of the surgeon performing the procedure [53,54]. In particular, for the severely burn patient, the immunologic derailment in the setting of systemic inflammatory response syndrome prohibits additional drug immunosuppression [55]. The immunologic rejection reaction of allogeneic skin grafts in severely burned patients has been intensively studied and described. To sum up, the allogeneic skin graft can cause a potent immune response involving both the innate and adaptive immune system of the host's organism. T cell mediated mechanism as well as B cell and NK cell activation play a significant role in the process of allograft rejection [56]. In conclusion, immunomodulation of allogeneic grafts would be a promising way to reduce rejection. Interference with the intrinsic alloreactivity of the whole organism by means of immunosuppressive drugs could thus be prevented. In particular, the application in immunocompromised patients, such as severely burned patients, would be extremely promising regarding the immuno-compatibility of transplants and would enable a diverse clinical use of, for example, allogeneic skin transplants without rejection.

1.3. Current Use of Allogeneic Skin Grafts in the Care of Severely Burned Patients

Despite the above-mentioned disadvantages of allotransplantations, allogeneic skin grafts have a place in the care of severely burned patients to a certain extent and are widely used for wound management in burn centers [57]. Autologous skin grafts are currently commercially available as cryopreserved and glycerol-preserved skin sheets via biobanks or skin banks all over the world [57,58]. The history of skin biobanking dates back until to the 1990s [59]. Transplantation of cryopreserved and glycerol-preserved and thus biologically unviable allogeneic skin from body donors is also clinically indicated in some cases because of the lack of autologous donor sites for split-thickness skin grafting [60]. Functional as biologic dressing, it can not only provide ideal temporary wound coverage in extensive burns when autologous skin grafting is not immediately available but also prepare the wound bed for definitive wound closure [57]. However, the use of allogeneic skin grafts are not promising. In particular, secondary graft rejection due to an immune reaction induced by the graft, as well as secondary infections and increased scarring, are disadvantages in their use as permanent skin substitutes [61]. The antigenic properties of the foreign skin can be reduced by glycerol preservation, resulting in the demise of cellular epidermal and dermal components [62]. Due to the immunocompromised state of the severely burn injured patients, delayed rejection may also occur during the course after the patient's immunocompetence is restored. The only advantage of using allogeneic material has been shown to be the immediate restoration of skin barrier function in terms of a biological dressing [62]. The aesthetic results after transplantation of allogeneic skin are usually unsatisfactory. Incongruent healing rates of allogeneic skin grafts have been reported in some cases [3]. To sum up, allogeneic skin grafting has its position in the clinical care of severely burned patients, but at the same time goes hand in hand with a plethora of limitations and disadvantages.

1.4. Current Use of Xenogeneic Skin Grafts in the Care of Severely Burned Patients

In addition to the gold standard of autologous skin grafting, xenogeneic materials, such as porcine skin and fish skin, are used for temporary defect coverage, particularly in large-scale burns [61,63]. It has been reported elsewhere that the use of porcine skin and fish skin in severely burned patients was associated with a significant reduction in intravenous fluid use, pain scores and pain medication. This allowed sufficient stabilization of the patient until definitive treatment of the skin defects by autologous skin grafting [64,65]. Other reports suggest, that the Nile tilapia skin (Orechromis niloticus) has noninfectious microbiota, a morphological structure similar to that of human skin, and therefore showed good outcomes when used as a xenograft for treatment of experimental burns [66]. A phase II randomized controlled trial even described complete re-epithelialization in burn wounds without autologous split-thickness skin grafting [67]. The research results in this regard appear promising, but further studies are needed to evaluate the potential use compared to autologous skin grafting as current gold standard in clinical routine. In conclusion, xenogeneic skin grafts have a place in the clinical care of severely burned patients, but at this time can only be considered as a temporary solution.

1.5. Skin Substitutes as an Alternative to Autologous Skin Transplantation

Over the years, a wide range of industrially manufactured skin substitutes have been established more or less successfully, so that a potpourri of purchasable skin substitutes are currently available on the market [3,68]. Each of these skin substitute materials plays a part in various research approaches and, in some cases, is also used in the clinical care of burn patients [69,70].

Dermal skin substitutes can be broadly categorized as decellularized dermis derived from human or animal sources, artificially constructed scaffolds comprised of highly purified biomaterials or entirely synthetic polymers. In view of the fact that there are dozens of different commercially available skin substitute matrices on the market, only MatriDerm® (MedSkin Solutions Dr. Suwelack AG, Billerbeck, Germany) and NovoSorb® Biodegredable Temporising Matrix (BTM) (PolyMedics Innovations, Denkendorf, Germany) will be presented here as examples in detail, since they are currently standard in clinical use and show promising results. However, Table 1 provides an overview of other dermal skin substitutes of biological and synthetic origin currently available on the market.

Table 1. Overview of dermal skin substitutes currently commercially available.

Name of Dermal Skin Substitute	Material	Literature
MatriDerm®	bovine collagen type I, collagen type III and elastin	[71]
Dermagraft®	neonatal-derived bioengineered tissue comprised of dermal fibroblasts	[72]
AlloDerm™	donated allograft human dermis, processed to remove cells while preserving biologic components and structure of the dermal matrix	[73]
Integra®	dermal component of bovine collagen type I and shark chondroitin-6-sulfate directed to the wound side and an outwardly directed silicone membrane	[74]
denovoSkin™	hydrogel from a dermo-epidermal component after cultivation from autologous skin tissue samples	[75]
NovoSorb® BTM	biodegradable polyurethane foam with a temporary non-biodegradable polyurethane seal	[76]

MatriDerm®, a dermal, cell-free skin substitute for deep-seated burns, has been commercially available for several years. The matrix consists of bovine collagen type I, collagen type III and elastin. As studied in animal models, MatriDerm® matrix is converted into endogenous matrix by the recipient organism over a period of weeks [71,77]. Similar biodegradable behavior has also been demonstrated in the human organism [78]. MatriDerm® is available in various thicknesses and can be stored at room temperature, making handling considerably easier than with other biomaterials [71]. In particular, the single-stage procedure with simultaneous autologous split-thickness skin grafting is clinically considered a significant advantage and showed no inferiority to allogeneic split-thickness skin grafting alone [3]. Better scar quality as well as reduced wound contraction were observed [79,80], so the results to date in clinical application are promising [80,81]. However, full-thickness skin replacement with MatriDerm® is so far only possible in combination with autologous split-thickness skin grafting.

NovoSorb® BTM is a fully synthetic dermal skin substitute that eliminates any risks of cross-species residual antigenicity. It consists of biodegradable polyurethane foam with a temporary non-biodegradable polyurethane seal. Thereby, it is easy and inexpensive to produce [76]. A further advantage is the avoidance of cross-species immune rejection or disease transmission as well as circumventing ethical and cultural objections to the use of animal derived products. A plethora of proof-of-concept studies using NovoSorb® BTM has been conducted to determine its safety and ability to provide permanent wound closure when combined with split-thickness skin grafts in a two-stage procedure in sheep, pigs and humans [82,83]. Furthermore, the particular abundance of host inflammatory cells in athymic nude mice receiving full-thickness skin excision followed by grafting of the dermal NovoSorb® BTM template, showed evidence that new collagen deposition and neovascularization with BTM had a more extensive vascular network compared to Integra® (Integra LifeSciences, Plainsboro, NJ, USA) [84]. NovoSorb® BTM demonstrates favorable properties as dermal skin substitute but further studies are needed to evaluate its position in clinical routine, especially for the treatment of burns.

1.6. Tissue Engineering for Skin Reconstruction

Tissue engineering of biologic skin substitutes has developed over the last few decades from individual applications of skin cells or biologic scaffolds to the combination of cells and scaffolds for treatment and healing of chronic skin wounds and burns. Several tissue engineered skin substitutes have overcome the disadvantages of autologous split-thickness skin grafting as well as the immunogenicity of skin allotransplantation. Most research approaches focus on the use of keratinocytes as a cell pool for tissue engineering approaches [20]. Autologous keratinocytes may persist indefinitely and provide permanent wound closure whereas allogeneic keratinocytes will only remain in the wound bed for days to weeks [85,86]. However, there are still remaining disadvantages such as high production costs, time consuming processes and culture conditions for each patient regarding the application of autologous keratinocytes [87]. Recently, major progress has been made in this field so that cultured autologous keratinocytes as a source for bioengineering can be produced in unlimited supplies by establishing cost-effective culture protocols and increasing their proliferative capacity [88,89]. Allogeneic keratinocytes can be provided off-the-shelf with less manufacturing challenges, but immune compatibility is a major concern with their use as mentioned above.

Despite single cellular tissue engineering approaches, combinations of keratinocytes and dermal skin substitutes have been investigated intensively to produce a skin substitute that is comparable to human healthy skin. For example, MatriDerm® was used as a matrix for cell-based studies to investigate its applicability as a carrier matrix for tissue engineering approaches due to its promising properties and effects on the human organism. Cells of various origins, such as pancreatic stem cells [90], preadipocytes [91], fibroblasts, and keratinocytes [92,93], have been shown to adhere and proliferate on the MatriDerm® matrix in vitro. This makes MatriDerm® suitable as a carrier matrix for further research approaches in the field of tissue engineering and regenerative medicine [92]. Since 2006, advanced models of tissue engineered skin substitutes have been described but all showed limited success [94–96]. With the growing field of skin tissue engineering, regulatory environments and requirements have expanded. Among the several determination of safety and efficacy, the determination of medical risks is a fundamental factor limiting the clinical applicability of novel tissue engineered skin constructs [97].

Despite the described disadvantages, allogeneic keratinocytes represent an important cell therapeutic tool, which could be further optimized by immunomodulation. With the establishment of viral vectors as a transfection method, efficient transfection of keratinocytes was achieved [98–100]. In this regard, viral transfection of keratinocytes represents a promising tool for gene therapy applications. For example, Vogt et al. demonstrated expression of growth factors and ß-galactosidase and regeneration of the epidermis after transplantation of retrovirally transfected keratinocytes in a porcine model [101]. Systemic expression of genes in bioreactor systems also offers multiple options with respect to gene therapy application of modified keratinocytes [102]. However, a careful risk-benefit analysis should be performed when using viral vectors. On the one hand, they can induce an uncontrolled immune response and, on the other hand, they only allow the transfer of genes of a limited size [103,104]. Despite intensive research and efforts, data on the application of genetically modified keratinocytes as skin substitutes in vivo remain insufficient. In conclusion, genetic modification of keratinocytes could provide the basis for the production of a universally applicable and immunologically compatible skin substitute [105].

Another potential approach for skin tissue engineering is the use of three-dimensional (3D) bioprinting. Bioprinting, involving computer-controlled deposition of scaffolds and cells in a plethora of shapes and patterns, can offer the potential to fully replicate native human skin [106]. As described in literature, multilayered approaches using fibroblast, keratinocytes as well as collagen have been made to bioprint human skin [107,108]. In comparison with traditional methods for skin engineering, 3D bioprinting offers several advantages in terms of shape- and form retention, flexibility, reproducibility, and high culture throughput. Therefore 3D bioprinting is a promising technology that can achieve rapid and reliable production of cellular skin substitutes, satisfying both clinical and industrial need [106,109]. Although 3D bioprinting shows promising results so far, the research is still in its infancy and further studies are needed to overcome the disadvantages such as vascularity, optimal cell and scaffold combinations and production costs [106,109].

1.7. Future Perspectives: Universal Off-the-Shelf Transplantable Skin Substitutes with Low Immunogenicity

Despite the wide range of skin substitutes available, autologous split-thickness skin grafting is still usually required for complete and sufficient wound closure. Although the ultimate treatment goal in plastic surgery is replacing "like with like", donor site tissue is often a limited source. Autologous skin grafts as above-mentioned have the advantages of living tissue allografts that derive from the patient itself and are not rejected. One of the most promising research approaches for future generations of patient-specific skin substitutes is the use of immunologically or genetically modified autologous keratinocytes due to their almost unlimited availability as they can overcome graft rejection and immune incompatibility. Morgan et al. first described the successful in vitro gene modification of keratinocytes by applying the method of retroviral gene transfer. They transferred a recombinant human growth hormone gene into cultured human keratinocytes, transplanted them into athymic mice and observed epithelial regeneration [110]. Especially during recent years, many different approaches have been made to generate a universal off-the-shelf transplantable skin substitute for cosmetic and reconstructive surgery [111]. However, gene therapy for the skin has been investigated intensively but showed limited success overall [112]. Several studies have demonstrated that modulation of MHC-I expression could significantly influence survival and acceptance of transplanted allogeneic organs. In a knockout mouse model lacking MHC-I and MHC-II expression, allogeneic skin grafts showed delayed rejection kinetics [113]. Auchincloss et al. demonstrated that MHC-II-deficient skin grafts exhibited graft rejection without delay in the mouse model [114]. The importance of MHC-I expression in allogeneic organ rejection was then investigated in further studies that focused on suppressing antigen presentation directly to the allograft. To achieve this, β2-microglobulin (β2M) and transporter-associated-with-antigen-processing (TAP)-deficient transplantation models were developed and further investigated. It was shown that in β2M-deficient mice, pancreatic islet allografts exhibited unlimited graft survival [115], whereas heart and liver allografts showed only delayed graft rejection [116]. Allografted kidneys showed significantly improved renal function of the graft [117]. In a further step, the rejection behavior of skin grafts in TAP- and in β2M-deficient mouse models was also investigated. This demonstrated delayed rejection of the allograft [118–120]. Despite intensive efforts, complete removal of the MHC class I molecule in the allograft has not yet been achieved by eliminating the β2-microglobulin or TAP transporter.

Genetic modification of cells to achieve better immuno-compatibility has been investigated in further in vitro studies. For example, using specific intrabodies in endothelial cells, a phenotypic knockout of MHC-I expression was achieved by retention of the molecules in the endoplasmic reticulum [121]. As another approach to allografting keratinocytes and skin, a significantly reduced MHC-I expression was demonstrated in human and monkey cell lines by using specific intrabodies. The cell lines showed different HLA-A, -B, and -C haplotypes [122]. However, due to the high genomic diversity of HLA genes, genotypic knockout of MHC-I molecules has not been feasible to date. To improve the acceptance of allogeneic skin grafts, it is desirable to suppress MHC-I expression and thus prevent rejection. Based on previous studies, the use of viral MHC-I modulatory proteins or vectors represents an innovative and promising research approach to modulate the expression of MHC-I molecules and thus prevent graft rejection. A plethora of experimental methods exists to create universal allogeneic keratinocytes that can overcome host cellular immune response.

In the course of coevolution, many viruses have developed the ability to suppress viral peptide presentation and thus, do not elicit an immune response from the infected organism [123,124]. A prominent example is human cytomegalovirus (HCMV), which, by reducing MHC-I expression on the cell surface of infected cells, does not elicit viral peptide presentation and no immune response from the infected organism [125,126]. Absence or reduction of MHC-I expression prevents activation of CD8+ cytotoxic T lymphocytes [127–129]. The underlying molecular mechanisms are well understood so far. For example, Ahn et al. demonstrated that HCMV uses various strategies to avoid being recognized by the immune system of the infected organism [130]. HCMV prevents MHC-I expression at the cell surface through various modulatory transmembrane glycoproteins called unique short glycoproteins (US). In particular, it has been shown that US2, US3, US6, and US11 glycoproteins are responsible for MHC-I modulation [126,131]. Thus, the use of US glycoproteins represents a promising approach to modulate the expression of MHC-I molecules in allografts and to prevent graft rejection. As published earlier by Schlottmann et al. human primary keratinocytes could be transfected using viral US11 vectors, resulting in a temporary reduction of MHC-I surface expression. Furthermore, they seeded transfected keratinocytes on MatriDerm® matrices and observed long-term cell survival as well as histological patterns comparable to healthy human skin [132]. The viral vector used was characterized by greater loading capacity while maintaining moderate immunogenicity and inflammatory components, thus representing a promising research approach. Nevertheless, vector tropism, the duration of transgene expression as well as vector immunogenicity are crucial issues and sometimes even disadvantages that have to be taken into account to allow efficient, specific and safe applications of viral vectors in transgene therapeutic approaches [133].

Gene editing can be another feasible approach for immunogenic modification of allogeneic keratinocytes. The significant advances in the field of gene therapy, especially using the Clustered Regularly Interspaced Short Palindromic Repeats/Cas9 (CRISPR/Cas9) system, could represent another promising research approach to generate an immunocompatible and universally applicable skin substitute. In this regard, research approaches using viral vectors could be replaced, so that the vector associated risks can be reduced. However, no approach to generate a skin construct using CRISPR/Cas9 has yet been sustainably established in the literature [134–136].

Another approach for a hypogenic skin graft engineered with universal cells has been recently described by Deuse et al. [137]. Endothelial cells, smooth muscle cells and cardiomyocytes derived from hypoimmunogenic mouse or human induced pluripotent stem cells showed inactivated MHC class I and II genes and an overexpression of CD47. Further experiments showed reliably immune evasive rejection in fully MHC-mismatched allogeneic recipients and long-term graft survival without the use of immunosuppressive medication [137].

However, the use of HLA silenced cells is not without clinical concerns as it remains uncertain as to what level HLA genes should be silenced in vivo or in vitro to evade host CD8+ cytotoxic T cell recognition or natural killer cell (NK cell) activation. Genetically modified allogeneic cells might therefore be invisible for T cell-based immune responses that are essential for the lysis of infected or oncogenically transformed cells as well as apoptosis. In addition, the results of Christinck et al. and Sykulev et al. have shown that 1 to 200 MHC-I molecules per cell can be sufficient to induce an immune response in the recipient organism after transplantation [138,139]. Therefore, there is a considerable need for further studies that investigate the immunological responses of allogeneic modified keratinocytes in vitro and in vivo.

2. Conclusions

Mankind's desire to replace whole organs and tissues with allogeneic transplants goes back over centuries. Significant successes, especially in burn surgery and consequently allogeneic skin transplantation for treatment of extensive burn wounds, could only be recorded in the last decades. As described in the preceding sections, despite intensive efforts, it has not yet been possible to produce a skin substitute that forms a full-fledged, universally applicable and immunologically compatible approach and whose application allows an appealing aesthetic result [140–144]. The first autologous skin graft was described in 1804. Since then, the autologous skin grafting procedure has been intensively researched and further developed, so that autologous split thickness skin grafting is nowadays the gold standard in the treatment of severely burn injured patients. However, as summarized in this review, allogeneic and xenogeneic skin grafts also have a place in the clinical care of severely burned patients. The first discoveries of transplantation immunology by Medawar et al. have led to far-reaching developments in the field of transplantation surgery, so that nowadays solid organs can finally be transplanted as well. However, allogeneic transplants still carry the risk of rejection, so that intervention in the intrinsic alloreactivity of the recipient organism, for example by immunosuppressive drugs, is necessary. To address these issues, a number of commercially available skin substitute matrices have been developed by the industry. In this review, MatriDerm® and NovoSorb® BTM were presented as examples of dermal skin substitute matrices. However, no commercially available skin substitute has achieved the properties of healthy human skin. An ideal skin substitute would have to ensure, if possible, an early restoration of the physiological and anatomical function of the skin. Currently, this ideal can only be provided by the use of full-thickness skin grafting or flap plasty [96]. An ideal skin substitute should sufficiently restore the function of the skin as a physical and chemical barrier against external influences [145]. In addition, it requires sufficient biomechanical stability as well as high biological functionality in order to allow sufficient loading capacity and to prevent a rejection reaction [146,147]. The process of thermoregulation should also be enabled by sufficient adhesion to the wound bed, sweating, and water diffusion [96,148]. Degradation of the skin substitute and remodeling into autologous tissue would also have to be present. The above-mentioned characteristics depend largely on the chosen skin substitute procedure. The biomaterials used require a basic framework that has neither antigenic nor toxic properties and can also ensure directed cell migration and proliferation [149,150]. Easy handling in application, rapid and inexpensive availability, and aesthetic results also play a decisive role in the use of skin substitute materials [148,151]. In addition to the industrial developments, the broad field of skin tissue engineering should not be ignored, which has been able to reveal many promising research approaches. Despite various scientific and industrial achievements during recent years as well as developments in burn care, there is no therapy with a skin substitute that shows promising aesthetic, functional, and immuno-compatible results based on acceptable and sufficient manufacturing. Therefore, forward-looking research approaches reveal immunological modification of allogeneic skin grafts. Thus, an ideal skin substitute with sufficient biomechanical properties would become available with comparable properties to healthy human skin and simultaneous immunological compatibility. The long-term goal remains the generation of an off-the-shelf transplantable skin substitute with high biological functionality and reduced immunogenicity. However, until this goal can be achieved, extensive research efforts are required to generate further results.

Author Contributions: Conceptualization, P.M.V., N.K. and F.S.; methodology, F.S., V.B. and N.K.; validation, P.M.V., N.K. and F.S.; investigation, N.K., V.B. and F.S.; resources, P.M.V.; data curation, P.M.V., N.K. and V.B.; writing—original draft preparation, F.S.; writing—review and editing, N.K., V.B. and P.M.V.; visualization, F.S.; supervision, N.K.; project administration, P.M.V.; funding acquisition, P.M.V. All authors have read and agreed to the published version of the manuscript.

Funding: This research received no external funding. We acknowledge support by the German Research Foundation (DFG) and the Open Access Publication Fund of Hannover Medical School (MHH).

Institutional Review Board Statement: Not applicable.

Informed Consent Statement: Not applicable.

Conflicts of Interest: The authors declare no conflict of interest.

References

1. Deutsche Gesellschaft für Verbrennungsmedizin. *Jahresbericht 2017 Verbrennungsmedizin*; Deutsche Gesellschaft für Verbrennungsmedizin: Berlin, Germany, 2017.
2. Vogt, P.M.; Mailänder, P.; Jostkleigrewe, F.; Reichert, B.; Adams, H.A. Centers for severely burned patients in Germany–management structure and needs. *Chirurg* **2007**, 411–413.
3. Vogt, P.M.; Kolokythas, P.; Niederbichler, A.; Knobloch, K.; Reimers, K.; Choi, C.Y. Innovative wound therapy and skin substitutes for burns. *Chirurg* **2007**, *78*, 335–342. [CrossRef]
4. Xiao, J.; Chai, B.R.; Kong, F.Y.; Peng, S.G.; Xu, S.H.; Wang, C.G.; Suo, H.B.; Huang, D.Q. Increased survival rate in patients with massive burns. *Burns* **1992**, *18*, 401–404. [CrossRef]
5. Finnerty, C.C.; Capek, K.D.; Voigt, C.; Hundeshagen, G.; Cambiaso-Daniel, J.; Porter, C.; Sousse, L.E.; El Ayadi, A.; Zapata-Sirvent, R.; Guillory, A.N.; et al. The P50 Research Center in Perioperative Sciences. *J. Trauma Acute Care Surg.* **2017**, *83*, 532–542. [CrossRef] [PubMed]
6. Haynes, B.W. Early excision and grafting in third degree burns. *Ann. Surg.* **1969**, *169*, 736–747. [CrossRef]
7. Hendren, W.H.; Constable, J.D.; Zawacki, B.E. Early partial excision of major burns in children. *J. Pediatr. Surg.* **1968**, *3*, 445–464. [CrossRef]
8. Pierer, H. Primary excision in burns. *Klin. Med. Osterr. Z. Wiss. Prakt. Med.* **1966**, *21*, 377–380.
9. Alrubaiy, L.; Al-Rubaiy, K.K. Skin substitutes: A brief review of types and clinical applications. *Oman Med. J.* **2009**, *24*, 4–6. [CrossRef]
10. Gibson, T.; Medawar, P.B. The fate of skin homografts in man. *J. Anat.* **1943**, *77*, 299–310.
11. Baronio, G. *Degli Innesti Animali*; Stamperia e Fonderia del Genio: Milano, Italy, 1804.
12. Jay, V. This month in history. *J. R. Soc. Med.* **1999**, *92*, 548. [CrossRef] [PubMed]
13. Alexander, J.W.; MacMillan, B.G.; Law, E.; Kittur, D.S. Treatment of severe burns with widely meshed skin autograft and meshed skin allograft overlay. *J. Trauma* **1981**, *21*, 433–438. [PubMed]
14. Rowan, M.P.; Cancio, L.C.; Elster, E.A.; Burmeister, D.M.; Rose, L.F.; Natesan, S.; Chan, R.K.; Christy, R.J.; Chung, K.K. Burn wound healing and treatment: Review and advancements. *Crit. Care* **2015**, *19*, 243. [CrossRef]
15. Karl, T.; Gussmann, A.; Storck, M. Chronic wounds—Perspective for integrated care. *Zentralbl. Chir.* **2007**, *132*, 232–235. [CrossRef] [PubMed]
16. Reinke, J.M.; Sorg, H. Wound repair and regeneration. *Eur. Surg. Res.* **2012**, *49*, 35–43. [CrossRef]
17. Rheinwald, J.G.; Green, H. Serial cultivation of strains of human epidermal keratinocytes: The formation of keratinizing colonies from single cells. *Cell* **1975**, *6*, 331–343. [CrossRef]
18. Rheinwald, J.G.; Green, H. Formation of a keratinizing epithelium in culture by a cloned cell line derived from a teratoma. *Cell* **1975**, *6*, 317–330. [CrossRef]
19. Wood, F.M.; Giles, N.; Stevenson, A.; Rea, S.; Fear, M. Characterisation of the cell suspension harvested from the dermal epidermal junction using a ReCell® kit. *Burns* **2012**, *38*, 44–51. [CrossRef]
20. Boyce, S.T.; Lalley, A.L. Tissue engineering of skin and regenerative medicine for wound care. *Burn. Trauma* **2018**, *6*, 4. [CrossRef]
21. Sood, R.; Roggy, D.; Zieger, M.; Balledux, J.; Chaudhari, S.; Koumanis, D.J.; Mir, H.S.; Cohen, A.; Knipe, C.; Gabehart, K.; et al. Cultured Epithelial Autografts for Coverage of Large Burn Wounds in Eighty-Eight Patients: The Indiana University Experience. *J. Burn Care Res.* **2010**, *31*, 559–568. [CrossRef]
22. Gravante, G.; Di Fede, M.C.; Araco, A.; Grimaldi, M.; De Angelis, B.; Arpino, A.; Cervelli, V.; Montone, A. A randomized trial comparing ReCell system of epidermal cells delivery versus classic skin grafts for the treatment of deep partial thickness burns. *Burns* **2007**, *33*, 966–972. [CrossRef]
23. Esteban-Vives, R.; Young, M.T.; Zhu, T.; Beiriger, J.; Pekor, C.; Ziembicki, J.; Corcos, A.; Rubin, P.; Gerlach, J.C. Calculations for reproducible autologous skin cell-spray grafting. *Burns* **2016**, *42*, 1756–1765. [CrossRef] [PubMed]
24. Gallico, G.G.; O'Connor, N.E.; Compton, C.C.; Kehinde, O.; Green, H. Permanent coverage of large burn wounds with autologous cultured human epithelium. *N. Engl. J. Med.* **1984**, *311*, 448–451. [CrossRef] [PubMed]

25. Munster, A.M. Cultured skin for massive burns. A prospective, controlled trial. *Ann. Surg.* **1996**, *224*, 372–375. [CrossRef] [PubMed]
26. Kopp, J.; Jeschke, M.G.; Bach, A.D.; Kneser, U.; Horch, R.E. Applied tissue engineering in the closure of severe burns and chronic wounds using cultured human autologous keratinocytes in a natural fibrin matrix. *Cell Tissue Bank.* **2004**, *5*, 89–96. [CrossRef]
27. Wallner, C.; Moormann, E.; Lulof, P.; Drysch, M.; Lehnhardt, M.; Behr, B. Burn Care in the Greek and Roman Antiquity. *Medicina* **2020**, *56*, 657. [CrossRef]
28. Tobin, G.R.; Breidenbach, W.C.; Ildstad, S.T.; Marvin, M.M.; Buell, J.F.; Ravindra, K.V. The History of Human Composite Tissue Allotransplantation. *Transpl. Proc.* **2009**, *41*, 466–471. [CrossRef]
29. Medawar, P.B. Immunity to homologous grafted skin; the fate of skin homografts transplanted to the brain, to subcutaneous tissue, and to the anterior chamber of the eye. *Br. J. Exp. Pathol.* **1948**, *29*, 58–69.
30. Brent, L.; Brooks, C.G.; Medawar, P.B.; Simpson, E.S. Transplantation tolerance. *Br. Med. Bull.* **1976**, *32*, 101–106. [CrossRef]
31. Brent, L.; Medawar, P.B. Cellular immunity and the homograft reaction. *Br. Med. Bull.* **1967**, *23*, 55–59. [CrossRef]
32. Medawar, P.B. Immunological Tolerance: The phenomenon of tolerance provides a testing ground for theories of the immune response. *Science* **1961**, *133*, 303–306. [CrossRef]
33. Horner, B.M.; Randolph, M.A.; Huang, C.A.; Butler, P.E.M. Skin tolerance: In search of the Holy Grail. *Transpl. Int.* **2007**, *21*, 101–112. [CrossRef]
34. Harrison, J.H.; Merrill, J.P.; Murray, J.E. Renal homotransplantation in identical twins. *Surg. Forum* **1956**, *6*, 432–436.
35. Knepper, M. Milestones in nephrology. *J. Am. Soc. Nephrol.* **2001**, 1788–1793.
36. Murphy, K.M.; Travers, P.; Walport, M. *Janeway Immunologie*, 7th ed.; Springer: Berlin/Heidelberg, Germany, 2009; ISBN 978-3-662-44227-2.
37. Rosenberg, A.S.; Singer, A. Cellular basis of skin allograft rejection: An in vivo model of immune-mediated tissue destruction. *Annu. Rev. Immunol.* **1992**, *10*, 333–358. [CrossRef] [PubMed]
38. Krenzien, F.; Keshi, E.; Splith, K.; Griesel, S.; Kamali, K.; Sauer, I.M.; Feldbrügge, L.; Pratschke, J.; Leder, A.; Schmelzle, M. Diagnostic Biomarkers to Diagnose Acute Allograft Rejection After Liver Transplantation: Systematic Review and Meta-Analysis of Diagnostic Accuracy Studies. *Front. Immunol.* **2019**, *10*, 758. [CrossRef] [PubMed]
39. Von Visger, J.; Cassol, C.; Nori, U.; Franco-Ahumada, G.; Nadasdy, T.; Satoskar, A.A. Complete biopsy-proven resolution of deposits in recurrent proliferative glomerulonephritis with monoclonal IgG deposits (PGNMIGD) following rituximab treatment in renal allograft. *BMC Nephrol.* **2019**, *20*, 53. [CrossRef]
40. Jang, J.K.; Kim, K.W.; Choi, S.H.; Jeong, S.Y.; Kim, J.H.; Yu, E.S.; Kwon, J.H.; Song, G.W.; Lee, S.G. CT of acute rejection after liver transplantation: A matched case–control study. *Eur. Radiol.* **2019**, *29*, 3736–3745. [CrossRef]
41. Opelz, G.; Wujciak, T. The influence of HLA compatibility on graft survival after heart transplantation. The Collaborative Transplant Study. *N. Engl. J. Med.* **1994**, *330*, 816–819. [CrossRef]
42. Opelz, G.; Wujciak, T.; Back, D.; Mytilineos, J.; Schwarz, V.; Albrecht, G. Effect of HLA compatibility on kidney transplantation. *Infusionsther. Transfusionsmed.* **1994**, *21*, 198–202.
43. Opelz, G. HLA matching in Asian recipients of kidney grafts from unrelated living or cadaveric donors. The Collaborative Transplant Study. *Hum. Immunol.* **2000**, *61*, 115–119. [CrossRef]
44. Opelz, G. Factors influencing long-term graft loss. The Collaborative Transplant Study. *Transplant. Proc.* **2000**, *32*, 647–649. [CrossRef]
45. Thorsby, E. The human major histocompatibility system. *Transplant. Rev.* **1974**, *18*, 51–129.
46. Bodmer, W.F. Evolution of HL-A and other major histocompatibility systems. *Genetics* **1975**, *79*, 293–304. [PubMed]
47. Hou, L.; Enriquez, E.; Persaud, M.; Steiner, N.; Oudshoorn, M.; Hurley, C.K. Next generation sequencing characterizes HLA diversity in a registry population from the Netherlands. *HLA* **2019**, *93*, 474–483. [CrossRef]
48. Wilke, M.; Pool, J.; den Haan, J.M.; Goulmy, E. Genomic identification of the minor histocompatibility antigen HA-1 locus by allele-specific PCR. *Tissue Antigens* **1998**, *52*, 312–317. [CrossRef]
49. den Haan, J.M.; Meadows, L.M.; Wang, W.; Pool, J.; Blokland, E.; Bishop, T.L.; Reinhardus, C.; Shabanowitz, J.; Offringa, R.; Hunt, D.F.; et al. The minor histocompatibility antigen HA-1: A diallelic gene with a single amino acid polymorphism. *Science* **1998**, *279*, 1054–1057. [CrossRef]
50. Mutis, T.; Gillespie, G.; Schrama, E.; Falkenburg, J.H.; Moss, P.; Goulmy, E. Tetrameric HLA class I-minor histocompatibility antigen peptide complexes demonstrate minor histocompatibility antigen-specific cytotoxic T lymphocytes in patients with graft-versus-host disease. *Nat. Med.* **1999**, *5*, 839–842. [CrossRef] [PubMed]
51. Opelz, G. Effect of the maintenance immunosuppressive drug regimen on kidney transplant outcome. *Transplantation* **1994**, *58*, 443–446. [CrossRef]
52. Weimer, R.; Melk, A.; Daniel, V.; Friemann, S.; Padberg, W.; Opelz, G. Switch from cyclosporine A to tacrolimus in renal transplant recipients: Impact on Th1, Th2, and monokine responses. *Hum. Immunol.* **2000**, *61*, 884–897. [CrossRef]
53. Opelz, G. Prognostic factors in the course of kidney transplantation. *Urologe A* **1994**, *33*, 377–382.
54. Murray, J.E. Human organ transplantation: Background and consequences. *Science* **1992**, *256*, 1411–1416. [CrossRef]
55. Manning, J. Sepsis in the Burn Patient. *Crit. Care Nurs. Clin. N. Am.* **2018**, *30*, 423–430. [CrossRef]
56. Benichou, G.; Yamada, Y.; Yun, S.-H.; Lin, C.; Fray, M.; Tocco, G. Immune recognition and rejection of allogeneic skin grafts. *Immunotherapy* **2011**, *3*, 757–770. [CrossRef]

57. Wang, C.; Zhang, F.; Lineaweaver, W.C. Clinical Applications of Allograft Skin in Burn Care. *Ann. Plast. Surg.* **2020**, *84*, S158–S160. [CrossRef]
58. Martínez-Flores, F.; Chacón-Gómez, M.; Madinaveitia-Villanueva, J.A.; Barrera-Lopez, A.; Aguirre-Cruz, L.; Querevalu-Murillo, W. El uso clínico de aloinjertos de piel humana criopreservados con fines de trasplante. *Cir. Cir.* **2015**, *83*, 485–491. [CrossRef] [PubMed]
59. Spence, R.J.; Ruas, E.J. The banking and clinical use of human skin allograft in trauma patients: Clinical use of allograft skin. *Md. Med. J.* **1986**, *35*, 205–212.
60. Fletcher, J.L.; Caterson, E.J.; Hale, R.G.; Cancio, L.C.; Renz, E.M.; Chan, R.K. Characterization of Skin Allograft Use in Thermal Injury. *J. Burn Care Res.* **2013**, *34*, 168–175. [CrossRef]
61. Cronin, H.; Goldstein, G. Biologic Skin Substitutes and Their Applications in Dermatology. *Dermatol. Surg.* **2013**, *39*, 30–34. [CrossRef]
62. Horch, R.; Stark, G.B.; Kopp, J.; Spilker, G. Cologne Burn Centre experiences with glycerol-preserved allogeneic skin: Part I: Clinical experiences and histological findings (overgraft and sandwich technique). *Burns* **1994**, *20* (Suppl. 1), S23–S26. [CrossRef]
63. Alam, K.; Jeffery, S.L.A. Acellular Fish Skin Grafts for Management of Split Thickness Donor Sites and Partial Thickness Burns: A Case Series. *Mil. Med.* **2019**, *184*, 16–20. [CrossRef]
64. Young, J.B.; Gondek, S.P.; Troche, M.; Summitt, J.B.; Rae, L.; Thayer, W.P.; Kahn, S.A. The use of porcine xenografts in patients with toxic epidermal necrolysis. *Burns* **2016**, *42*, 1728–1733. [CrossRef]
65. Hermans, M.H.E. Porcine xenografts vs. (cryopreserved) allografts in the management of partial thickness burns: Is there a clinical difference? *Burns* **2014**, *40*, 408–415. [CrossRef]
66. Costa, B.A.; Lima Júnior, E.M.; de Moraes Filho, M.O.; Fechine, F.V.; de Moraes, M.E.A.; Silva Júnior, F.R.; do Nascimento Soares, M.F.A.; Rocha, M.B.S. Use of Tilapia Skin as a Xenograft for Pediatric Burn Treatment: A Case Report. *J. Burn Care Res.* **2019**, *40*, 714–717. [CrossRef]
67. Lima Júnior, E.M.; De Moraes Filho, M.O.; Costa, B.A.; Rohleder, A.V.P.; Sales Rocha, M.B.; Fechine, F.V.; Forte, A.J.; Alves, A.P.N.N.; Silva Júnior, F.R.; Martins, C.B.; et al. Innovative Burn Treatment Using Tilapia Skin as a Xenograft: A Phase II Randomized Controlled Trial. *J. Burn Care Res.* **2020**, *41*, 585–592. [CrossRef]
68. Halim, A.S.; Khoo, T.L.; Mohd Yussof, S.J. Biologic and synthetic skin substitutes: An overview. *Indian J. Plast. Surg.* **2010**, *43*, S23–S28. [CrossRef]
69. Felder, J.M.; Hechenbleikner, E.; Jordan, M.; Jeng, J. Increasing the Options for Management of Large and Complex Chronic Wounds With a Scalable, Closed-System Dressing for Maggot Therapy. *J. Burn Care Res.* **2012**, *33*, e170–e176. [CrossRef]
70. Atherton, D.D.; Tang, R.; Jones, I.; Jawad, M. Early Excision and Application of Matriderm with Simultaneous Autologous Skin Grafting in Facial Burns. *Plast. Reconstr. Surg.* **2010**, *125*, 60e–61e. [CrossRef]
71. Böttcher-Haberzeth, S.; Biedermann, T.; Schiestl, C.; Hartmann-Fritsch, F.; Schneider, J.; Reichmann, E.; Meuli, M. Matriderm® 1 mm versus Integra® Single Layer 1.3 mm for one-step closure of full thickness skin defects: A comparative experimental study in rats. *Pediatr. Surg. Int.* **2012**, *28*, 171–177. [CrossRef] [PubMed]
72. Marston, W.A. Dermagraft®, a bioengineered human dermal equivalent for the treatment of chronic nonhealing diabetic foot ulcer. *Expert Rev. Med. Devices* **2004**, *1*, 21–31. [CrossRef]
73. Yim, H.; Cho, Y.S.; Seo, C.H.; Lee, B.C.; Ko, J.H.; Kim, D.; Hur, J.; Chun, W.; Kim, J.H. The use of AlloDerm on major burn patients: AlloDerm prevents post-burn joint contracture. *Burns* **2010**, *36*, 322–328. [CrossRef]
74. Burke, J.F.; Yannas, I.V.; Quinby, W.C.; Bondoc, C.C.; Jung, W.K. Successful use of a physiologically acceptable artificial skin in the treatment of extensive burn injury. *Ann. Surg.* **1981**, *194*, 413–428. [CrossRef]
75. Meuli, M.; Hartmann-Fritsch, F.; Hüging, M.; Marino, D.; Saglini, M.; Hynes, S.; Neuhaus, K.; Manuel, E.; Middelkoop, E.; Reichmann, E.; et al. A Cultured Autologous Dermo-epidermal Skin Substitute for Full-Thickness Skin Defects. *Plast. Reconstr. Surg.* **2019**, *144*, 188–198. [CrossRef] [PubMed]
76. Li, A.; Dearman, B.L.; Crompton, K.E.; Moore, T.G.; Greenwood, J.E. Evaluation of a Novel Biodegradable Polymer for the Generation of a Dermal Matrix. *J. Burn Care Res.* **2009**, *30*, 717–728. [CrossRef]
77. Michael, S.; Sorg, H.; Peck, C.-T.; Reimers, K.; Vogt, P.M. The mouse dorsal skin fold chamber as a means for the analysis of tissue engineered skin. *Burns* **2013**, *39*, 82–88. [CrossRef] [PubMed]
78. Shevchenko, R.V.; James, S.L.; James, S.E. A review of tissue-engineered skin bioconstructs available for skin reconstruction. *J. R. Soc. Interface* **2010**, *7*, 229–258. [CrossRef] [PubMed]
79. de Vries, H.J.; Middelkoop, E.; van Heemstra-Hoen, M.; Wildevuur, C.H.; Westerhof, W. Stromal cells from subcutaneous adipose tissue seeded in a native collagen/elastin dermal substitute reduce wound contraction in full thickness skin defects. *Lab. Investig.* **1995**, *73*, 532–540.
80. De Vries, H.J.; Zeegelaar, J.E.; Middelkoop, E.; Gijsbers, G.; Van Marle, J.; Wildevuur, C.H.; Westerhof, W. Reduced wound contraction and scar formation in punch biopsy wounds. Native collagen dermal substitutes. A clinical study. *Br. J. Dermatol.* **1995**, *132*, 690–697. [CrossRef]
81. Haslik, W.; Kamolz, L.-P.; Nathschläger, G.; Andel, H.; Meissl, G.; Frey, M. First experiences with the collagen-elastin matrix Matriderm as a dermal substitute in severe burn injuries of the hand. *Burns* **2007**, *33*, 364–368. [CrossRef]
82. Greenwood, J.E.; Dearman, B.L.; Li, A.; Moore, T.G. Evaluation of NovoSorb novel biodegradable polymer for the generation of a dermal matrix. Part 1: In-vitro studies. *Wound Pr. Res.* **2010**, *18*, 14–22.

83. Greenwood, J.E.; Li, A.; Dearman, B.L.; Moore, T.G. Evaluation of NovoSorb novel biodegradable polymer for the generation of a dermal matrix. Part 2: In-vivo studies. *Wound Pr. Res.* **2010**, *18*, 24–34.
84. Cheshire, P.A.; Herson, M.R.; Cleland, H.; Akbarzadeh, S. Artificial dermal templates: A comparative study of NovoSorb™ Biodegradable Temporising Matrix (BTM) and Integra® Dermal Regeneration Template (DRT). *Burns* **2016**, *42*, 1088–1096. [CrossRef]
85. Falanga, V.; Sabolinski, M. A bilayered living skin construct (APLIGRAF®) accelerates complete closure of hard-to-heal venous ulcers. *Wound Repair Regen.* **1999**, *7*, 201–207. [CrossRef] [PubMed]
86. Centanni, J.M.; Straseski, J.A.; Wicks, A.; Hank, J.A.; Rasmussen, C.A.; Lokuta, M.A.; Schurr, M.J.; Foster, K.N.; Faucher, L.D.; Caruso, D.M.; et al. StrataGraft Skin Substitute Is Well-tolerated and Is Not Acutely Immunogenic in Patients with Traumatic Wounds. *Ann. Surg.* **2011**, *253*, 672–683. [CrossRef]
87. Kogan, S.; Halsey, J.; Agag, R.L. Biologics in Acute Burn Injury. *Ann. Plast. Surg.* **2019**, *83*, 26–33. [CrossRef]
88. Radtke, C.; Reimers, K.; Allmeling, C.; Vogt, P.M. Efficient production of transfected human keratinocytes under serum-free and feeder layer-free conditions. *Handchir. Mikrochir. Plast. Chir.* **2009**, *41*, 333–340. [CrossRef]
89. Chapman, S.; Liu, X.; Meyers, C.; Schlegel, R.; McBride, A.A. Human keratinocytes are efficiently immortalized by a Rho kinase inhibitor. *J. Clin. Investig.* **2010**, *120*, 2619–2626. [CrossRef]
90. Salem, H.; Ciba, P.; Rapoport, D.H.; Egana, J.T.; Reithmayer, K.; Kadry, M.; Machens, H.G.; Kruse, C. The influence of pancreas-derived stem cells on scaffold based skin regeneration. *Biomaterials* **2009**, *30*, 789–796. [CrossRef]
91. Keck, M.; Haluza, D.; Selig, H.F.; Jahl, M.; Lumenta, D.B.; Kamolz, L.-P.; Frey, M. Adipose Tissue Engineering. *Ann. Plast. Surg.* **2011**, *67*, 484–488. [CrossRef]
92. Killat, J.; Reimers, K.; Choi, C.; Jahn, S.; Vogt, P.; Radtke, C. Cultivation of Keratinocytes and Fibroblasts in a Three-Dimensional Bovine Collagen-Elastin Matrix (Matriderm®) and Application for Full Thickness Wound Coverage In Vivo. *Int. J. Mol. Sci.* **2013**, *14*, 14460–14474. [CrossRef]
93. Golinski, P.A.; Zöller, N.; Kippenberger, S.; Menke, H.; Bereiter-Hahn, J.; Bernd, A. Development of an engraftable skin equivalent based on matriderm with human keratinocytes and fibroblasts. *Handchir. Mikrochir. Plast. Chir.* **2009**, *41*, 327–332. [CrossRef]
94. Duranceau, L.; Genest, H.; Bortoluzzi, P.; Moulin, V.; Auger, F.A.; Germain, L. Successful grafting of a novel autologous engineered skin substitutes (epidermis and dermis) on twelve burn patients. *J. Burn Care Res.* **2014**, *35*, 121.
95. Boyce, S.T. Design principles for composition and performance of cultured skin substitutes. *Burns* **2001**, *27*, 523–533. [CrossRef]
96. Boyce, S.T.; Simpson, P.S.; Rieman, M.T.; Warner, P.M.; Yakuboff, K.P.; Bailey, J.K.; Nelson, J.K.; Fowler, L.A.; Kagan, R.J. Randomized, Paired-Site Comparison of Autologous Engineered Skin Substitutes and Split-Thickness Skin Graft for Closure of Extensive, Full-Thickness Burns. *J. Burn Care Res.* **2017**, *38*, 61–70. [CrossRef] [PubMed]
97. Witten, C.M.; McFarland, R.D.; Simek, S.L. Concise Review: The U.S. Food and Drug Administration and Regenerative Medicine. *Stem Cells Transl. Med.* **2015**, *4*, 1495–1499. [CrossRef]
98. Garlick, J.A.; Katz, A.B.; Fenjves, E.S.; Taichman, L.B. Retrovirus-mediated transduction of cultured epidermal keratinocytes. *J. Investig. Dermatol.* **1991**, *97*, 824–829. [CrossRef]
99. Braun-Falco, M.; Doenecke, A.; Smola, H.; Hallek, M. Efficient gene transfer into human keratinocytes with recombinant adeno-associated virus vectors. *Gene Ther.* **1999**, *6*, 432–441. [CrossRef] [PubMed]
100. Chen, M.; Li, W.; Fan, J.; Kasahara, N.; Woodley, D. An efficient gene transduction system for studying gene function in primary human dermal fibroblasts and epidermal keratinocytes. *Clin. Exp. Dermatol.* **2003**, *28*, 193–199. [CrossRef]
101. Vogt, P.M.; Thompsont, S.; Andree, C.; Liu, P.; Breuing, K.; Hatzis, D.; Brown, H.; Mulligant, R.C.; Eriksson, E.; Murray, J.E. Genetically modified keratinocytes transplanted to wounds reconstitute the epidermis. *Proc. Natl. Acad. Sci. USA* **1994**, *91*, 9307–9311. [CrossRef] [PubMed]
102. Meng, X.; Sawamura, D.; Ina, S.; Tamai, K.; Hanada, K.; Hashimoto, I. Keratinocyte gene therapy: Cytokine gene expression in local keratinocytes and in circulation by introducing cytokine genes into skin. *Exp. Dermatol.* **2002**, *11*, 456–461. [CrossRef]
103. Collins, D.E.; Reuter, J.D.; Rush, H.G.; Villano, J.S. Viral Vector Biosafety in Laboratory Animal Research. *Comp. Med.* **2017**, *67*, 215–221. [PubMed]
104. David, R.M.; Doherty, A.T. Viral Vectors: The Road to Reducing Genotoxicity. *Toxicol. Sci.* **2017**, *155*, 315–325. [CrossRef] [PubMed]
105. Eming, S.A.; Krieg, T.; Davidson, J.M. RETRACTED: Gene therapy and wound healing. *Clin. Dermatol.* **2007**, *25*, 79–92. [CrossRef]
106. Tarassoli, S.P.; Jessop, Z.M.; Al-Sabah, A.; Gao, N.; Whitaker, S.; Doak, S.; Whitaker, I.S. Skin tissue engineering using 3D bioprinting: An evolving research field. *J. Plast. Reconstr. Aesthetic Surg.* **2018**, *71*, 615–623. [CrossRef]
107. Cubo, N.; Garcia, M.; del Cañizo, J.F.; Velasco, D.; Jorcano, J.L. 3D bioprinting of functional human skin: Production and in vivo analysis. *Biofabrication* **2016**, *9*, 015006. [CrossRef] [PubMed]
108. Lee, V.; Singh, G.; Trasatti, J.P.; Bjornsson, C.; Xu, X.; Tran, T.N.; Yoo, S.-S.; Dai, G.; Karande, P. Design and Fabrication of Human Skin by Three-Dimensional Bioprinting. *Tissue Eng. Part C Methods* **2014**, *20*, 473–484. [CrossRef]
109. Vijayavenkataraman, S.; Lu, W.F.; Fuh, J.Y.H. 3D bioprinting of skin: A state-of-the-art review on modelling, materials, and processes. *Biofabrication* **2016**, *8*, 032001. [CrossRef]
110. Morgan, J.R.; Barrandon, Y.; Green, H.; Mulligan, R.C. Expression of an Exogenous Growth Hormone Gene by Transplantable Human Epidermal Cells. *Cell Scince Virolgy Mol. CeU Bid* **1984**, *81*, 1421–1465. [CrossRef]

111. Kardeh, S.; Mazloomrezaei, M.; Dianatpour, M.; Farjadian, S. Universal off-the-shelf skin substitutes for cosmetic and reconstructive surgery. *Burns* **2020**, *46*, 741–743. [CrossRef] [PubMed]
112. Eming, S.A.; Krieg, T.; Davidson, J.M. Gene transfer in tissue repair: Status, challenges and future directions. *Expert Opin. Biol. Ther.* **2004**, *4*, 1373–1386. [CrossRef]
113. Grusby, M.J.; Auchincloss, H.; Lee, R.; Johnson, R.S.; Spencer, J.P.; Zijlstra, M.; Jaenisch, R.; Papaioannou, V.E.; Glimcher, L.H. Mice lacking major histocompatibility complex class I and class II molecules. *Proc. Natl. Acad. Sci. USA* **1993**, *90*, 3913–3917. [CrossRef] [PubMed]
114. Auchincloss, H.; Lee, R.; Shea, S.; Markowitzt, J.S.; Grusbytt, M.J.; Glimchert, L.H. The role of "indirect" recognition in initiating rejection of skin grafts from major histocompatibility complex class I-deficient mice. *Immunology* **1993**, *90*, 3373–3377. [CrossRef] [PubMed]
115. Markmann, J.F.; Bassiri, H.; Desai, N.M.; Odorico, J.S.; Kim, J.I.; Koller, B.H.; Smithies, O.; Barker, C.F. Indefinite survival of MHC class I-deficient murine pancreatic islet allografts. *Transplantation* **1992**, *54*, 1085–1089. [CrossRef]
116. Qian, S.; Fu, F.; Li, Y.; Lu, L.; Rao, A.S.; Starzl, T.E.; Thomson, A.W.; Fung, J.J. Impact of donor MHC class I or class II antigen deficiency on first-and second-set rejection of mouse heart or liver allografts. *Immunology* **1996**, *88*, 124–129. [CrossRef] [PubMed]
117. Coffman, T.; Geier, S.; Ibrahim, S.; Griffiths, R.; Spurney, R.; Smithies, O.; Koller, B.; Sanfilippo, F. Improved renal function in mouse kidney allografts lacking MHC class I antigens. *J. Immunol.* **1993**, *151*, 425–435. [PubMed]
118. Lee, R.S.; Grusby, M.J.; Laufer, T.M.; Colvin, R.; Glimcher, L.H.; Auchincloss, H. CD8+ effector cells responding to residual class I antigens, with help from CD4+ cells stimulated indirectly, cause rejection of "major histocompatibility complex-deficient" skin grafts. *Transplantation* **1997**, *63*, 1123–1133. [CrossRef]
119. Ljunggren, H.G.; Van Kaer, L.; Sabatine, M.S.; Auchincloss, H.; Tonegawa, S.; Ploegh, H.L. MHC class I expression and CD8+ T cell development in TAP1/beta 2-microglobulin double mutant mice. *Int. Immunol.* **1995**, *7*, 975–984. [CrossRef]
120. Zijlstra, M.; Auchincloss, H.; Loring, J.M.; Chase, C.M.; Russell, P.S.; Jaenisch, R. Skin graft rejection by beta 2-microglobulin-deficient mice. *J. Exp. Med.* **1992**, *175*, 885–893. [CrossRef]
121. Beyer, F.; Doebis, C.; Busch, A.; Ritter, T.; Mhashilkar, A.; Marasco, W.M.; Laube, H.; Volk, H.-D.; Seifert, M. Decline of surface MHC I by adenoviral gene transfer of anti-MHC I intrabodies in human endothelial cells-new perspectives for the generation of universal donor cells for tissue transplantation. *J. Gene Med.* **2004**, *6*, 616–623. [CrossRef]
122. Mhashilkar, A.; Doebis, C.; Seifert, M.; Busch, A.; Zani, C.; Hoo, J.S.; Nagy, M.; Ritter, T.; Volk, H.-D.; Marasco, W. Intrabody-mediated phenotypic knockout of major histocompatibility complex class I expression in human and monkey cell lines and in primary human keratinocytes. *Gene Ther.* **2002**, *9*, 307–319. [CrossRef]
123. Hill, A.; Ploegh, H. Getting the inside out: The transporter associated with antigen processing (TAP) and the presentation of viral antigen. *Proc. Natl. Acad. Sci. USA* **1995**, *92*, 341–343. [CrossRef]
124. Powers, C.; DeFilippis, V.; Malouli, D.; Früh, K. Cytomegalovirus immune evasion. *Curr. Top. Microbiol. Immunol.* **2008**, *325*, 333–359.
125. Tortorella, D.; Gewurz, B.E.; Furman, M.H.; Schust, D.J.; Ploegh, H.L. Viral subversion of the immune system. *Annu. Rev. Immunol.* **2000**, *18*, 861–926. [CrossRef]
126. Loenen, W.A.; Bruggeman, C.A.; Wiertz, E.J. Immune evasion by human cytomegalovirus: Lessons in immunology and cell biology. *Semin. Immunol.* **2001**, *13*, 41–49. [CrossRef]
127. Barnes, P.D.; Grundy, J.E. Down-regulation of the class I HLA heterodimer and beta 2-microglobulin on the surface of cells infected with cytomegalovirus. *J. Gen. Virol.* **1992**, *73 Pt 9*, 2395–2403. [CrossRef]
128. Del Val, M.; Münch, K.; Reddehase, M.J.; Koszinowski, U.H. Presentation of CMV immediate-early antigen to cytolytic T lymphocytes is selectively prevented by viral genes expressed in the early phase. *Cell* **1989**, *58*, 305–315. [CrossRef]
129. Schwartz, R.H. T-lymphocyte recognition of antigen in association with gene products of the major histocompatibility complex. *Annu. Rev. Immunol.* **1985**, *3*, 237–261. [CrossRef]
130. Ahn, K.; Angulot, A.; Ghazalt, P.; Peterson, P.A.; Yang, Y.; Froh, K.; The, T.; Johnson, R.W. Human cytomegalovirus inhibits antigen presentation by a sequential multistep process. *Immunology* **1996**, *93*, 10990–10995. [CrossRef]
131. Jones, T.R.; Hanson, L.K.; Sun, L.; Slater, J.S.; Stenberg, R.M.; Campbell, A.E. Multiple independent loci within the human cytomegalovirus unique short region down-regulate expression of major histocompatibility complex class I heavy chains. *J. Virol.* **1995**, *69*, 4830–4841. [CrossRef]
132. Schlottmann, F.; Strauss, S.; Hake, K.; Vogt, P.M.; Bucan, V. Down-Regulation of MHC Class I Expression in Human Keratinocytes Using Viral Vectors Containing US11 Gene of Human Cytomegalovirus and Cultivation on Bovine Collagen-Elastin Matrix (Matriderm®): Potential Approach for an Immune-Privileged Skin Substitute. *Int. J. Mol. Sci.* **2019**, *20*, 2056. [CrossRef]
133. Thomas, C.E.; Ehrhardt, A.; Kay, M.A. Progress and problems with the use of viral vectors for gene therapy. *Nat. Rev. Genet.* **2003**, *4*, 346–358. [CrossRef]
134. Komor, A.C.; Badran, A.H.; Liu, D.R. CRISPR-Based Technologies for the Manipulation of Eukaryotic Genomes. *Cell* **2017**, *168*, 20–36. [CrossRef]
135. Go, D.E.; Stottmann, R.W. The Impact of CRISPR/Cas9-Based Genomic Engineering on Biomedical Research and Medicine. *Curr. Mol. Med.* **2016**, *16*, 343–352. [CrossRef]
136. Peng, R.; Lin, G.; Li, J. Potential pitfalls of CRISPR/Cas9-mediated genome editing. *FEBS J.* **2016**, *283*, 1218–1231. [CrossRef]

137. Deuse, T.; Hu, X.; Gravina, A.; Wang, D.; Tediashvili, G.; De, C.; Thayer, W.O.; Wahl, A.; Garcia, J.V.; Reichenspurner, H.; et al. Hypoimmunogenic derivatives of induced pluripotent stem cells evade immune rejection in fully immunocompetent allogeneic recipients. *Nat. Biotechnol.* **2019**, *37*, 252–258. [CrossRef] [PubMed]
138. Christinck, E.R.; Luscher, M.A.; Barber, B.H.; Williams, D.B. Peptide binding to class I MHC on living cells and quantitation of complexes required for CTL lysis. *Nature* **1991**, *352*, 67–70. [CrossRef]
139. Sykulev, Y.; Joo, M.; Vturina, I.; Tsomides, T.J.; Eisen, H.N. Evidence that a single peptide-MHC complex on a target cell can elicit a cytolytic T cell response. *Immunity* **1996**, *4*, 565–571. [CrossRef]
140. Odessey, R. Addendum: Multicenter experience with cultured epidermal autograft for treatment of burns. *J. Burn Care Rehabil.* **1992**, *13*, 174–180. [CrossRef]
141. Pittelkow, M.R.; Scott, R.E. New techniques for the in vitro culture of human skin keratinocytes and perspectives on their use for grafting of patients with extensive burns. *Mayo Clin. Proc.* **1986**, *61*, 771–777. [CrossRef]
142. Desai, M.H.; Mlakar, J.M.; McCauley, R.L.; Abdullah, K.M.; Rutan, R.L.; Waymack, J.P.; Robson, M.C.; Herndon, D.N. Lack of long-term durability of cultured keratinocyte burn-wound coverage: A case report. *J. Burn Care Rehabil.* **1991**, *12*, 540–545. [CrossRef]
143. Williamson, J.S.; Snelling, C.F.; Clugston, P.; Macdonald, I.B.; Germann, E. Cultured epithelial autograft: Five years of clinical experience with twenty-eight patients. *J. Trauma* **1995**, *39*, 309–319. [CrossRef]
144. Rue, L.W.; Cioffi, W.G.; McManus, W.F.; Pruitt, B.A. Wound closure and outcome in extensively burned patients treated with cultured autologous keratinocytes. *J. Trauma* **1993**, *34*, 662–667. [CrossRef]
145. Cuono, C.B.; Langdon, R.; Birchall, N.; Barttelbort, S.; McGuire, J. Composite autologous-allogeneic skin replacement: Development and clinical application. *Plast. Reconstr. Surg.* **1987**, *80*, 626–637. [CrossRef]
146. Elias, P.M. Stratum corneum architecture, metabolic activity and interactivity with subjacent cell layers. *Exp. Dermatol.* **1996**, *5*, 191–201. [CrossRef]
147. Elias, P.M. Epidermal lipids, barrier function, and desquamation. *J. Investig. Dermatol.* **1983**, *80*, 44s–49s. [CrossRef]
148. Hansbrough, J.F.; Doré, C.; Hansbrough, W.B. Clinical Trials of a Living Dermal Tissue Replacement Placed Beneath Meshed, Split-Thickness Skin Grafts on Excised Burn Wounds. *J. Burn Care Rehabil.* **1992**, *13*, 519–529. [CrossRef] [PubMed]
149. Metcalfe, A.D.; Ferguson, M.W.J. Bioengineering skin using mechanisms of regeneration and repair. *Biomaterials* **2007**, *28*, 5100–5113. [CrossRef]
150. Metcalfe, A.D.; Ferguson, M.W.J. Tissue engineering of replacement skin: The crossroads of biomaterials, wound healing, embryonic development, stem cells and regeneration. *J. R. Soc. Interface* **2007**, *4*, 413–437. [CrossRef]
151. Pruitt, B.A.; Levine, N.S. Characteristics and uses of biologic dressings and skin substitutes. *Arch. Surg.* **1984**, *119*, 312–322. [CrossRef]

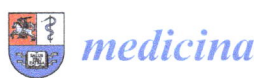

Article

Historical Perspectives on the Development of Current Standards Enzymatic Debridement

Wolfram Heitzmann *, Paul Christian Fuchs and Jennifer Lynn Schiefer *

Clinic of Plastic, Reconstructive, Hand and Burn Surgery, Hospital Cologne Merheim, University of Witten-Herdecke, 51109 Cologne, Germany; fuchsp@kliniken-koeln.de
* Correspondence: heitzmannw@kliniken-koeln.de (W.H.); schiefer.jennifer@gmail.com (J.L.S.)

Received: 11 November 2020; Accepted: 15 December 2020; Published: 17 December 2020

Abstract: *Background and Objective:* The use of plant-based products for burn treatment dates back to 1600 BC. Enzymatic debridement, which can be achieved as non-surgical or conservative debridement, has recently gained increasing attention. Several reviews have been published thus far. However, there has been no historical article including the achievements of the last 20 years, and this is the first review to present the achievements made in the field of enzymatic debridement in the last 20 years. This study aimed to present a historical overview of the development of enzymatic debridement until the present day. *Methods*: Enzymes from bacteria and plants were initially used for full-thickness burn treatment; however, they did not gain attention. Papain-derived products were the first plant-based products used for enzymatic debridement. Sutilains gained broad use in the 70s and 80s but came off market in the 1990s. Bromelain has been used for burn treatment owing to its strong debriding properties. NexoBrid™ is used as a minimally invasive approach for enzymatic debridement of deep dermal burns. However, its use has been limited due to commercially available bromelain and the presence of four distinct cysteine proteinases. NexoBrid™ involves faster eschar removal together with reduced blood loss, leading to improved long-term outcomes. However, research on nonoperative enzymatic debridement of burns has taken decades and is still ongoing. *Results*: Overall, the results of our study indicate that necrectomy, which has been used for a long time, remains the standard of care for burns. However, enzymatic debridement has several advantages, such as faster eschar removal, reduced blood loss, and reduced need for skin grafting, especially in cases of facial and hand burns. Enzymatic debridement cannot replace surgical intervention, as the enzyme only works on the surface of the eschar. Enzymatic debridement is not recommended in the early phase of scald burns. *Conclusions*: Enzymatic debridement has become an integral part of burn therapy and the standard of care in specific burn centers.

Keywords: burn therapy; enzymatic debridement; bromelain; NexoBrid™

1. Introduction

Burn injuries have always been and remain frequent, and burn therapy is a highly challenging field of medicine. In 2004, nearly 11 million burn injuries reported worldwide were severe, requiring medical attention [1]. Fortunately, a vast majority of burns are not fatal because of high standards of medical care and progress in modern burn therapy. The first and most important step in burn therapy is the total removal of eschar to avoid critical complications such as wound infections or compartment syndromes and to initiate wound healing. The first reference to debridement dates back to 25 AD, when the Roman encyclopedist Aulus Cornelius Celsus described a surgical wound treatment with operative removal of the burned skin [2]. Since 1970, early excision of burns has been considered the standard therapy [3].

However, this debridement method had disadvantages such as causing huge trauma and excessive bleeding, as well as having insufficient and selective removal from the burned region [4]. Therefore, a search for alternative debridement methods was initiated, and techniques such as laser-induced thermotherapy and the use of water jet surgical tools (e.g., Versajet) entered the domain of eschar removal. With these new debridement techniques, the vital dermal tissue and, more importantly, stem cells could be preserved to a greater extent. This, in turn, could lead to higher rates of spontaneous re-epithelialization and improved healing and scar quality. The most selective form of debridement can be achieved by non-surgical or conservative debridement. Among the techniques used for this method, enzymatic debridement has gained the most attention in recent decades. The first products used for enzymatic debridement were plant-based ones, starting with Papain-derived products in 1940. Others like Ficin or Debricin, enzymes made of ficus carica, and Bromelain, made of ananas comosus, followed. On the other hand, efforts were made to use products of bacterial origin such as Streptokinase from Hemolytic streptococci, Santyl from *Clostridium histolyticum*, or Travase from Bacillus subtilis.

The use of bromelain-based enzymatic debridement (NexoBrid™, Mediwound, Isreal) has become an integral part of burn therapy and the standard of care (SOC) in specific burn centers, especially in cases of facial and hand burns [5]. In light of the above, it is worth looking back on the history of enzymatic debridement to understand its role in modern medicine and simultaneously glance forward to the promising prospects that lie ahead in the field of burn therapy. Thus far, several reviews have been published. However, this study is the first to include the achievements made in the field of enzymatic debridement in the last 20 years. This study aims to present a historical overview of the developments in enzymatic debridement until the present day.

2. Different Sources of Enzymes

The use of plant-based products for burn treatment dates back to 1600 BC. The Egyptian Smith Papyrus describes the use of resin and honey for treating burn wounds. By 1500 BC, other herbal remedies such as *Cyperus esculentus* had been added to the list of substances for treating burns [6]. However, it was not until 1940 that enzymes of plant origin were used for eschar removal. At first, papain was extracted from the juice made using the fruits and leaves of *Carica papaya*. Papain was activated by adding either triethanolamine [7] or cysteine hydrochloride with sodium salicylate [8]. All of these solutions had a strong debriding effect. Guzman et al. used papain solution on wet surgical gauze for dressing burn wounds without any additional activator and achieved satisfactory debridement results [9]. In addition, an enzyme made from fig tree latex (debricin) showed a rapid debridement effect on second-degree burns; however, no further investigation was performed due to lack of standardization [10]. Currently, bromelain-based products are commonly used in most parts of the world. (Appendix A).

Another group of enzymes with debriding properties has bacterial origin. In 1951, Altemeier et al. described enzymes derived from *Clostridium histolyticum*, *Escherichia coli*, *Pseudomonas aeruginosa*, and *Bacillus proteus*. In vitro and in vivo collagenase made from *Clostridium histolyticum* showed the most potent effects [11]. The only such product with Food and Drug Administration approval in the USA is clostridial collagenase ointment (CCO) (Santyl). There is evidence for CCOs' positive effect on burn wounds [12]. The findings suggest that CCO can be used to debride burn wounds with less pain and nursing labor than traditional therapy with other silver-impregnated products. However, large randomized controlled trials are needed in the future to draw definitive conclusions. In contrast, streptokinase and streptodornase (Varidase) showed disappointing results, especially in the case of debridement of full-thickness burns. This is why they have not gained acceptance in burn therapy [13].

Garret was the first to publish a study on neutral proteases made from *Bacillus subtilis* (sutilains) in 1969. Over 100 patients were treated efficiently using sutilains [14]. Under the tradename Travase, sutilains gained increasing attention in the 1970s and 1980s. However, treatment with Travase led to an increasing number of wound infections soon after the application of the enzyme. A possible postulated reason for this side effect was the need for a moist environment, which stimulates bacterial growth [15,16]. To compensate for this adverse effect, simultaneous treatment with antiseptic substances such as silver sulfadiazine or mafenide is recommended. Moreover, depending on the debriding effect in that case, the patient needs to be treated in a moist environment for 3–10 days, which is a long treatment time. The debridement effect can be accelerated by applying Travase twice a day instead of once and by starting application on day 1 postburn. Using this process, full debridement can be obtained within 24 h. Wound closure can be achieved faster by autologous skin grafting than with standard conservative treatment. This made Travase the most commonly used enzyme in American burn units until it came off market in the 1990s [17,18].

Another non-surgical method for the debridement of eschar involved the use of acids, mainly pyrovic acid and phosphoric acid, until the 1960s [19,20]. An obvious disadvantage of this therapy was uncomfortable, painful, and long-lasting debridement. Therefore, this approach was abandoned and replaced by early surgical eschar removal in the 1970s.

During 1965–1979, several scientific groups examined additional enzymes such as trypsins, chymotrypsins, and fibroylsin-desoxyribonuclease. These enzymes prevented wound infection but did not reach relevant clinical use [21]. Vibriolysin extracted from *Vibrio histolyticus* and blowfly larvae extracts met the same fate [22,23].

Searching for an agent that could supersede surgical debridement, Klasen et al. reported in 2000 that chemical or enzymatic debridement had not yet achieved the status of general application. The main reasons were poor quality, high variability of composition, and lack of standardization of enzymatic treatment [24]. With the help of novel technologies in enzyme extraction and processing, these obstacles have now been overcome.

In the field of burn research, bromelain has gained the most attention during the last decade. Thus, it is the only enzyme that has achieved general application in Europe. Therefore, it is worth taking a closer look at its past, present, and future.

3. The Discovery of Bromelain

The preparation of a new protease mixture from the pineapple plant was described for the first time by Heinicke and Gortner in 1957. Batting of hides, tenderizing of meat, or chill-proofing of beer were the initially considered non-medical areas of application. Furthermore, these authors coined the term "bromelain", indicating any protease made from any member of the Bromeliaceae family [25].

The rise of the use of bromelain for burn treatment was noted in 1971, when Levine et al. tested the debriding effect of several different enzyme mixtures in vitro. They found that bromelain had the strongest debriding properties when assessed on the basis of hydroxyproline release. Further, they observed that adding mafenide did not inactivate bromelain's debriding effect, whereas sulfadiazine did [26]. They continued their experiments on bromelain in 1973 on a porcine model with third-degree burns. Again, bromelain showed a good debriding effect without converting second-degree burns into third-degree burns and without having any local toxic effects on the pigs [27].

Levenson et al. also studied bromelain using different animal models [28]. However, the bromelain available at the time consisted of a mixture of proteolytic enzymes with an unknown chemical composition. Thus, there was no reproducibility or standardization [29]. Different substances were then added to reinforce the debriding effect of bromelain. Therefore, bromelain was combined with several mercaptans, such as N-acetyl cysteine, penicillamine, and cysteine ethyl ester. Application of N-acetyl cysteine to deep burns resulted in faster healing than applying conventional treatment to burns in rats. They concluded that mercaptans have debriding properties, act quickly, are not toxic, and reinforce the debriding effect of bromelain when combined with it [24,30,31]. However, the use of this combination has not prevailed.

Klein et al. published the first relevant clinical trial investigating the treatment of burn patients with bromelain in 1985. They described varying debridement success, most likely due to the differences in the composition of the preparations because of botanical variations [24,32]. At the same time, Boswick et al. investigated enzymatic debridement with bromelain in a multi-center study in the USA. At three burn centers, 36 patients were debrided with bromelain. Adequate debridement took up to 24 h in nearly half of the patients. The rest required additional surgery because of insufficient enzymatic debridement. The possible reasons for debridement failure were delayed application of the enzymes and pretreatment with silver sulfadiazine [33].

4. Pitfalls during the Implementation of Enzymatic Debridement with Bromelain

After being tested in several in vitro models and animal models, bromelain finally reached clinical trials in 1985. However, these first clinical findings were less promising than expected, showing insufficient debriding effects. One cause worth mentioning was the inactivation of bromelain by the commonly used silver sulfadiazine [26]. However, the most important reason for inconsistent findings in these studies was the use of commercially available bromelain that was not standardized, and there was no measurable enzyme composition. The presence of at least four distinct cysteine proteinases, namely, ananain1, ananain2, stem bromelain, and comosain, has been described [34]. Therefore, each patient within a trial was treated with an agent with different proteolytic enzyme composition with different debriding properties, leading to variations in debriding intensity. With the commercial production of NexoBrid™, made from pineapple stems, a product with a standardized bromelain composition was finally available.

5. Enzymatic Debridement with NexoBrid™

5.1. First Advantages of Nexobrid over SOC

Since 18 December 2012, NexoBrid™ has gained approval as a minimally invasive technique for enzymatic debridement of deep dermal burns in Europe. The first multicenter study on the product was published in 2014 by Rosenberg et al. They showed that enzymatic debridement with NexoBrid™ resulted in faster eschar removal with reduced blood loss than the SOC. Furthermore, a reduction in the need for autografting was achieved because of more selective debridement, which spared the vital dermis. This again led to a reduction in donor site morbidities while achieving comparable long-term results of wound healing in esthetics, function, and quality of life [35].

5.2. The Learning Curve

In 2017, Schulz et al. demonstrated their initial learning curve in the enzymatic debridement of severely burned hands using NexoBrid™. Twenty patients with deeply burned hands were treated with NexoBrid™. The treatment was efficient in 90% of the cases. Correct wound-bed evaluation was described to be challenging, and wound-bed appearance was found to be different from surgical excision. Therefore, surprisingly, the majority of the burn surface areas were overestimated. Treatment was performed under plexus anesthesia by one burn surgeon and one nurse. With this new process, the treatment costs could be significantly reduced. Although these patients had sustained deep burns on their hands, there was no need for skin grafting after enzymatic debridement. Suprathel was used as a wound dressing. In this study, the mean number of days required for complete wound healing was 28 [36].

5.3. Less Need of Autografting at Same Scar Quality Compared to SOC

Thus far, excisional debridement with autografting has remained the SOC for burn therapy. Because of the promising findings on enzymatic debridement for burned hands, Schulz et al. compared the SOC to enzymatic debridement with bromelain (NexoBrid™, EDNX). Therefore, 20 patients with deep-dermal or full-thickness burns on the hands were treated with surgical excision of the necrotic tissue, whereas 20 patients with similar burns were treated with NexoBrid™. EDNX was superior in burn-depth evaluation, tissue preservation, completeness of debridement, and wound closure. The number of wounds requiring autograft was reduced for those treated with NexoBrid™. However, scar quality after 3 months did not differ substantially between the two groups [37].

5.4. European Guidelines

To summarize, there is increasing evidence that enzymatic debridement is a powerful method for eschar removal in burn wounds, reducing blood loss, need for autologous skin grafting, and need for surgical excision. To assess the role and clinical advantages of NexoBrid™ beyond the scope of the literature and in view of the users' experience, a European consensus meeting was scheduled. The first European guidelines on the use of NexoBrid™ were set in 2017 by Hirche et al. based on their experience of applying this enzymatic debridement in more than 500 patients [38].

In 2017, Loo et al. evaluated the evidence in published studies on the benefits of using NexoBrid™ compared with the use of traditional surgical excision (the SOC) for burn wound debridement. Studies published from 1986 to 2017 were considered. They confirmed strong supporting evidence of the superior effect of NexoBrid™, based on the time needed for complete debridement, need for surgery, area of burn excised, and need for autografting. Anecdotal and refuting evidence was found only for the proposed improvement in scar quality and reduced time needed for wound healing [39].

With growing experience in the use of enzymatic debridement, especially for burns of the hand, face, and the genital area, Hirche et al. released a consensus guideline update in 2020 based on the clinical experience of and practice patterns followed for 1232 summarized cases. The degree of consensus (97.7%) was remarkably high. This alone shows the success and significance of enzymatic debridement therapy in burn treatment. However, Hirche et al. reported that surgical excision with tangential knives and/or hydro-surgery remains the SOC [5]. In addition to all these positive effects, it must be outlined that in case of long-term results, such as esthetics, function, and quality of life, the effects of SOC and enzymatic debridement are comparable.

5.5. Limitations of the Use of Nexobrid

With increasing experience in enzymatic debridement, some limitations have also been uncovered.

There have been implications that enzymatic debridement does not work well on burned feet within cases of established diabetic foot disease. In a study on such cases, all patients experienced wound deepening post enzymatic debridement and needed additional surgical necrectomy, most likely due to microangiopathy [40]. To date, there is no concrete knowledge about the effects of enzymatic debridement in chemical burns, which requires further research. Furthermore, there is a consensus that enzymatic debridement should not be used as therapy for high-voltage injuries. In patients with this injury pattern, deep muscle damage with increasing compartment pressure is likely if enzymatic debridement is performed. Enzymatic debridement cannot replace surgical intervention with compartment release in these cases, as the enzyme works only on the surface of the eschar. Additionally, enzymatic debridement is not recommended in the early phase of scald burns, as poor results have been shown in these cases. Finally, there have been only a few instances of enzymatic debridement performed on large surfaces. Thus far, this attempt seems to be realizable, but the systemic effects of bromelain on patients with large-surface burns and the effects of enzymatic debridement on water loss and volume management should first be evaluated [5].

6. Conclusions

Since the Second World War, investigation into nonoperative enzymatic debridement of burns has been ongoing. Several enzymes and other chemical agents have been tested worldwide for their debriding properties [24]. However, results have been highly variable because enzyme compositions have been neither constant nor reproducible. Additionally, enzyme quality has been low, as the production methods have not been technologically advanced enough. Therefore, it was not until 2013 that with NexoBrid™, the first agent with a well-known and constant composition of enzyme preparation, that enzymatic debridement of burns achieved general application within Europe [35].

The most important advantage of enzymatic debridement is that the selectivity of enzymes toward damaged and unsalvageable tissue is greater than that of mechanical eschar removal. By saving the vital dermis and stem cells, higher rates of spontaneous re-epithelialization have been achieved and the need for autografting has been reduced. This leads to reduced donor site morbidity. Particularly in areas with thin subcutaneous tissue, where relevant structures are left vulnerable, the advantages of NexoBrid™ are essential. To achieve the best results, enzymatic debridement is followed by the use of resorbable skin substitutes, such as Suprathel. However, further investigation in the field of wound treatment after enzymatic debridement is awaited. Another advantage of enzymatic debridement of burns is the prevention of operative escharotomy in circumferential deep burns of the distal upper extremity [41]. For this, the NexoBrid™ treatment must be initialized immediately, omitting the presoaking phase [5].

Limitations: It must be mentioned that this study represents a review of literature. The articles included in the study were selected according to the PRISMA flow diagram. Several records found in the database search were excluded due to lack of relevance in the historical overall context or lack of availability. This could be considered as a limitation of this study.

Taking the whole history of enzymatic debridement into consideration, we can draw conclusions that research on its application has already gained increasing attention. Enzymatic debridement has become an integral part of burn therapy and the SOC in specific burn centers. However, further investigations into some of the areas mentioned above is needed to allow enzymatic debridement to reach its full potential.

Author Contributions: W.H.: Conceptualization; Investigation; Methodology; Writing-original draft. P.C.F.: Writing—review and editing. J.L.S.: Conceptualization; Supervision; Project administration; Writing—review and editing. All authors have read and agreed to the published version of the manuscript.

Funding: MediWound Germany paid the publishing fee. No further external funding was received.

Conflicts of Interest: Jennifer Lynn Schiefer has a consulting relationship with MediWound. The other authors declare no conflict of interest.

Appendix A

Table A1. Overview of debriding enzymes [7,10,11,13,14,25].

	Most Important Enzymes	Publication Date	Author	Enzyme Source	Advantages	Disadvantages
Plant origin	Papain	1940	Glasser	*Carica papaya*	Strong debriding effect	Activator substance needed (e.g., triethanolamine)
Plant origin	Ficin/Debricin	1949	Connel	*Ficus carica*	Rapid debriding effect	Lack of standardization
Plant origin	Bromelain	1957;1985	Heinicke, Klein	*Ananas comosus*	Fastest debriding effect, high level of standardization approval as a medical product (NexoBrid™)	Expensive treatment standard use only in burn centers due to the learning curve
Bacterial origin	Clostridial collagenase ointment/CCO/Santyl	1951	Altemeier	*Clostridium histolyticum*	Effective debridement of human eschar	Lack of randomized trials
Bacterial origin	Streptokinase/ Streptodornase/Varidase	1952;1957	Teitelman, Connel	Hemolytic streptococci	-	Insufficient debridement of full-thickness burns

Table A1. *Cont.*

	Most Important Enzymes	Publication Date	Author	Enzyme Source	Advantages	Disadvantages
Bacterial origin	Sutilains/Travase	1969	Garett	*Bacillus subtilis*	Wound closure by autologous skin grafting is achieved faster than that with SOC approval as a medical product in the US	Increase in wound infections when used time consuming therapy (full debridement within 24 h)

References

1. Peck, M.D. Epidemiology of burns throughout the World. Part I: Distribution and risk factors. *Burns* **2011**, *37*, 1087–1100. [CrossRef] [PubMed]
2. Meissel, G. *Die Verbrennungsbehandlung—Ein Historischer Überblick*; Springer: Wien, Austria, 2009; pp. 1–4.
3. Janzekowic, Z. A new concept in the early excision and immediate grafting of burns. *J. Trauma* **1970**, *10*, 1103–1108. [CrossRef]
4. Gurfinkel, R.; Rosenberg, L.; Cohen, S.; Barezovsky, A.; Cagnano, E.; Singer, A.J. Histological assessment of tangentially excised burn eschars. *Can. J. Plast. Surg.* **2010**, *18*, 33–36. [CrossRef]
5. Hirche, C.; Almeland, S.K.; Dheansa, B.; Fuchs, P.; Governa, M.; Hoeksema, H.; Korzeniowski, T.; Lumenta, D.B.; Marinescu, S.; Martinez-Mendez, J.R.; et al. Eschar removal by bromelain based enzymatic debridement (Nexobrid®) in burns: European consensus guidelines update. *Burns* **2020**, *46*, 782–796. [CrossRef] [PubMed]
6. Hartmann, A. Back to the roots—Dermatology in ancient Egyptian medicine. *JDDG* **2016**, *14*, 389–396. [CrossRef]
7. Glasser, S.R. A new treatment for sloughing wounds: Preliminary report. *Am. J. Surg.* **1940**, *40*, 320–322. [CrossRef]
8. Cooper, G.R.; Hodge, G.B.; Beard, J.W. Enzymatic debridement in the local treatment of burns. *Am. J. Dis. Child.* **1943**, *65*, 909. [CrossRef]
9. Guzman, A.V.; De Guzman, M.G.S. The enzymatic debridement of suppurations, necrotic lesions and burns with papain. *J. Int. Coll. Surg.* **1953**, *20*, 695–702.
10. Connell, J.F., Jr.; Del Guercio, L.R.; Rousselot, L.M. Debricin: Clinical experiences with a new proteolytic enzyme in surgical wounds. *Surg. Gynecol. Obstet.* **1959**, *108*, 93–99. [CrossRef]
11. Altemeier, W.A.; Coith, R.; Culbertson, W.; Tytell, A. Enzymatic debridement of burns. *Ann. Surg.* **1951**, *134*, 581–587. [CrossRef]
12. Pham, C.H.; Collier, Z.J.; Fang, M.; Howell, A.; Gillenwater, T.J. The role of collagenase ointment in acute burns: A systematic review and meta-analysis. *J. Wound. Care* **2019**, *28* (Suppl. S2), S9–S15. [CrossRef] [PubMed]
13. Teitelman, S.L.; Movitz, D.; Zimmerman, L.M. Enzymatic debridement of necrotic surfaces. *Ann. Surg.* **1952**, *136*, 267–271. [CrossRef] [PubMed]
14. Garret, T.A. Bacillus subtilis protease: A new topical agent for debridement. *Clin. Med.* **1969**, *76*, 11–15.
15. Krizek, T.J.; Robson, M.C.; Groskin, M.G. Experimental burn wound sepsis—Evaluation of enzymatic debridement. *J. Surg. Res.* **1974**, *17*, 219–227. [CrossRef]
16. Hummel, R.P.; Kautz, P.D.; Macmillan, B.G.; Altemeier, W.A. The continuing problem of sepsis following enzymatic debridement of burns. *J. Trauma* **1974**, *14*, 572–579. [CrossRef]
17. Pennisi, V.R.; Capozzi, A. Travase: Observations and controlled study of the effectiveness in burn débridement. *Burns* **1975**, *1*, 274–278. [CrossRef]
18. Dimick, A.R. Experience with the use of proteolytic enzyme (Travase) in burn patients. *J. Trauma* **1977**, *17*, 948–955. [CrossRef]
19. Connor, G.J.; Harvey, S.C. The pyruvic acid method in deep clinical burns. *Ann. Surg.* **1946**, *124*, 799–810. [CrossRef]
20. Schweitzer, R.J.; Bradsher, J.T. Acid Débridement of Burns with Phosphoric-Acid Gel. *N. Engl. J. Med.* **1951**, *244*, 705–709. [CrossRef]
21. Rodeheaver, G.; Marsh, D.; Edgerton, M.T.; Edlich, R.F. Proteolytic enzymes as adjuncts to antimicrobial prophylaxis of contaminated wounds. *Am. J. Surg.* **1975**, *129*, 537–544. [CrossRef]

22. Durham, D.R.; Fortney, D.Z.; Nanney, L.B. Preliminary evaluation of vibriolysin, a novel proteolytic enzyme compound suitable for the derbridement of burn wound eschar. *J. Burn Care Rehabil.* **1993**, *13*, 544–551. [CrossRef] [PubMed]
23. Vistnes, L.M.; Lee, R.; Ksander, G.A. Proteolytic activity of blow fly larvae secretions in experimental burns. *Surgery* **1981**, *90*, 835–841. [PubMed]
24. Klasen, H. A review on the nonoperative removal of necrotic tissue from burn wounds. *Burns* **2000**, *26*, 207–222. [CrossRef]
25. Heinicke, R.M.; Gortner, W.A. Stem bromelain—A new protease preparation from pineapple plants. *Econ. Bot.* **1957**, *11*, 225–234. [CrossRef]
26. Levine, N.; Seifter, E.; Levenson, S.M. Enzymatic debridement of burns. *Surg. Forum* **1971**, *22*, 57–58. [CrossRef] [PubMed]
27. Levine, N.; Seifter, E.; Connerton, C.; Levenson, S.M. Debridement of experimental skin burns of pigs with bromelain, a pineapple-stem enzyme. *Plast. Reconstr. Surg.* **1973**, *52*, 412–424. [CrossRef]
28. Levenson, S.M.; Kan, D.; Gruber, C.; Crowley, L.V.; Lent, R.; Watford, A.; Seifter, E. Chemical Debridement of Burns. *Ann. Surg.* **1974**, *180*, 670–704. [CrossRef]
29. Levenson, S.M. Supportive therapy in burn care. Debriding agents. *J. Trauma* **1979**, *19*, 928–930.
30. Levenson, S.M.; Gruber, D.K.; Gruber, C.; Lent, R.; Seifter, E. Chemical debridement of burns: Mercaptans. *J. Trauma* **1981**, *21*, 632–644. [CrossRef]
31. Kan, D.; Gruber, C.; Watford, A.; Seifter, E.; Levenson, S.M. Chemical debridement of burns with N-acetylcysteine. *Surg. Forum* **1979**, *30*, 48–50.
32. Klein, G.K.V. Historical Development of Bromelain in the Treatment of Burn Wounds. In *Care of the Burn Wound*; May, S.R., Dogo, G., Eds.; Karger: Basel, Switzerland, 1985; pp. 90–96.
33. Boswick, J.A. Clinical Experience with a New Enzymatic Debriding Agent. In *Care of the Burn Wound*; May, S.R., Dogo, G., Eds.; Karger: Basel, Switzerland, 1985; pp. 97–100.
34. Rowan, A.; Christopher, C.; Kelley, S.; Buttle, D.; Ehrlich, H. Debridement of experimental full-thickness skin burns of rats with enzyme fractions derived from pineapple stem. *Burns* **1990**, *16*, 243–246. [CrossRef]
35. Rosenberg, L.; Krieger, Y.; Bogdanov-Berezovski, A.; Silberstein, E.; Shoham, Y.; Singer, A.J. A novel rapid and selective enzymatic debridement agent for burn wound management: A multi-center RCT. *Burns* **2014**, *40*, 466–474. [CrossRef] [PubMed]
36. Schulz, A.; Perbix, W.; Shoham, Y.; Daali, S.; Charalampaki, C.; Fuchs, P.; Schiefer, J. Our initial learning curve in the enzymatic debridement of severely burned hands—Management and pit falls of initial treatments and our development of a post debridement wound treatment algorithm. *Burns* **2017**, *43*, 326–336. [CrossRef] [PubMed]
37. Schulz, A.; Shoham, Y.; Rosenberg, L.; Rothermund, I.; Perbix, W.; Fuchs, P.C.; Lipensky, A.; Schiefer, J.L. Enzymatic Versus Traditional Surgical Debridement of Severely Burned Hands: A Comparison of Selectivity, Efficacy, Healing Time, and Three-Month Scar Quality. *J. Burn Care Res.* **2017**, *38*, e745–e755. [CrossRef]
38. Hirche, C.; Citterio, A.; Hoeksema, H.; Koller, J.; Lehner, M.; Martinez, J.R.; Monstrey, S.; Murray, A.; Plock, J.A.; Sander, F.; et al. Eschar removal by bromelain based enzymatic debridement (Nexobrid®) in burns: An European consensus. *Burns* **2017**, *43*, 1640–1653. [CrossRef]
39. Loo, Y.L.; Goh, B.K.L.; Jeffery, S. An Overview of the Use of Bromelain-Based Enzymatic Debridement (Nexobrid®) in Deep Partial and Full Thickness Burns: Appraising the Evidence. *J. Burn Care Res.* **2018**, *39*, 932–938. [CrossRef]
40. Berner, J.; Keckes, D.; Pywell, M.; Dheansa, B. Limitations to the use of bromelain-based enzymatic debridement (NexoBrid®) for treating diabetic foot burns: A case series of disappointing results. *Scars Burn. Heal.* **2018**, *4*, 2059513118816534. [CrossRef]
41. Fischer, S.; Haug, V.; Diehm, Y.; Rhodius, P.; Cordts, T.; Schmidt, V.J.; Kotsougiani, D.; Horter, J.; Kneser, U.; Hirche, C. Feasability and safety of enzymatic debridement for the prevention of operative escharotomy in circumferential deep burns of the distal upper extremity. *Surgery* **2019**, *165*, 19–24. [CrossRef]

Publisher's Note: MDPI stays neutral with regard to jurisdictional claims in published maps and institutional affiliations.

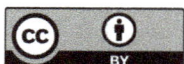

© 2020 by the authors. Licensee MDPI, Basel, Switzerland. This article is an open access article distributed under the terms and conditions of the Creative Commons Attribution (CC BY) license (http://creativecommons.org/licenses/by/4.0/).

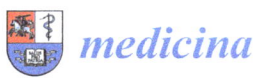

Review

A History of Fluid Management—From "One Size Fits All" to an Individualized Fluid Therapy in Burn Resuscitation

Dorothee Boehm * and Henrik Menke

Department of Plastic, Aesthetic and Hand Surgery, Specialized Burn Center, Sana Klinikum Offenbach, Starkenburgring 66, 63069 Offenbach, Germany; henrik.menke@sana.de
* Correspondence: dorothee.boehm@sana.de; Tel.: +69-8405-5141; Fax: +69-8405-5144

Abstract: Fluid management is a cornerstone in the treatment of burns and, thus, many different formulas were tested for their ability to match the fluid requirements for an adequate resuscitation. Thereof, the Parkland-Baxter formula, first introduced in 1968, is still widely used since then. Though using nearly the same formula to start off, the definition of normovolemia and how to determine the volume status of burn patients has changed dramatically over years. In first instance, the invention of the transpulmonary thermodilution (TTD) enabled an early goal directed fluid therapy with acceptable invasiveness. Furthermore, the introduction of point of care ultrasound (POCUS) has triggered more individualized schemes of fluid therapy. This article explores the historical developments in the field of burn resuscitation, presenting different options to determine the fluid requirements without missing the red flags for hyper- or hypovolemia. Furthermore, the increasing rate of co-morbidities in burn patients calls for a more sophisticated fluid management adjusting the fluid therapy to the actual necessities very closely. Therefore, formulas might be used as a starting point, but further fluid therapy should be adjusted to the actual need of every single patient. Taking the developments in the field of individualized therapies in intensive care in general into account, fluid management in burn resuscitation will also be individualized in the near future.

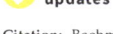

Citation: Boehm, D.; Menke, H. A History of Fluid Management—From "One Size Fits All" to an Individualized Fluid Therapy in Burn Resuscitation. *Medicina* **2021**, *57*, 187. https://doi.org/10.3390/medicina57020187

Academic Editor: Lars P. Kamolz

Received: 30 December 2020
Accepted: 14 February 2021
Published: 23 February 2021

Publisher's Note: MDPI stays neutral with regard to jurisdictional claims in published maps and institutional affiliations.

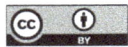

Copyright: © 2021 by the authors. Licensee MDPI, Basel, Switzerland. This article is an open access article distributed under the terms and conditions of the Creative Commons Attribution (CC BY) license (https://creativecommons.org/licenses/by/4.0/).

Keywords: fluid management; resuscitation volume; transpulmonary thermodilution; ultrasound; burn resuscitation

1. Introduction

1.1. The Use of Formulas as a Starting Point

Burn patients in the initial resuscitation phase typically require large volumes to restore adequate perfusion pressure and prevent organ failure. To estimate the actual fluid requirements, Baxter and Shires introduced the Parkland formula in 1968 and thus enabled a better outcome of burn patients [1]. Their formula originally proposes a resuscitation volume between 3.5 mL and 4 mL/kg body weight/% TBSA/24 h with half of the fluid volume given early, i.e., in the first 8 h post-burn. Baxter and Shires therefore used several animal studies to determine the decrease in extracellular fluid and fluid loss via the burned surface and subsequently examined the optimal amount of resuscitation fluid as well as the optimal time of fluid administration. Clinically, they showed an adequate urine output using this fluid regimen. In the following years, this study of Baxter and Shires was reduced to the "Parkland formula", i.e., 4 mL/kg body weight/% TBSA/24 h achieving a urine output of 50 mL/h. However, the second part of the clinical studies of Baxter and Shires is not commonly mentioned in the present discussion on burn resuscitation, and will be discussed later on in this review.

Apart from the Parkland formula, many other formulas have been proposed to estimate the necessary resuscitation volume more closely, e.g., Evans formula [2] or the modified Brooke formula (2 mL/kg/%TBSA) [3]. Those formulas as well as the Parkland formula have been tested in various studies [4,5]. Neither was a more accurate formula found for burn injuries ranging up to 60% TBSA [3] nor has any other formula gained the same popularity as the Parkland formula still has [6,7]. In a recent study with 90 burn patients by Ete et al. [5], the necessary resuscitation volume was 3.14 mL/kg/% TBSA and 3.36 mL/kg/%TBSA for burn patients with concomitant inhalational injury and, therefore, close to the 3.5 mL/kg/%TBSA of the original Parkland formula.

1.2. The Hazard of Over-Resuscitation

Though hypovolemia was initially the predominant cause for mortality of burn shock [8] and still increases the risk of acute kidney injury [9], formula-based fluid resuscitation led, in some cases, to hypervolemia, which also provoked adverse effects and increased mortality [10]. In the following years, the symptoms and hazards of over-resuscitation were discussed in the literature. The basic reason for adverse effects of over-resuscitation is the phenomenon of "fluid creep", which was first described by Pruitt et al. [11]. The excessive fluid does, therefore, not optimize the volumetric status of the patient but rather increases the tissue edema and thus worsens edema-associated complications. Chung et al. stated that the volume given in excess to the initial estimation necessitates even more fluid intake in the following hours [12].

Beside an incline in pulmonary function because of lung edema, the abdominal compartment syndrome (ACS) is one of the most devastating complications with a mortality of over 80% in burn patients [13,14]. Due to hypervolemia and increasing abdominal edema with consequently rising intra-abdominal pressure (IAP), the inferior vena cava (IVC) blood flow and thus cardiac output decrease in first instance with consecutive decreasing urine output and also mechanical ventilation and pulmonary function worsen as early warning signs [15]. Since an increasing abdominal edema and intra-abdominal hypertension (i.e., over 12 mmHg) are not rarely seen, the IAP should be monitored during the resuscitation phase through measurement of the bladder pressure and beyond according to the guidelines of the World Society of Abdominal Compartment Syndrome [16,17].

Still, the discussion about the most suitable method to estimate the adequate resuscitation volumes and how to keep the golden middle of normovolemia is going on. This review will provide an overview of different analyzing methods and parameters to assess fluid requirements. The question of how and when to use colloids or which kind of resuscitation fluid should be used will not be covered by this review. We rather focus on the evolution from a goal-directed resuscitation with the use of different parameters to the most recent development of an individualized resuscitation taking individual organ function into account.

2. Early Goal-Directed Resuscitation

To avoid under- and over-resuscitation, different parameters were analyzed in the past to guide fluid management. This "goal-directed" therapy was discussed early in the history of burn resuscitation. As early as 1968, Baxter and Shires used not only urinary output but also a pulmonary catheter (PAC) in the clinical part of their study to measure the cardiac output as an additional parameter [1]. In contrast to a formula-based fluid therapy, the goal-directed approach uses early and regular adjustments of the fluid intake, though a formula-based estimation is also used to start off initially. Thus, the initially estimated fluid intake could be over- or under-estimated in comparison to the given volume. In fact, the comparison of estimated fluid requirements using Parkland or Brooke formula with the real fluid administration showed in several studies an over-resuscitation in 50 to 100% of burn patients [3,18–20]. In most cases, the fluid administration was increased to match the goal of adequate urine output (UO).

Therefore, a vital point for sensible goal-directed fluid therapy is which parameters to choose and how to combine them. The different parameters to guide fluid therapy are discussed in this section.

2.1. Vital Signs, Urine Output and Serum Lactate/Base Deficit as Parameters

The most widely used parameters are urinary output and vital signs such as blood pressure or mean arterial blood pressure (MAP) and heart rate since they are measurable with minimal effort and in most circumstances and locations worldwide.

Additionally, Baxter and Shires used urine output (UO) as target parameter in their formula-based resuscitation of burn patients. In the following years, urine output remained the leading parameter for goal-directed resuscitation. Though UO can be used easily as an indicator for sufficient resuscitation, it is not a reliable parameter if adequate tissue perfusion and oxygen delivery are the ultimate goals. Furthermore, oliguria or anuria may also be signs for multiple pathologies—not only hypovolemia. In the aforementioned abdominal compartment syndrome, for example, oliguria is a common sign with rising IAP. In fact, UO should not be used as sole parameter to guide resuscitation. However, still it is one of the most popular parameters and still recommended by the American Burn Association [21]. Dries and Waxmann retrospectively compared vital signs and UO with PAC monitoring in their response to fluid administration. Whereas PAC measurements closely reacted after fluid intake with increased cardiac output (CO) and oxygen consumption, vital signs and UO showed no significant change [22]. Saffle et al. demonstrated that UO increased after additional fluid intake with a delay of several hours. Although fluid administration was increased after a decline in UO 8 h after burn, a significant incline of UO was not detectable until 12 h later [23]. At this point, UO peaked up 250 mL/h until 36 h post-burn, though fluid administration was reduced rapidly and thus lagging nearly 12 h behind the initial increase in fluid intake. Therefore, vital signs are not reliable enough and UO as slow reacting parameter inefficient in highly dynamic situations as the burn shock. Hence, these parameters could lead to over-resuscitation when used as goals to guide fluid therapy [11,24].

Of note, serum lactate and arterial base deficit are reliable markers of tissue perfusion. Both parameters indicate uncompensated shock and cell death also in burn patients [25]. However, a rapid lactate clearance shows an adequate resuscitation and subsequently improves survival. As marker of cell death, both parameters rise after the damage of poor organ perfusion is done. Therefore, both parameters should not be used as a goal but rather to confirm adequate resuscitation by rapid correction of initially increased serum lactate and base deficit and to predict a positive outcome.

2.2. Static Parameters—CVP and Inferior Vena Cava Diameter

Static parameters, e.g., the central venous pressure (CVP) were often used in the past, though the volumetric status is influenced by many dynamic processes such as changing intrathoracic pressure during in- and expiration with alterations of blood flow and thus changing stroke volume. Therefore, static parameters in general show low reliability to reflect the actual volumetric status of the patient [26]. Multiple studies showed that the CVP does not represent the volumetric status of the patient and also failed to predict the response to fluid intake [27,28].

Accordingly, the sole determination of the diameter of the inferior vena cava (IVC) is not reliable enough and cut-off values depend on the patients' height. However, the changes in IVC diameter during in- and expiration—i.e., the respiratory variation—proved an adequate tool that can be easily determined via ultrasound bedside [29,30] and will be discussed in Section 3.3.

2.3. Thermodilution and Arterial Pressure Wave Analysis

In the last few years, the transpulmonal thermodilution (TTD) has gained popularity as a useful method to determine volumetric parameters as well as cardiac output (CO) and systemic vascular resistance (SVR). The TTD technique (PiCCO©, PulseCO©) uses volume boluses of 10–20 mL of ice cold saline and measures the time between the injection site (central venous catheter) and an arterial catheter (in the femoral or brachial artery). Therefore, it is less invasive than the formerly used pulmonary artery catheter (PAC), which has been replaced by the TTD-technique. TTD enables the calculation of volumetric parameters such as the global enddiastolic volume (GEDV) or intrathoracic blood volume (ITBV) which reliably reflect the actual preload [31].

The increasing pulmonary edema with ongoing resuscitation is represented by the extra-vascular lung water (ELW). Branski et al. could show that an increasing mortality is linked to increased ELW-values [32]. This matches the experience that increasing lung edema prolongs mechanical ventilation as well as length of stay [33]. This parameter is, therefore, recommended as a red flag to stop or reduce further fluid administration.

As a drawback, the TTD- technique and arterial pressure wave analysis presumes a normal cardiac function without cardiac valve dysfunction and excludes patients with arrhythmia. Additionally, a pre-existing history of pulmonary diseases influences the calculation and interpretation of the ELW.

In general, TTD and arterial pressure wave analysis show their greatest reliability not in single measurements, but in detecting changes in the course of ongoing resuscitation.

2.4. Thermodilution and "Permissive Hypovolemia"

Initially, goal-directed therapy was used to achieve normal or supra-normal parameters. However, when normal or even supra-normal values of preload parameters (GEDV and ITBV) are targeted, resuscitation volumes estimated by the Parkland formula are exceeded regularly [34–37]. Surprisingly, no significant change in renal failure, vasopressor use or mortality could be demonstrated in the group of increased resuscitation volumes and with normal preload values in these studies [38]. Thus, optimizing preload parameters to normal or even supra-normal values showed no advantage. As a consequence, Arlati et al. stated that "permissive hypovolemia" was also feasible without the danger of poor organ perfusion and consecutive tissue damage [39]. The goals in this study were defined as a minimum cardiac index (CI = CO/body surface area) of 2 L/min/m^2 and an hourly urine output of at least 0.5 mL/kg. Arlati and his group showed reduced resuscitation volumes in the first 12 h post-burn, i.e., 3.2 mL/kg/%TBSA, compared to the estimated Parkland formula (4.6 mL/kg/%TBSA). The permissive hypovolemia group even showed an optimized lactate clearance compared to the control group. ITBV as preload parameter ranged between 650 and 750 mL/m^2 and, therefore, significantly below normal values (900 mL/m^2). Despite the size of the study (n = 12), Arlati could show significant decreased multiple organ dysfunction scores (MODS) in the permissive hypovolemia group.

In a larger study by Sanchez et al. (n = 132), the cardiac index was also used as primary goal to guide burn fluid therapy [40]. Goals were set as a CI of at least 2,5 L/min/m^2, ITBV > 600 mL/m^2 and rapid lactate clearance. The mean volume given was 4.05 mL/kg/%TBSA confirming the results of Charles Baxter. Of note, urine output was not used as resuscitation parameter and the authors reported no correlation between CI and urine output. However, in some cases with a UO of >0.5 mL/kg/h, severe hypovolemia with elevated lactate levels were found and vice versa. Hence, both studies demonstrated the CI to be superior as parameter for goal-directed therapy compared to the widely used urine output or preload parameter alone.

3. Individualized Fluid Management

In contrast to the goal-directed therapy, which uses a preset goal for every patient, the individualized approach considers co-morbidities and defines the goals in concordance to the individual organ function of every patient. As a consequence of increasing life expectancy, the average age as well as the incidence of co-morbidities has been rising significantly over the last few decades. Whereas occupational health and safety increased over the last years and occupation associated burns are decreasing likewise, the percentage of elderly and morbid patients rises continuously in developed countries [41].

3.1. Cardiac Function and Fluid Responsiveness

In the course of burn resuscitation, cardiac function is a limiting factor for fluid administration. Thus, it is important to understand the pathophysiologic response to fluid challenges. In short, the myocardium is able to optimize its contractility in a certain range, i.e., within the steep part of the Frank–Starling curve. In this optimum range the myocardium is stretched by adequate preload without over-stretching in case of volume overload [42]. Unfortunately, this optimum range is decreased by several cardiac diseases leading to poor fluid responsiveness. In these patients, low CO will not rise after fluid administration but rather deteriorate with increasing resuscitation volume. Thus, the preset goal of normalized CO is achievable for patients with normal cardiovascular responsiveness to fluid challenge. In contrast, further volume administration and increased preload have no benefit in non-responders. The assessment of cardiac function and fluid responsiveness is therefore a cornerstone of individualized resuscitation.

3.2. Parameters of Fluid Responsiveness

The transpulmonary thermodilution (TTD) technique as mentioned above can also be used to analyze the arterial pressure wave (PiCCO©, PulseCO©, FloTrac©). The variation of the pulse pressure variation (PPV) and stroke volume variation (SVV) reliably predict the fluid responsiveness with a sensitivity of 80% [43]. Furthermore, the analysis of the arterial pulse curve enables a continuous measurement and promptly demonstrates changes after increased fluid intake. Thus, the combination of TTD and pulse curve analysis (PiCCO©, PulseCO©) not only displays hypovolemia via preload parameters (GEDV and ITBV) but also predicts fluid responsiveness [44]. Unfortunately, arrhythmia, head of bed elevation [45] as well as the settings of mechanical ventilation, low or changing tidal volume, spontaneous breathing and positive end-expiratory pressure (PEEP) especially, strongly influence SVV and PPV parameters [46]. Further parameters of fluid responsiveness are discussed in the following sections.

3.3. Point of Care Ultrasound—POCUS

The use of ultrasound as point of care diagnostic is now widely used. The most intriguing points are its rapid availability and non-invasive use. Additionally, the broad spectrum of applications ranges from identification of different causes of shock (hypovolemia versus pulmonary embolism etc.), examination of potential complications or combined injuries (pneumothorax, Focused Assessment with Sonography in Trauma/FAST), lung ultrasound, cardiac function, volumetric status and fluid responsiveness [47]. Lung ultrasound is useful to estimate lung edema which is a stop sign for fluid administration similar to raised ELW values using the TTD technique.

As mentioned above, the diameter of the inferior vena cava (IVC) is an easily assessed but unreliable parameter for the actual volumetric status. However, the respiratory variation of the IVC—i.e., the dynamic changes in diameter during the respiratory cycle—reliably reflects the volumetric status [48]. The respiratory variation can be expressed as:

$$\text{IVC variability} = 100 \times \frac{\text{IVC}_{maximum} - \text{IVC}_{minimum}}{\text{IVC}_{mean}}$$

The cut-off point for the calculated IVC variability lies at 12% and, thus, measurements over 12% are predictive of fluid responsiveness [48].

Though the variation is influenced by ventilator settings and respiration efforts in spontaneously breathing patients [49], a recent meta-analysis by Zhang et al. showed a high specificity of the respiratory variation of the IVC of 87% and 85% in mechanical ventilation and spontaneous breathing, respectively. Additionally, sensitivity in mechanically ventilated patients was reliable with 81% but moderate in spontaneously breathing patients with 70% [50]. Therefore, additional parameters are useful to assess fluid responsiveness, especially in spontaneously breathing patients.

3.4. Echocardiography

Focused cardiac ultrasound includes measurement of contractility of the left and right ventricle, stroke volume, valve dysfunction as well as respiratory changes (stroke volume variation) or changes after fluid challenges [51,52]. Therefore, an initial assessment can be done and the responsiveness to fluid administration can be assessed in the course of resuscitation. Focused echocardiography can be done as transthoracic echocardiography (TTE) or transesophageal (TEE) the latter being more invasive and requiring sedation, yet being independent from mechanical ventilation or thoracic (burn) wounds.

Whereas overt hypovolemia can be determined quickly by visual assessment of the left ventricle ("kissing ventricles" as a typical sign), estimation of contractility and fluid responsiveness makes further measurements necessary. Herein, ejection fraction (EF) and stroke volume should be assessed as parameters for left ventricle contractility. The stroke volume (measured as velocity time index of the left ventricular outflow tract) is used to derive cardiac output [53] and measurement of stroke volume variation during the respiratory cycle is equally to the SVV measured by TTD using the same cut-off values [54]. Therefore, a SVV of 12–14% is highly predictive of a positive fluid response, whereas values below 10% reliably identify fluid non-responders [55].

Recently, the contractility of the right ventricle has been focused on since it is crucial for fluid responsiveness. Therefore, the tricuspid annular plane systolic excursion (TAPSE) should be measured as parameter for right ventricular contractility and right ventricle dilatation and flattening of the septum as the "red flags" for fluid administration should not be missed [56]. Echocardiography of the right ventricle also contributes to the interpretation of IVC measurements. Herein, a wide IVC diameter with low respiratory variation suggests a fluid non-responder. In combination with right ventricle dilatation, this constitutes a red flag for any further fluid administration.

3.5. Fluid Responsiveness and Fluid Challenge

Additionally, these parameters can be re-assessed after a fluid challenge. Therefore, mini-fluid challenges of 100 mL of colloids are sufficient to certify fluid responsiveness by optimizing cardiac output by at least 10% [57]. Instead of fluid administration, the passive leg raise (PLR) maneuver also enables a fluid challenge of 250–300 mL by autotransfusion. In contrast to intravenous fluid administration, the volume effect after PLR persists for 20–45 min and is, thus, reversible. When PLR test is conducted correctly (change patient's position from semirecumbent to supine with legs 45° elevated) and CO or SVV are measured before and 1–2 min after changing the patient's position, this test is easy to perform and highly reliable. A meta-analysis of Cherpanath and colleagues found a pooled sensitivity of 86% and specificity of 92% with a summary AUROC of 0.95 [58]. Contraindications for PLR maneuver are raised intracranial pressure, intra-abdominal hypertension and lower limb amputations, the last two conditions attenuating the effect of PLR maneuver and therefore leading to unreliable results.

In contrast to single measurements of SVV or cardiac output, the change after volume challenge—nevertheless, via fluid administration or PLR—is independent from ventilator settings, spontaneous breathing or arrhythmia [58]. Thus, the dynamic analysis of fluid responsiveness using PLR/fluid challenge results in more robust measurements and are therefore useful in a variety of clinical settings.

4. Discussion—How to Find the Golden Middle

In 1968, Baxter and Shires proposed 3.5–4.5 mL/kg/% TBSA to estimate fluid requirements in burn patients. Still widely used, this formula seems to match the actual fluid requirements adequately in the majority of patients with moderate burn injuries. However in severely burned patients exceeding 60% TBSA, fluid requirements increase disproportionally. Thus, a formula-based resuscitation will predict fluid requirements more inaccurately with rising TBSA. Cancio et al. showed fluid requirements of 6 mL/kg/%TBSA in burn patients exceeding 80% TBSA [3]. In the history of burn resuscitation, fluid administration was adjusted to different parameters as goal directed fluid management. As an easy to handle parameter, urine output is still widely used to guide resuscitation of burn patients. Though the initial goal of 1 mL/kg/h urine output also used by Baxter and Shires was reduced to 0.5 mL/kg/h in the following years, most burn patients seemed to call for higher resuscitation volumes, named as "fluid creep". However, major burn injuries are highly dynamic situations calling for close adjustment of fluid therapy. Because of the rapid dynamic in the acute phase of severe burns, static parameters such as CVP cannot be recommended. Even slowly reacting parameters such as UO or lactate and base deficit are not reliable enough to guide the actual fluid administration. They should rather be used to verify adequate resuscitation [23].

The development of transpulmonary thermodilution (TTD) enabled the measurement of preload parameters (GEDV and ITBV), cardiac output (CO/CI) and ELW as a parameter of increasing lung edema with limited invasiveness compared to the pulmonary artery catheter (PAC). Herein, recent studies have shown that preload parameters should be used with caution to guide resuscitation in the acute burn shock since normal values are only achievable by significant over-resuscitation. In contrast, cardiac output or cardiac index proved to be reliable to guide fluid administration and enable a closer adjustment of resuscitation to the actual fluid requirements of the patient. Hereby, goal directed resuscitation using cardiac output allows for permissive hypovolemia and concurrently optimized oxygen delivery [39].

Baxter and Shires transferred their findings in different animal experiments to the clinical setting [1]. The first 11 burn patients were resuscitated with 4 mL/kg/%TBSA lactated Ringer solution and their haemodynamics were analyzed, especially CO measured with PAC. Though the loss of extracellular volume was restored in all cases applying the formula of 4 mL/kg/%TBSA, the authors found three groups of cardiac response to fluid therapy. Young burn patients with up to 50% TBSA showed an increasing CO after fluid administration achieving normal cardiac function after 24 h post-burn. In burn patients exceeding 80% TBSA, CO could be restored after 24 h but thereafter showed a continuous decrease unresponsive to fluid administration. As a third group, Baxter and Shires identified burn patients with low CO early after burn trauma without cardiac response to fluid administration. They defined this group as patients "over 45 years of age". In a subsequent series of 277 burn patients, these different types of cardiovascular response were confirmed. Though it was not the authors' conclusion, this study demonstrated that not only resuscitation volume and preset goals but also individual organ function, especially fluid responsiveness, are equally important to optimize resuscitation.

Therefore, the goal directed resuscitation should be refined to an individualized resuscitation. Herein, focused echocardiography plays a vital role to assess cardiac function initially and cardiovascular response to fluid administration in the course of resuscitation. Furthermore, the analysis of fluid responsiveness (SVV, IVC variability, CO) demonstrates the potential improvement of increased volume administration beforehand and thus avoids the hazards of over-resuscitation [56]. Moreover, TTD and echocardiography can be used equally to assess SVV and CO but both techniques are complementary concerning the analysis of volumetric status and lung edema. Additionally, point-of-care ultrasound offers a variety of options concerning differentiating the possible causes of shock or enabling ultrasound guided interventions.

5. Conclusions

The difference between the goal-directed and individualized approach is an adjustment of fluid therapy to the preset goals in the first case and an adjustment of multiple target parameters to the organ function of the individual patient in the second case. In short, a "one size fits all" approach sets the criteria to be met by the patient, whereas an individualized approach relies on the assessment of cardiac, pulmonary and kidney function in the first step and consecutively defines reliable goals and necessary fluid administration for this patient in the second step. Thus, individualization can be seen as a future development of the goal-directed therapy.

As Kevin Chung stated: "The complex nature of the body's response to burn injury compounded by the variable response to resuscitation likely makes the starting point almost irrelevant." [12]. Therefore, the actual discussion should move on from the question about the most exact formula to the question about the most reliable parameters to estimate individual organ function and to define adequate resuscitation.

Author Contributions: Conceptualization and original draft preparation: D.B.; validation and formal analysis: H.M. All authors have read and agreed to the published version of the manuscript.

Funding: This research received no external funding.

Institutional Review Board Statement: Not applicable.

Informed Consent Statement: Not applicable.

Data Availability Statement: Not applicable.

Conflicts of Interest: The authors have no conflict of interest to declare.

References

1. Baxter, C.R.; Shires, T. Physiological response to crystalloid resuscitation of severe burns. *Ann. N Y Acad. Sci.* **1968**, *150*, 874–894. [CrossRef] [PubMed]
2. Evans, E.I.; Purnell, O.J.; Robinett, P.W.; Batchelor, A.; Martin, M. Fluid and electrolyte requirements in severe burns. *Ann. Surg.* **1952**, *135*, 804–817. [CrossRef]
3. Cancio, L.C.; Chavez, S.; Alvarado-Ortega, M.; Barillo, D.J.; Walker, S.C.; McManus, A.T.; Goodwin, C.W. Predicting increased fluid requirements during the resuscitation of thermally injured patients. *J. Trauma Acute Care Surg.* **2004**, *56*, 404–413. [CrossRef]
4. Blumetti, J.; Hunt, J.L.; Arnoldo, B.D.; Parks, J.K.; Purdue, G.F. The Parkland formula under fire: Is the criticism justified? *J. Burn Care Res.* **2008**, *29*, 180–186. [CrossRef]
5. Ete, G.; Chaturvedi, G.; Barreto, E.; Paul, M.K. Effectiveness of Parkland formula in the estimation of resuscitation fluid volume in adult thermal burns. *Chin. J. Traumatol.* **2019**, *22*, 113–116. [CrossRef] [PubMed]
6. Baker, R.H.; Akhavani, M.A.; Jallali, N. Resuscitation of thermal injuries in the United Kingdom and Ireland. *J. Plast. Reconstr. Aesthet. Surg.* **2007**, *60*, 682–685. [CrossRef] [PubMed]
7. Greenhalgh, D.G. Burn resuscitation: The results of the ISBI/ABA survey. *Burns* **2010**, *36*, 176–182. [CrossRef]
8. Kumar, P. Fluid resuscitation for burns: A double edge weapon. *Burns* **2002**, *28*, 613–614. [CrossRef]
9. Mason, S.A.; Nathens, A.B.; Finnerty, C.C.; Gamelli, R.L.; Gibran, N.S.; Arnoldo, B.D.; Tompkins, R.G.; Herndon, D.N.; Jeschke, M.G.; Inflammation, and the Host Response to Injury Collaborative Research Program. Hold the Pendulum: Rates of Acute Kidney Injury are Increased in Patients Who Receive Resuscitation Volumes Less than Predicted by the Parkland Equation. *Ann. Surg.* **2016**, *264*, 1142–1147. [CrossRef]
10. Klein, M.B.; Hayden, D.; Elson, C.; Nathens, A.B.; Gamelli, R.L.; Gibran, N.S.; Herndon, D.N.; Arnoldo, B.; Silver, G.; Schoenfeld, D.; et al. The association between fluid administration and outcome following major burn: A multicenter study. *Ann. Surg.* **2007**, *245*, 622–628. [CrossRef] [PubMed]
11. Pruitt, B.A., Jr. Protection from excessive resuscitation: "pushing the pendulum back". *J. Trauma Acute Care Surg.* **2000**, *49*, 567–568. [CrossRef]
12. Chung, K.K.; Wolf, S.E.; Cancio, L.C.; Alvarado, R.; Jones, J.A.; McCorcle, J.; King, B.T.; Barillo, D.J.; Renz, E.M.; Blackbourne, L.H. Resuscitation of severely burned military casualties: Fluid begets more fluid. *J. Trauma Acute Care Surg.* **2009**, *67*, 231–237. [CrossRef] [PubMed]
13. Strang, S.G.; Van Lieshout, E.M.; Breederveld, R.S.; Van Waes, O.J. A systematic review on intra-abdominal pressure in severely burned patients. *Burns* **2014**, *40*, 9–16. [CrossRef]
14. Boehm, D.; Schroder, C.; Arras, D.; Siemers, F.; Siafliakis, A.; Lehnhardt, M.; Dadras, M.; Hartmann, B.; Kuepper, S.; Czaja, K.U.; et al. Fluid Management as a Risk Factor for Intra-abdominal Compartment Syndrome in Burn Patients: A Total Body Surface Area-Independent Multicenter Trial Part, I.J. *Burn Care Res.* **2019**, *40*, 500–506. [CrossRef] [PubMed]
15. Boehm, D.; Arras, D.; Schroeder, C.; Siemers, F.; Corterier, C.C.; Lehnhardt, M.; Dadras, M.; Hartmann, B.; Kuepper, S.; Czaja, K.U.; et al. Mechanical ventilation as a surrogate for diagnosing the onset of abdominal compartment syndrome (ACS) in severely burned patients (TIRIFIC-study Part II). *Burns* **2020**, *46*, 1320–1327. [CrossRef] [PubMed]
16. Kirkpatrick, A.W.; Ball, C.G.; Nickerson, D.; D'Amours, S.K. Intraabdominal hypertension and the abdominal compartment syndrome in burn patients. *World J. Surg.* **2009**, *33*, 1142–1149. [CrossRef] [PubMed]
17. Kirkpatrick, A.W.; Roberts, D.J.; De Waele, J.; Jaeschke, R.; Malbrain, M.L.; De Keulenaer, B.; Duchesne, J.; Bjorck, M.; Leppaniemi, A.; Ejike, J.C.; et al. Intra-abdominal hypertension and the abdominal compartment syndrome: Updated consensus definitions and clinical practice guidelines from the World Society of the Abdominal Compartment Syndrome. *Intensive Care Med.* **2013**, *39*, 1190–1206. [CrossRef]
18. Kaups, K.L.; Davis, J.W.; Dominic, W.J. Base deficit as an indicator or resuscitation needs in patients with burn injuries. *J. Burn Care Rehabil.* **1998**, *19*, 346–348. [CrossRef] [PubMed]

19. Ivy, M.E.; Atweh, N.A.; Palmer, J.; Possenti, P.P.; Pineau, M.; D'Aiuto, M. Intra-abdominal hypertension and abdominal compartment syndrome in burn patients. *J. Trauma Acute Care Surg.* **2000**, *49*, 387–391. [CrossRef]
20. Cartotto, R.C.; Innes, M.; Musgrave, M.A.; Gomez, M.; Cooper, A.B. How well does the Parkland formula estimate actual fluid resuscitation volumes? *J. Burn Care Rehabil.* **2002**, *23*, 258–265. [CrossRef]
21. Pham, T.N.; Cancio, L.C.; Gibran, N.S.; American Burn, A. American Burn Association practice guidelines burn shock resuscitation. *J. Burn Care Res.* **2008**, *29*, 257–266. [CrossRef]
22. Dries, D.J.; Waxman, K. Adequate resuscitation of burn patients may not be measured by urine output and vital signs. *Crit. Care Med.* **1991**, *19*, 327–329. [CrossRef]
23. Saffle, J.I. The phenomenon of "fluid creep" in acute burn resuscitation. *J. Burn Care Res.* **2007**, *28*, 382–395. [CrossRef] [PubMed]
24. Cartotto, R.; Zhou, A. Fluid creep: The pendulum hasn't swung back yet! *J. Burn Care Res.* **2010**, *31*, 551–558. [CrossRef] [PubMed]
25. Cartotto, R.; Choi, J.; Gomez, M.; Cooper, A. A prospective study on the implications of a base deficit during fluid resuscitation. *J. Burn Care Rehabil.* **2003**, *24*, 75–84. [CrossRef] [PubMed]
26. Bellomo, R.; Uchino, S. Cardiovascular monitoring tools: Use and misuse. *Curr. Opin. Crit. Care* **2003**, *9*, 225–229. [CrossRef] [PubMed]
27. Kumar, A.; Anel, R.; Bunnell, E.; Habet, K.; Zanotti, S.; Marshall, S.; Neumann, A.; Ali, A.; Cheang, M.; Kavinsky, C.; et al. Pulmonary artery occlusion pressure and central venous pressure fail to predict ventricular filling volume, cardiac performance, or the response to volume infusion in normal subjects. *Crit. Care Med.* **2004**, *32*, 691–699. [CrossRef] [PubMed]
28. Marik, P.E.; Cavallazzi, R. Does the central venous pressure predict fluid responsiveness? An updated meta-analysis and a plea for some common sense. *Crit. Care Med.* **2013**, *41*, 1774–1781. [CrossRef] [PubMed]
29. Barbier, C.; Loubieres, Y.; Schmit, C.; Hayon, J.; Ricome, J.L.; Jardin, F.; Vieillard-Baron, A. Respiratory changes in inferior vena cava diameter are helpful in predicting fluid responsiveness in ventilated septic patients. *Intensive Care Med.* **2004**, *30*, 1740–1746. [CrossRef] [PubMed]
30. Marik, P.E.; Monnet, X.; Teboul, J.L. Hemodynamic parameters to guide fluid therapy. *Ann. Intensive Care* **2011**, *1*, 1. [CrossRef] [PubMed]
31. Sakka, S.G.; Bredle, D.L.; Reinhart, K.; Meier-Hellmann, A. Comparison between intrathoracic blood volume and cardiac filling pressures in the early phase of hemodynamic instability of patients with sepsis or septic shock. *J. Crit. Care* **1999**, *14*, 78–83. [CrossRef]
32. Branski, L.K.; Herndon, D.N.; Byrd, J.F.; Kinsky, M.P.; Lee, J.O.; Fagan, S.P.; Jeschke, M.G. Transpulmonary thermodilution for hemodynamic measurements in severely burned children. *Crit. Care* **2011**, *15*, R118. [CrossRef] [PubMed]
33. Mitchell, J.P.; Schuller, D.; Calandrino, F.S.; Schuster, D.P. Improved outcome based on fluid management in critically ill patients requiring pulmonary artery catheterization. *Am. Rev. Respir. Dis.* **1992**, *145*, 990–998. [CrossRef] [PubMed]
34. Holm, C.; Melcer, B.; Horbrand, F.; Worl, H.; von Donnersmarck, G.H.; Muhlbauer, W. Intrathoracic blood volume as an end point in resuscitation of the severely burned: An observational study of 24 patients. *J. Trauma Acute Care Surg.* **2000**, *48*, 728–734. [CrossRef] [PubMed]
35. Holm, C.; Mayr, M.; Tegeler, J.; Horbrand, F.; Henckel von Donnersmarck, G.; Muhlbauer, W.; Pfeiffer, U.J. A clinical randomized study on the effects of invasive monitoring on burn shock resuscitation. *Burns* **2004**, *30*, 798–807. [CrossRef] [PubMed]
36. Csontos, C.; Foldi, V.; Fischer, T.; Bogar, L. Arterial thermodilution in burn patients suggests a more rapid fluid administration during early resuscitation. *Acta. Anaesthesiol. Scand.* **2008**, *52*, 742–749. [CrossRef] [PubMed]
37. Aboelatta, Y.; Abdelsalam, A. Volume overload of fluid resuscitation in acutely burned patients using transpulmonary thermodilution technique. *J. Burn Care Res.* **2013**, *34*, 349–354. [CrossRef]
38. Guilabert, P.; Usua, G.; Martin, N.; Abarca, L.; Barret, J.P.; Colomina, M.J. Fluid resuscitation management in patients with burns: Update. *Br. J. Anaesth.* **2016**, *117*, 284–296. [CrossRef]
39. Arlati, S.; Storti, E.; Pradella, V.; Bucci, L.; Vitolo, A.; Pulici, M. Decreased fluid volume to reduce organ damage: A new approach to burn shock resuscitation? A preliminary study. *Resuscitation* **2007**, *72*, 371–378. [CrossRef] [PubMed]
40. Sanchez, M.; Garcia-de-Lorenzo, A.; Herrero, E.; Lopez, T.; Galvan, B.; Asensio, M.; Cachafeiro, L.; Casado, C. A protocol for resuscitation of severe burn patients guided by transpulmonary thermodilution and lactate levels: A 3-year prospective cohort study. *Crit. Care* **2013**, *17*, R176. [CrossRef] [PubMed]
41. Jeschke, M.G.; Peck, M.D. Burn Care of the Elderly. *J. Burn Care Res.* **2017**, *38*, e625–e628. [CrossRef] [PubMed]
42. Patterson, S.W.; Starling, E.H. On the mechanical factors which determine the output of the ventricles. *J. Physiol.* **1914**, *48*, 357–379. [CrossRef] [PubMed]
43. Zhang, Z.; Lu, B.; Sheng, X.; Jin, N. Accuracy of stroke volume variation in predicting fluid responsiveness: A systematic review and meta-analysis. *J. Anesth.* **2011**, *25*, 904–916. [CrossRef] [PubMed]
44. Hofer, C.K.; Muller, S.M.; Furrer, L.; Klaghofer, R.; Genoni, M.; Zollinger, A. Stroke volume and pulse pressure variation for prediction of fluid responsiveness in patients undergoing off-pump coronary artery bypass grafting. *Chest* **2005**, *128*, 848–854. [CrossRef] [PubMed]
45. Daihua, Y.; Wei, C.; Xude, S.; Linong, Y.; Changjun, G.; Hui, Z. The effect of body position changes on stroke volume variation in 66 mechanically ventilated patients with sepsis. *J. Crit. Care* **2012**, *27*, 416–417. [CrossRef]
46. Slama, M.; Maizel, J. Pulse Pressure Variations in Acute Respiratory Distress Syndrome: "Fifty Shades of Grey". *Crit. Care Med.* **2016**, *44*, 452–453. [CrossRef]

47. Lee, L.; DeCara, J.M. Point-of-Care Ultrasound. *Curr. Cardiol. Rep.* **2020**, *22*, 149. [CrossRef] [PubMed]
48. Feissel, M.; Michard, F.; Faller, J.P.; Teboul, J.L. The respiratory variation in inferior vena cava diameter as a guide to fluid therapy. *Intensive Care Med.* **2004**, *30*, 1834–1837. [CrossRef] [PubMed]
49. Gignon, L.; Roger, C.; Bastide, S.; Alonso, S.; Zieleskiewicz, L.; Quintard, H.; Zoric, L.; Bobbia, X.; Raux, M.; Leone, M.; et al. Influence of Diaphragmatic Motion on Inferior Vena Cava Diameter Respiratory Variations in Healthy Volunteers. *Anesthesiology* **2016**, *124*, 1338–1346. [CrossRef]
50. Zhang, Z.; Xu, X.; Ye, S.; Xu, L. Ultrasonographic measurement of the respiratory variation in the inferior vena cava diameter is predictive of fluid responsiveness in critically ill patients: Systematic review and meta-analysis. *Ultrasound Med. Biol.* **2014**, *40*, 845–853. [CrossRef] [PubMed]
51. Spencer, K.T.; Kimura, B.J.; Korcarz, C.E.; Pellikka, P.A.; Rahko, P.S.; Siegel, R.J. Focused cardiac ultrasound: Recommendations from the American Society of Echocardiography. *J. Am. Soc. Echocardiogr.* **2013**, *26*, 567–581. [CrossRef] [PubMed]
52. Porter, T.R.; Shillcutt, S.K.; Adams, M.S.; Desjardins, G.; Glas, K.E.; Olson, J.J.; Troughton, R.W. Guidelines for the use of echocardiography as a monitor for therapeutic intervention in adults: A report from the American Society of Echocardiography. *J. Am. Soc. Echocardiogr.* **2015**, *28*, 40–56. [CrossRef] [PubMed]
53. Orde, S.; Slama, M.; Hilton, A.; Yastrebov, K.; McLean, A. Pearls and pitfalls in comprehensive critical care echocardiography. *Crit. Care* **2017**, *21*, 279. [CrossRef] [PubMed]
54. Boyd, J.H.; Sirounis, D.; Maizel, J.; Slama, M. Echocardiography as a guide for fluid management. *Crit. Care* **2016**, *20*, 274. [CrossRef] [PubMed]
55. Marik, P.E.; Cavallazzi, R.; Vasu, T.; Hirani, A. Dynamic changes in arterial waveform derived variables and fluid responsiveness in mechanically ventilated patients: A systematic review of the literature. *Crit. Care Med.* **2009**, *37*, 2642–2647. [CrossRef] [PubMed]
56. Miller, A.; Mandeville, J. Predicting and measuring fluid responsiveness with echocardiography. *Echo. Res. Pract.* **2016**, *3*, G1–G12. [CrossRef]
57. Muller, L.; Toumi, M.; Bousquet, P.J.; Riu-Poulenc, B.; Louart, G.; Candela, D.; Zoric, L.; Suehs, C.; de La Coussaye, J.E.; Molinari, N.; et al. An increase in aortic blood flow after an infusion of 100 mL colloid over 1 min can predict fluid responsiveness: The mini-fluid challenge study. *Anesthesiology* **2011**, *115*, 541–547. [CrossRef]
58. Cherpanath, T.G.; Hirsch, A.; Geerts, B.F.; Lagrand, W.K.; Leeflang, M.M.; Schultz, M.J.; Groeneveld, A.B. Predicting Fluid Responsiveness by Passive Leg Raising: A Systematic Review and Meta-Analysis of 23 Clinical Trials. *Crit. Care Med.* **2016**, *44*, 981–991. [CrossRef]

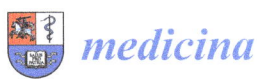

Review

The History of Carbon Monoxide Intoxication

Ioannis-Fivos Megas [1], Justus P. Beier [2] and Gerrit Grieb [1,2,*]

1. Department of Plastic Surgery and Hand Surgery, Gemeinschaftskrankenhaus Havelhoehe, Kladower Damm 221, 14089 Berlin, Germany; fivos.megas@gmail.com
2. Burn Center, Department of Plastic Surgery and Hand Surgery, University Hospital RWTH Aachen, Pauwelsstrasse 30, 52074 Aachen, Germany; jbeier@ukaachen.de
* Correspondence: gerritgrieb@gmx.de

Abstract: Intoxication with carbon monoxide in organisms needing oxygen has probably existed on Earth as long as fire and its smoke. What was observed in antiquity and the Middle Ages, and usually ended fatally, was first successfully treated in the last century. Since then, diagnostics and treatments have undergone exciting developments, in particular specific treatments such as hyperbaric oxygen therapy. In this review, different historic aspects of the etiology, diagnosis and treatment of carbon monoxide intoxication are described and discussed.

Keywords: carbon monoxide; CO intoxication; COHb; inhalation injury

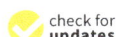

Citation: Megas, I.-F.; Beier, J.P.; Grieb, G. The History of Carbon Monoxide Intoxication. *Medicina* **2021**, *57*, 400. https://doi.org/10.3390/medicina57050400

Academic Editors: Lars P. Kamolz and Bernd Hartmann

Received: 24 March 2021
Accepted: 19 April 2021
Published: 21 April 2021

Publisher's Note: MDPI stays neutral with regard to jurisdictional claims in published maps and institutional affiliations.

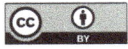

Copyright: © 2021 by the authors. Licensee MDPI, Basel, Switzerland. This article is an open access article distributed under the terms and conditions of the Creative Commons Attribution (CC BY) license (https://creativecommons.org/licenses/by/4.0/).

1. Introduction and Overview

Intoxication with carbon monoxide in organisms needing oxygen for survival has probably existed on Earth as long as fire and its smoke. Whenever the respiratory tract of living beings comes into contact with the smoke from a flame, CO intoxication and/or inhalation injury may take place. Although the therapeutic potential of carbon monoxide has also been increasingly studied in recent history [1], the toxic effects historically dominate a much longer period of time.

As a colorless, odorless and tasteless gas, CO is produced by the incomplete combustion of hydrocarbons and poses an invisible danger. CO enters the human body through the inhalation of flue gases and can cause tissue hypoxia due to its affinity for the hemoglobin molecule, i.e., about 240 times higher than that of oxygen [2]. The oxygen is replaced and carboxyhemoglobin (COHb) is formed [3]. Organs that have a high oxygen demand and thus depend on high blood flow can be severely affected [4]. For example, due to its affinity for myoglobin, which is also 60 times greater than that of oxygen, the replacement of oxygen leads to cardiac depression and hypotension [5]. The exact pathophysiological mechanism is not yet fully understood. However, the toxic effect is attributed to the binding of CO to cytochrome oxidase and the inhibition of the electron transport chain [6].

Intoxication with CO causes thousands of deaths each year, as shown by a large number of the most recent studies published to date [7–9]. A brief overview of symptoms caused by CO poisoning includes nausea (40%), headache (46%), dyspnea (20%) and tachycardia (41%). Many patients also complain of dizziness and vomiting [9,10].

The diagnosis of CO intoxication involves several parameters. The basis is the measurement of the percentage of COHb, which can be detected by arterial blood gas examination. Alternatively, non-invasive CO-oximetry can be performed, especially in a preclinical setting [11]. Using these techniques, highly elevated values can be measured that differ greatly from the normal ratio of carboxyhemoglobin to hemoglobin of 2–3% in non-smokers and 5-9% in smokers [12]. However, this basic diagnosis must be supported, especially in severe cases, by further investigations such as thorough clinical examination, different laboratory markers and radiological diagnostics [13–15].

2. Literature Research

The literature search for this review was conducted with PubMed and Google Scholar using the following keywords: "carbon monoxide intoxication history", "inhalation injury history" and "burns history". In addition, we cross-checked reference lists from eligible publications and relevant review articles to identify additional studies. Our search in the relevant literature revealed 38 PubMed entries up to the year 1945, about 1850 entries from 1946 to 1975, about 2035 entries from 1976 to 2000 and the current literature from 2001 to 2020 has about 2564 entries. A time bar of the available publications on PubMed is shown in Figure 1.

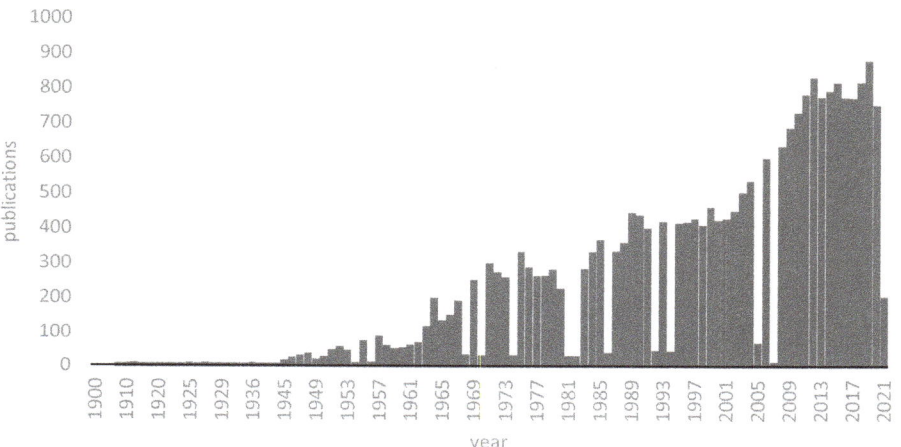

Figure 1. A time bar of the publications on Co intoxication available on PubMed across time.

Further, the search in PubMed revealed that there are some publications concerning the reproduction of burn medicine in antiquity [16,17] but none dealing specifically with CO intoxication. This, however, could be observed for the first time in the early 20th century [18].

3. 1900 to 1945

A total of 38 PubMed entries dealing with CO intoxications could be found in the period up to 1945. The first published article from 1906 involved animal experiments. The authors Nasmith and Graham investigated the hematology of carbon monoxide poisoning [18]. The methodology of their experiments is described in the following paragraph:

Twelve guinea pigs were taken, six males and six females, and placed in two cages in the gas chamber after making careful estimations of the white and red blood corpuscles and haemoglobin. Gas was then allowed to mix with the air drawn through the chamber until the mixture was of such a strength that 250/0 of the haemoglobin of the guinea-pigs was saturated with carbon monoxide.

The authors discovered that carbon monoxide prevents the normal supply of oxygen to the tissue and thus disrupts the metabolism of cells. They concluded a massive toxic effect of CO. The guinea pigs that lived constantly in a diluted carbon monoxide atmosphere during this experiment showed a reduced oxygen transport capacity of the blood. However, their organisms were able to compensate for the lack of oxygen by increasing the hemoglobin concentration and the number of erythrocytes. Furthermore, they found that the effect of carbon monoxide on increasing the number of erythrocytes was similar to the effect of high altitudes [18].

Another article from this period described the problems of military mining in cases when explosive charges do not detonate completely and continue to burn. Thus, very highly concentrated CO vapors were produced, which could have devastating consequences in a narrow mine [19]. The symptoms of CO intoxication were described for the first time in humans. The medical term used here for the clinical picture is "gassing". In addition, this article also describes the first therapeutic approaches for CO intoxication [19].

Treatment is summed up in warmth, oxygen, artificial respiration, rest. Circulatory stimulants, such as hot coffee, are valuable. Strychnine has been found useful for stimulating the respiratory centre, but chief reliance is to be placed upon artificial respiration by Schäfer's method [20], combined with the administration of oxygen [19].

Of course, some of these therapeutic approaches are outdated nowadays, but the central aspect of the therapy of CO intoxication was already recognized at that time, namely the administration of highly concentrated oxygen [19].

4. 1945 to 1980

During this time, due to industrial innovations such as the switch from coal to natural gas for the domestic supply, the number of CO intoxications began to decrease [21]. Apart from this aspect, this may also have been due to a growing number of alternative methods to commit suicide, in particular by using tranquilizers and antidepressants developed at that time [21]. However, cases of CO intoxication were still associated with high morbidity and mortality, resulting in more research into therapeutic options during this period. One of these new therapeutic methods was hyperbaric oxygen therapy (HBO), which will be discussed in a separate section due to its great importance [22,23]. Diagnostics also expanded in the 1970s, with the first devices, such as the Dräger test tube, that could accurately measure CO concentrations in exhaled breath [24]. This was certainly a significant innovation pre-clinically and in emergency situations. The initial clinical algorithm in 1970 is very similar to that used today.

In selecting a form of therapy there are two aspects to consider: firstly, the prevention of death and, secondly, the reduction of neuropsychiatric sequelae such as those described by H. Garland and J. Pearce. Carboxyhaemoglobin should be eliminated as quickly as possible because its presence alters the dissociation curve of the remaining oxyhaemoglobin, impeding oxygen release to the tissues [21].

Furthermore, it was first observed that long-term psychiatric sequelae could occur after CO intoxication. A follow-up study of 74 patients by Smith et al. in 1973 showed that the state of consciousness upon admission to hospital in the acute phase of poisoning correlated significantly with the development of severe neuropsychiatric sequelae. These findings underpin the importance of prompt and effective treatment of carbon monoxide poisoning and the need to follow up all clinical cases in anticipation of a recurrent course or the development of sequelae [25].

Nevertheless, Barret et al. indicated that, during this time, CO intoxications were often overlooked [2]. They conducted a trial in Grenoble, France, to determine the true incidence of missed or misdiagnosed CO intoxications. Misdiagnoses were unusually high, resulting in the launch of a public information campaign. The initial high rate of misdiagnosis (30% in 1975–1977) declined after the campaign (12% in 1978 and 5% in 1980), although the rate of hospitalization for confirmed CO poisoning increased substantially [2].

5. From 1980 to Present

Today, it is known that immediate intervention in CO intoxication is crucial. Triage and transfer to specialized hospitals as soon as possible after stabilization of the patient's cardiopulmonary status are essential. For this purpose, vital parameters such as heart rate, blood pressure and percutaneous oxygen/CO-saturation are continuously monitored. In case of respiratory insufficiency, immediate intubation and ventilation with 100% O_2 are required until further therapy can be initiated in an intensive care unit [9,12]. As described above, the administration of highly concentrated oxygen in the prehospital setting is essential in cases of suspected CO intoxication [26,27]. The Glasgow Coma Scale (GCS) is the most suitable way to immediately assess the neurological status of the patient [9,28]. These algorithms have existed since and even before the 1990s and have not changed much since then [26].

Innovations in recent years that have contributed significantly to the improvement of therapeutic options for patients with CO intoxication and inhalation trauma include the improvement of ventilation of intensive care patients. For example, it was shown that the use of lower tidal volumes (TVs) when ventilating patients with acute lung injury and acute respiratory distress syndrome reduces mortality in these patients by 22% [29]. The corresponding study was discontinued, as mortality in the group treated with lower tidal volumes was highly significantly lower than that of the group treated with high tidal volumes [29]. New standards like this were also adopted for the treatment of CO intoxication.

Furthermore, the long-term effects, such as inflammatory changes in the airway, are nowadays closely scrutinized in order to further reduce morbidity and mortality after CO intoxication [30].

6. History of Hyperbaric Oxygen Therapy for CO Intoxication

The first hyperbaric oxygen (HBO) chamber applied for medical purposes was described in 1622 [31]. In the 19th century, HBO chambers were used for the therapy of diseases such as tuberculosis, anemia and cholera [31]. Today, HBO chambers are also very promising in experimental settings, such as, e.g., conditioning cells for tissue engineering [32]. However, in the late 19th century, the first application of an HBO chamber was used in connection with CO intoxication. In 1895, Haldane could not poison a mouse in a chamber with a high oxygen concentration and a low CO concentration [33].

The chief aim of the present investigation has been to determine experimentally the causes of the symptoms produced in man by carbonicoxide, and particularly the relation of the changes in the blood to the symptoms, to the percentage of carbonic oxide breathed, and to the period during which the inhalation is continued [33].

It took several years for the idea of using HBO in CO intoxication to be revived. Smith et al. and Churchill-Davidson et al. first described the benefits of HBO therapy in CO intoxicated patients [34]. Since then, HBO therapy has remained a controversial topic and a definite recommendation cannot be made, as Buckley et al. show in their systematic review [35]. The first major studies concerning this topic were performed in the 1980s. A clinical trial by Raphael et al. compared the use of normobaric oxygen (NBO) with HBO. The results of this study showed that HBO therapy was not beneficial in patients who did not lose consciousness during carbon monoxide intoxication, regardless of their carboxyhemoglobin level. In this study, neither a positive effect nor a negative effect of HBO therapy could be demonstrated [36].

Further large randomized trials followed in the 1990s. Scheinkestel et al. showed that, in comparison with NBO, HBO therapy had no benefits and may have even worsened the outcome and was therefore not recommended by the authors [37]. Another randomized controlled trial with 179 patients by Annane et al. in 2011 also showed critical results regarding HBO therapy. No evidence of superiority of HBO over NBO in patients with a transient loss of consciousness could be shown. Furthermore, a second HBO session in comatose patients was associated with a worse outcome [38].

In contrast to these results, other studies have shown that a large majority of patients benefit from hyperbaric oxygen therapy by effectively minimizing late neurological sequelae as well as the development of brain edema and pathological changes to the central nervous system [39–41]. In 2002, Weaver et al. published a double-blind, randomized trial in the New England Journal of Medicine. In this study, NBO was compared with HBO therapy with respect to cognitive sequelae after acute carbon monoxide poisoning. The results showed that, six weeks after CO poisoning, neurological pathologies detected by neuropsychological testing were significantly less frequent in the HBO group (25 vs. 46.1%; $p = 0.007$) [42].

Currently, there are only a few national and no international guidelines on how to treat CO intoxication. For example, according to the "Clinical Guidance for Carbon Monoxide (CO) Poisoning", as published by the U.S. CDC (The Centers for Disease Control and Prevention), HBO therapy shall *"be considered when the patient has a COHgb level of more than 25–30%, there is evidence of cardiac involvement, severe acidosis, transient or prolonged unconsciousness, neurological impairment, abnormal neuropsychiatric testing, or the patient is ≥36 years in age. HBO is also administered at lower COHgb (<25%) levels if suggested by clinical condition and/history of exposure"* [43].

According to the recommendations of the U.K. Department of Health and the NHS England, a *"COHb concentration of >20% should be an indication to consider hyperbaric oxygen and the decision should be taken on the basis of specific indications, i.e., loss of consciousness at any stage, neurological signs or symptoms other than headache, myocardial ischaemia/arrhythmia diagnosed by ECG, or pregnancy"* [44,45].

In Germany, a national guideline is currently under development under the auspices of the DIVI (German Interdisciplinary Association for Intensive Care and Emergency Medicine) which shall be finished and published soon (May 2021) [46].

In summary, a common opinion nowadays seems to be that routine HBO treatment cannot be recommended in general, but may be beneficial in patients with severe intoxication [35].

7. Conclusions

CO intoxication can occur in all living beings and has been a problem since fire and its vapors have existed on Earth. The etiology, diagnosis and specific treatment for CO intoxications have been studied very carefully over the years. Recovery, healing and therapeutic strategies of affected patients have been developed only in the 20th century and have been refined since then. As the controversial debate of HBO therapy shows, the destination of this journey has not been reached even today.

Author Contributions: Conceptualization: I.-F.M. and G.G.; methodology: I.-F.M., J.P.B. and G.G.; validation: J.P.B. and G.G.; formal analysis I.-F.M., J.P.B. and G.G.; investigation, I.-F.M., J.P.B. and G.G.; resources, I.-F.M., J.P.B. and G.G.; writing—original draft preparation: I.-F.M.; writing—reviewing and editing: I.-F.M., J.P.B. and G.G.; supervision: J.P.B. and G.G.; project administration: G.G.; All authors have read and agreed to the published version of the manuscript.

Funding: This research received no external funding.

Institutional Review Board Statement: Not applicable.

Informed Consent Statement: Not applicable.

Data Availability Statement: Not applicable.

Conflicts of Interest: The authors declare no conflict of interest.

References

1. Kim, H.-H.; Choi, S. Therapeutic Aspects of Carbon Monoxide in Cardiovascular Disease. *Int. J. Mol. Sci.* **2018**, *19*, 2381. [CrossRef] [PubMed]
2. Barret, L.; Danel, V.; Faure, J. Carbon Monoxide Poisoning, a Diagnosis Frequently Overlooked. *J. Toxicol. Clin. Toxicol.* **1985**, *23*, 309–313. [CrossRef]
3. Silver, S.; Smith, C.; Worster, A.; BEEM (Best Evidence in Emergency Medicine) Team. Should hyperbaric oxygen be used for carbon monoxide poisoning? *CJEM* **2006**, *8*, 43–46. [CrossRef]
4. Llano, A.L.; Raffin, T.A.; Ilano, A.L. Management of Carbon Monoxide Poisoning. *Chest* **1990**, *97*, 165–169. [CrossRef]
5. Jaffe, F.A. Pathogenicity of Carbon Monoxide. *Am. J. Forensic Med. Pathol.* **1997**, *18*, 406–410. [CrossRef] [PubMed]
6. Goldbaum, L.R.; Ramirez, R.G.; Absalon, K.B. What is the mechanism of carbon monoxide toxicity? *Aviat. Space Environ. Med.* **1975**, *46*, 1289–1291.
7. Hampson, N.B. Emergency department visits for carbon monoxide poisoning in the Pacific Northwest. *J. Emerg. Med.* **1998**, *16*, 695–698. [CrossRef]

8. Thom, S.R. Hyperbaric-oxygen therapy for acute carbon monoxide poisoning. *N. Engl. J. Med.* **2002**, *347*, 1105–1106. [CrossRef]
9. Grieb, G.; Simons, D.; Schmitz, L.; Piatkowski, A.; Grottke, O.; Pallua, N. Glasgow Coma Scale and laboratory markers are superi-or to COHb in predicting CO intoxication severity. *Burns* **2011**, *37*, 610–615. [CrossRef]
10. Garland, H.; Pearce, J. Neurological complications of carbon monoxide poisoning. *Q. J. Med.* **1967**, *36*, 445–455.
11. Piatkowski, A.; Ulrich, D.; Grieb, G.C.; Pallua, N. A new tool for the early diagnosis of carbon monoxide intoxication. *Inhal. Toxicol.* **2009**, *21*, 1144–1147. [CrossRef] [PubMed]
12. Schimmel, J.; George, N.; Schwarz, J.; Yousif, S.; Suner, S.; Hack, J.B. Carboxyhemoglobin Levels Induced by Cigarette Smoking Outdoors in Smokers. *J. Med. Toxicol.* **2018**, *14*, 68–73. [CrossRef]
13. Buehler, J.H.; Berns, A.S.; Webster, J.R.; Addington, W.W.; Cugell, D.W. Lactic acidosis from carboxyhemoglobinemia after smoke inhalation. *Ann. Intern. Med.* **1975**, *82*, 803–805. [CrossRef] [PubMed]
14. Sokal, J.A. The effect of exposure duration on the blood level of glucose, pyruvate and lactate in acute carbon monoxide in-toxication in man. *J. Appl. Toxicol.* **1985**, *5*, 395–397. [CrossRef]
15. Sokal, J.A.; Kralkowska, E. The relationship between exposure duration, carboxyhemoglobin, blood glucose, pyruvate and lactate and the severity of intoxication in 39 cases of acute carbon monoxide poisoning in man. *Arch. Toxicol.* **1985**, *57*, 196–199. [CrossRef] [PubMed]
16. Wallner, C.; Moormann, E.; Lulof, P.; Drysch, M.; Lehnhardt, M.; Behr, B. Burn Care in the Greek and Roman Antiquity. *Medicina* **2020**, *56*, 657. [CrossRef] [PubMed]
17. Moiemen, N.S.; Lee, K.C.; Joory, K. History of burns: The past, present and the future. *Burn. Trauma* **2014**, *2*, 169–180. [CrossRef] [PubMed]
18. Nasmith, G.G.; Graham, D.A.L. The haematology of carbon-monoxide poisoning. *J. Physiol.* **1906**, *35*, 32–52. [CrossRef]
19. Gas in Military Mines: The Symptoms of Carbon Monoxide Poisoning. *Hospital* **1916**, *60*, 169.
20. Schäfer, E.A. Description of a Simple and Efficient Method of Performing Artificial Respiration in the Human Subject, espe-cially in Cases of Drowning; to which is appended Instructions for the Treatment of the Apparently Drowned. *Med. Chir. Trans.* **1904**, *87*, 609–623.
21. Carbon monoxide poisoning. *Br. Med. J.* **1970**, *3*, 180. [CrossRef]
22. Smith, G.; Ledingham, I.; Sharp, G.; Norman, J.; Bates, E. Treatment of coal-gas poisoning with oxygen at 2 atmospheres pressure. *Lancet* **1962**, *279*, 816–819. [CrossRef]
23. Lawson, D.D.; Mcallister, R.A.; Smith, G. Treatment of acute experimental carbon-monoxide poisoning with oxygen under pressure. *Lancet* **1961**, *1*, 800–802. [CrossRef]
24. Davis, N. Carbon monoxide poisoning. *Br. Med. J.* **1979**, *2*, 1584. [CrossRef]
25. Smith, J.S.; Brandon, S. Morbidity from Acute Carbon Monoxide Poisoning at Three-year Follow-up. *BMJ* **1973**, *1*, 318–321. [CrossRef]
26. Ernst, A.; Zibrak, J.D. Carbon monoxide poisoning. *N. Engl. J. Med.* **1998**, *339*, 1603–1608. [CrossRef]
27. Weaver, L.K.; Howe, S.; Hopkins, R.; Chan, K.J. Carboxyhemoglobin half-life in carbon monoxide-poisoned patients treated with 100% oxygen at atmospheric pressure. *Chest* **2000**, *117*, 801–808. [CrossRef]
28. Weaver, L.K. Clinical practice. Carbon monoxide poisoning. *N. Engl. J. Med.* **2009**, *360*, 1217–1225. [CrossRef] [PubMed]
29. Acute Respiratory Distress Syndrome Network; Brower, R.G.; Matthay, M.A.; Morris, A.; Schoenfeld, D.; Thompson, B.T.; Wheeler, A. Ventilation with lower tidal volumes as compared with traditional tidal volumes for acute lung injury and the acute respiratory distress syndrome. *N. Engl. J. Med.* **2000**, *342*, 1301–1308. [PubMed]
30. Park, G.Y.; Park, J.W.; Jeong, D.H.; Jeong, S.H. Prolonged airway and systemic inflammatory reactions after smoke inhalation. *Chest* **2003**, *123*, 475–480. [CrossRef] [PubMed]
31. Danesh-Sani, S.A.; Shariati-Sarabi, Z.; Feiz, M.R. Comprehensive Review of Hyperbaric Oxygen Therapy. *J. Craniofacial Surg.* **2012**, *23*, e483–e491. [CrossRef] [PubMed]
32. Yoshinoya, Y.; Böcker, A.H.; Ruhl, T.; Siekmann, U.; Pallua, N.; Beier, J.P.; Kim, B.-S. The Effect of Hyperbaric Oxygen Therapy on Human Adipose-Derived Stem Cells. *Plast. Reconstr. Surg.* **2020**, *146*, 309–320. [CrossRef] [PubMed]
33. Haldane, J. The Action of Carbonic Oxide on Man. *J. Physiol.* **1895**, *18*, 430–462. [CrossRef] [PubMed]
34. Churchill-Davidson, I. Therapeutic uses of hyperbaric oxygen. *Ann. R. Coll. Surg. Engl.* **1966**, *39*, 164–168.
35. Buckley, N.A.; Juurlink, D.N.; Isbister, G.; Bennett, M.H.; Lavonas, E.J. Hyperbaric oxygen for carbon monoxide poisoning. *Cochrane Database Syst. Rev.* **2011**, CD002041. [CrossRef] [PubMed]
36. Raphael, J.C.; Elkharrat, D.; Jars-Guincestre, M.C.; Chastang, C.; Chasles, V.; Vercken, J.B.; Gajdos, P. Trial of normobaric and hyper-baric oxygen for acute carbon monoxide intoxication. *Lancet* **1989**, *2*, 414–419. [CrossRef]
37. Scheinkestel, C.D.; Myles, P.S.; Cooper, D.J.; Millar, I.L.; Tuxen, D.V.; Bailey, M.; Jones, K. Hyperbaric or normobaric oxygen for acute carbon monoxide poisoning: A randomised controlled clinical trial. *Med. J. Aust.* **1999**, *170*, 203–210. [CrossRef]
38. Annane, D.; Chadda, K.; Gajdos, P.; Jars-Guincestre, M.-C.; Chevret, S.; Raphael, J.-C. Hyperbaric oxygen therapy for acute domestic carbon monoxide poisoning: Two randomized controlled trials. *Intensiv. Care Med.* **2010**, *37*, 486–492. [CrossRef]
39. Sinkovic, A.; Smolle-Juettner, F.M.; Krunic, B.; Marinšekz, M. Severe Carbon Monoxide Poisoning Treated by Hyperbaric Oxygen Therapy—A Case Report. *Inhal. Toxicol.* **2006**, *18*, 211–214. [CrossRef]
40. Stoller, K.P. Hyperbaric oxygen and carbon monoxide poisoning: A critical review. *Neurol. Res.* **2007**, *29*, 146–155. [CrossRef]

41. Juurlink, D.N.; Buckley, N.; Stanbrook, M.B.; Isbister, G.; Bennett, M.H.; McGuigan, M. Hyperbaric oxygen for carbon monoxide poisoning. *Cochrane Database Syst. Rev.* **2005**, *24*, 75–92. [CrossRef]
42. Weaver, L.K.; Hopkins, R.O.; Chan, K.J.; Churchill, S.; Elliott, C.G.; Clemmer, T.P.; Orme, J.F.; Thomas, F.O.; Morris, A.H. Hyperbaric oxygen for acute carbon monoxide poisoning. *N. Engl. J. Med.* **2002**, *347*, 1057–1067. [CrossRef] [PubMed]
43. U.S. CDC (The Centers for Disease Control and Prevention): Clinical Guidance for Carbon Monoxide Poisoning | Natural Disasters and Severe Weather. 2020. Available online: https://www.cdc.gov/disasters/co_guidance.html (accessed on 11 March 2021).
44. Mutluoglu, M.; Metin, S.; Arziman, I.; Uzun, G.; Yildiz, S. The use of hyperbaric oxygen therapy for carbon monox-ide poisoning in Europe. *Undersea Hyperb Med.* **2016**, *43*, 49–56. [PubMed]
45. U. K. Department of Health and the NHS England: Carbon Monoxide Poisoning. GOV.UK. Available online: https://www.gov.uk/government/publications/carbon-monoxide-poisoning (accessed on 11 March 2021).
46. DIVI (German Interdisciplinary Association for Intensive Care and Emergency Medicine): AWMF. Available online: https://www.awmf.org/leitlinien/detail/anmeldung/1/ll/040-012.html (accessed on 11 March 2021).

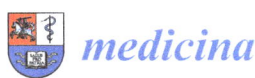

Review

The History and Development of Hyperbaric Oxygenation (HBO) in Thermal Burn Injury

Christian Smolle [1,2], Joerg Lindenmann [1,2,*], Lars Kamolz [1,2] and Freyja-Maria Smolle-Juettner [1,2,*]

[1] Division of Plastic, Aesthetic and Reconstructive Surgery, Division of Thoracic and Hyperbaric Surgery, Medical University Graz, Auenbruggerplatz 29, A-8036 Graz, Austria; christian.smolle@medunigraz.at (C.S.); lars.kamolz@medunigraz.at (L.K.)

[2] Division of Thoracic and Hyperbaric Surgery, Medical University Graz, Auenbruggerplatz 29, A-8036 Graz, Austria

* Correspondence: joerg.lindenmann@medunigraz.at (J.L.); freyja.smolle@medunigraz.at (F.-M.S.-J.)

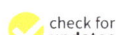

Citation: Smolle, C.; Lindenmann, J.; Kamolz, L.; Smolle-Juettner, F.-M. The History and Development of Hyperbaric Oxygenation (HBO) in Thermal Burn Injury. *Medicina* 2021, 57, 49. https://doi.org/10.3390/medicina57010049

Received: 19 December 2020
Accepted: 4 January 2021
Published: 8 January 2021

Publisher's Note: MDPI stays neutral with regard to jurisdictional claims in published maps and institutional affiliations.

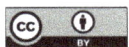

Copyright: © 2021 by the authors. Licensee MDPI, Basel, Switzerland. This article is an open access article distributed under the terms and conditions of the Creative Commons Attribution (CC BY) license (https://creativecommons.org/licenses/by/4.0/).

Abstract: *Background and Objectives:* Hyperbaric oxygenation (HBO) denotes breathing of 100% oxygen under elevated ambient pressure. Since the initiation of HBO for burns in 1965, abundant experimental and clinical work has been done. Despite many undisputedly positive and only a few controversial results on the efficacy of adjunctive HBO for burn injury, the method has not yet been established in clinical routine. *Materials and Methods:* We did a retrospective analysis of the literature according to PRISMA—guidelines, from the very beginning of HBO for burns up to present, trying to elucidate the question why HBO is still sidelined in the treatment of burn injury. *Results:* Forty-seven publications (32 animal experiments, four trials in human volunteers and 11 clinical studies) fulfilled the inclusion criteria. Except four investigators who found little or no beneficial action, all were able to demonstrate positive effects of HBO, most of them describing less edema, improved healing, less infection or bacterial growth and most recently, reduction of post-burn pain. Secondary enlargement of burn was prevented, as microvascular perfusion could be preserved, and cells were kept viable. The application of HBO, however, concerning pressure, duration, frequency and number of treatment sessions, varied considerably. Authors of large clinical studies underscored the intricate measures required when administering HBO in severe burns. *Conclusions:* HBO unquestionably has a positive impact on the pathophysiological mechanisms, and hence on the healing and course of burns. The few negative results are most likely due to peculiarities in the administration of HBO and possibly also to interactions when delivering the treatment to severely ill patients. Well-designed studies are needed to definitively assess its clinical value as an adjunctive treatment focusing on relevant outcome criteria such as wound healing time, complications, length of hospital stay, mortality and scar quality, while also defining optimal HBO dosage and timing.

Keywords: hyperbaric oxygenation; history; review; burn injury

1. Introduction

1.1. History of Hyperbaric Oxygenation

In 1662, Henshaw, a British physician first utilized hyperbaric therapy, placing patients in a steel container that was pressurized with air. Though John Priestly discovered oxygen as soon as 1775, the marginally effective compressed air therapy was only cautiously replaced by breathing of 100% oxygen under increased ambient pressure, thus initiating "hyperbaric oxygenation". The reason for the delay was the fear of side effects based on the work of Lavoisier and Seguin who had suspected toxic effects of highly concentrated oxygen in 1789. It took almost 100 years until in 1878 Paul Bert, who is considered the "father of the hyperbaric physiology", documented the toxic effects of hyperbaric oxygen on the central nervous system that were manifested as seizures [1]. Yet, his findings took time to settle in the hyperbaric medical community. About half a century later in 1937, Behnke and Shaw first used hyperbaric oxygen successfully for the treatment of decompression sickness. In 1955, Churchill-Davidson [2] applied HBO to potentiate the effects of radiation therapy in cancer patients, while at the same time Boerema developed HBO as an adjunct to cardiac surgery, thus prolonging the time for circulatory arrest [3]. Since that time, HBO has been applied for a variety of medical conditions, as the pathophysiological and molecular mechanisms of hyperbaric oxygen treatment were increasingly understood.

1.2. Principle and Mechanisms of Hyperbaric Oxygenation

HBO denotes breathing of 100% oxygen under elevated ambient pressure between 2 and 3 atmospheres absolute (ATA) in a hyperbaric chamber. In direct correlation to the pressure level, oxygen physically dissolves in the plasma increasing arterial pO_2. At a pressure of 2 ATA oxygen dissolves in the plasma resulting in an arterial pO_2 of about 1400 mmHg, which can be further raised to 2000 mmHg at a pressure of 3 ATA. At 3 ATA, the sheer amount of dissolved oxygen obviates the need for erythrocytes for oxygenation [4]. Additionally, tissue oxygen tensions rise in accordance to arterial oxygen pressure and elevated levels may persist for several hours [5]. However, the mechanism of action of HBO is not mere hyper-oxygenation counteracting tissue hypoxia but is based on the fact that hyperbaric oxygen is a highly potent drug.

HBO redistributes blood flow causing vasoconstriction in regions with increased perfusion and vasodilation in hypoxic ones. On the molecular level HBO effectuates preservation of ATP, downregulation of complex molecular cascades involving ß-2 Integrin and pro-inflammatory cytokines, upregulation of anti-inflammatory cytokines and growth factors as well as mobilization of stem cells. Since microorganisms are unable to compensate for the high levels of oxygen, HBO exerts an unspecific antibacterial action. In addition, a reduction in leukocyte chemotaxis and an increase of phagocytosis enhance the efficiency of antibiotic treatment [6–8]. While problems in the middle ear and the nasal sinuses may be encountered during pressurization if there is obstruction due to swelling, side effects of the hyperbaric oxygen (paraesthesia, seizures) are very uncommon, if a pressure of 3 ATA is not exceeded. Even if they occur, they are quickly reversible if hyperbaric oxygen is switched to pressurized air [9].

1.3. HBO in Burn Injury

The use of HBO in burns was based on a serendipitous finding. In 1965, Japan, Wada and Ikeda [10] applied HBO treatment for severe CO intoxication to a group of coal miners who had also sustained second-degree burns during an explosion. In the HBO-treated miners the burns healed remarkably better than in other victims. Since then, HBO for burns has been dealt with in experimental and clinical trials and in numerous reviews [11–16].

When delving into the history of HBO for burn injury reviewing experimental and clinical work, one finds a considerable heterogeneity of study designs, and of injury characteristics such as type, extent, and depth as well as a variety of different species used in experimental settings. Additionally, the dose of HBO deriving from the factors magnitude of pressure, duration of the individual treatment session and total number of sessions varies considerably [17–19], as does the interval between the burn injury and the first HBO session. Since downregulation of mediator cascades is most effective if done as early as possible, this timespan has proved to be a crucial parameter in a variety of other indications [14,20–22].

We established a synopsis about the original animal and human experimental or clinical studies on HBO in burns published since 1965.

2. Materials and Methods

Literature Search and Evaluation

We proceeded according to PRISMA guidelines [23]. For the terms "hyperbaric oxygen" and "burn" dating back to 1965, 314 articles were identified in Pubmed, 15 in Embase advanced and 5 in Cochrane databases. In addition, we found six relevant publications in proceedings of large international hyperbaric meetings. We included only publications the full-text of which was available. We excluded papers not providing sufficient information and redundant work. (For the PRISMA selection process, see Figure 1).

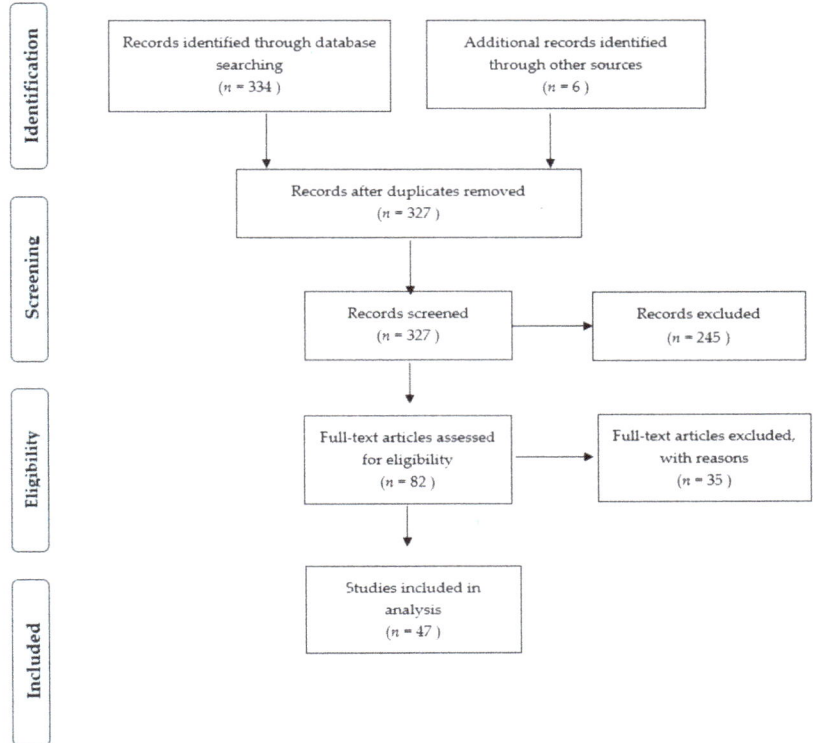

Figure 1. PRISMA selection process.

We evaluated species, number of individuals, type of study, % of total body surface area (TBSA), depth of burn, and pressure applied during HBO. As outcome parameters we documented metabolic effects, edema formation/fluid requirement, inflammation, micro-vessel patency/regrowth, infection, scarring, epithelization, pain, requirement for surgery, morbidity, mortality, duration of in-hospital stay and cost.

For descriptive statistics, each experiment was recorded as a statistical entity.

3. Results
3.1. General Considerations

Forty-seven publications (32 animal studies, four trials in human volunteers and 11 clinical studies or case series) fulfilled the inclusion criteria.

The total number of animals amounted to more than 3000, while there were 58 human volunteers and clinical studies in 2208 patients. Animal experiments were based on complex designs with up to 15 arms. On the contrary, only one out of four human volunteers [13] and two out of 11 clinical studies were prospectively randomized [24,25]. Three volunteer studies [26–28] used a crossover design, three clinical studies included matched pairs [29–31], four non-randomized controls [12,32–34] and two were case series [35,36].

The HBO regimens (pressure in ATA, duration of single session, frequency per day, total number of sessions) differed considerably. In clinical studies the interval between the injury and the first HBO was also inconsistent, and some authors gave no or incomplete information about the abovementioned factors. The same was true for the type of local treatment.

For the details of both experimental and clinical studies see Tables 1 and 2, for the descriptive statistics see Tables 3 and 4.

Table 1. Depth of burns: PT: partial thickness, FT: full thickness, S: superficial; HBO: hyperbaric oxygenation; NBO: normobaric oxygenation; THAM: Tris (hydroxymethyl) aminomethane buffer.

Author/Year	Species	Nr. Individuals	Study Design	% TBSA	Depth of Burn	Local Treatment
Marchal/1966	Rats	187	no burn/HBO: 10			
			burn/untreated: 15; burn/HBO: 15	20	FT	
			7 arm (at least 21 each;) burn/no treatment burn/HBO only burn/saline burn/saline, HBO burn/THAM burn/THAM, HBO (each day) burn/THAM, HBO (every other day)	75	PT	
Nelson/1966	Dogs	24	2 arm; burn/untreated: 12 burn/HBO: 12	75	PT	
Ketchum/1967	Rabbits	26	2 arm; burn/untreated: 13; burn/HBO: 13	5	FT, PT	
Ketchum/1970	Rats	30	2 arm; burn/untreated: 15 burn/HBO: 15	20	FT	
Benichoux/1968	Rats	160	8 arm; no burn/HBO: 10 burn/no treatment: 25 burn/HBO only: 25 burn/saline: 25 burn/saline, HBO: 25 burn/THAM: 25 burn/THAM, HBO every day: 25 burn/THAM, HBO every second day: 25	75	PT	
		200	8 arm; no burn/HBO; burn/THAM; burn/HBO every second day; burn/colmycine, penicilline; burn/THAM, HBO; burn/penicilline, colimycin, HBO; burn/THAM, penicilline, colimycine burn/THAM, penicillin, colimycine, HBO	30	PT	

Table 1. Cont.

Author/Year	Species	Nr. Individuals	Study Design	% TBSA	Depth of Burn	Local Treatment
Perrins/1969	Pigs	8	2 arm; burn/untreated: 4 burn/HBO: 4	12	FT	
		4	2 arm; burn/untreated: 2 burn/HBO: 2	8	PT	
Spinadel/1969	Guinea pigs	99	3 arm; burn/untreated: 33 burn/antibiotics 33 burn/HBO & antibiotics: 33	25	PT	Gentamycin-powder
	Hamsters	75	3 arm; burn/untreated: 25 burn/antibiotics: 25 burn/HBO & antibiotics: 25	25	PT	Gentamycin-powder
Gruber/1970	Rats	24	3 arm; pedicled flap, replanted/HBO: 8 composite skin graft, replanted/HBO: 8; burn/HBO: 8	10	FT	
Bleser/1971	Rats	520	3 arm; no burn/untreated: 20 burn/untreated: 250 burn/HBO, THAM, penicillin, colimycine: 250	32	PT	
Bleser/1973	Rats	100	2 arm; burn/untreated: 50 burn/HBO: 50	5	FT	
Härtwig/1974	Rats	100	2 arm; burn/untreated: 50 burn/HBO: 50	2	FT	
Korn/1977	Guinea pigs	117	Series I: 3 arm; burn/HBO: 52 burn/Hyperbaric normoxia: 27 burn/untreated: 38	5	PT	open/pro-tected
		54	Series II: 2 arm; burn/HBO: 30 burn/untreated: 24	5	PT	open/pro-tected
		40	Series III: 4 arm; no burn/control: 8 no burn/HBO: 8 burn/untreated: 12 burn/HBO: 12	5	PT	open/pro-tected
Niccole/1977	Rats	80	4 arm; burn/untreated: 20 burn/HBO: 20 burn/sliver-sulfadiazine: 20 burn/HBO/silver-sulfadiazine: 20	20	40 PT 40 FT	sulfadiazine (removed before HBO); no dressings

Table 1. Cont.

Author/Year	Species	Nr. Individuals	Study Design	% TBSA	Depth of Burn	Local Treatment
Wells/1977	Dogs	24	3 arm; burn/no fluid: 8 burn/no fluid, NBO: 8 burn/fluid, HBO: 8	40	FT	
Arzinger-Jonasch/1978	Guinea pigs	120	5 arm; burn/HBO: 10	15	PT	
			burn/HBO: 10		FT	
			burn/HBO: 20; necrectomy at various time points		FT	necrectomy
			burn/HBO: 20; necrectomy, full-thickness grafts at various time points		FT	necrectomy/skin graft
			burn/necrectomy, full-thickness grafts at various time time points: 60;		FT	necrectomy/skin graft
Nylander/1984	Mice	54	2 arm; burn/untreated: 27 burn/HBO: 27	6	PT	
Kaiser/1985	Guinea pig	102	5 arm: burn not infected/untreated: 21 burn not infected/HBO: 21 burn infected (pseudomonas)/untreated: 30 burn infected (pseudomonas)/primary HBO: 15 burn infected (pseudomonas)/secondary HBO: 15	5	FT	
Kaiser/1988	Guinea pigs	75	2 arm; burn/untreated: 43 burn/HBO: 32	5	PT	
Stewart/1989	Rats	90	15 arm; no burn/untreated: 6			
			burn/untreated, biopsy at 12 h: 6	5	PT	silver sulfadiazine
			burn/1 HBO, biopsy at 12 h: 6		PT	
			burn/2 HBO, biopsy at 12 h: 6		PT	
			burn/1HBO biopsy at 36 h: 6		PT	
			burn/untreated, biopsy; 5 groups of 6 animals each at 36, 48, 72, 96 or 120 h		PT	
			burn/2 HBO, biopsy; 5 groups of 6 animals each at 36, 48, 72, 96 or 120 h		PT	

Table 1. Cont.

Author/Year	Species	Nr. Individuals	Study Design	% TBSA	Depth of Burn	Local Treatment
Saunders/1989	Guinea pigs	30	2 arm; burn/untreated: 15 burn/HBO: 15 (3 different times of evaluation: 6, 24, 48 h)		PT	
Tenenhaus/1994	Mice	125	5 arm; no burn/fluid, food: 22 burn/fluid, food: 32 burn/fluid, food, compressed air: 15 burn/, fluid, food, NBO: 24 burn/fluid, food, HBO: 32	32	FT	
		139	4 arm; no burn/fluid, no food: 22 burn/fluid, no food: 51 burn/fluid, no food, HBO 2 × 120 min: 57 burn/fluid, no food, HBO 3 × 120 min: 9	32	FT	
Espinosa/1995	Guinea pigs	20	3 arm; burn/untreated: 6 burn/HBO: 7 burn/HBO, antibiotic: 7	10	PT	
Hussmann/1996	Rats	74	11 arm; no burn/untreated: 4	10	FT	
			no burn/anaesthesia, untreated: 7			
			burn/untreated: 7		FT	
			excision of 10% TBSA/suture: 7			excision
			no burn/HBO (acute): 7			
			no burn/HBO (chronical): 7			
			burn/excision after 4 h: 7		FT	excision
			burn/HBO (once): 7		FT	
			burn/HBO (repeated): 7		FT	
			burn/excision after 4 h and HBO (once): 7		FT	excision
			burn/excision after 4 h and HBO (repeated): 7		FT	excision
Germonpré/1996	Rats	46	3 arm; burn/untreated: 10 burn/HBO: 17 burn/Piracetam: 19	5	PT	mafenide gauze; Op-Site
Shoshani/1998	Guinea pigs	54	3 arm; burn/silversulfadiazine: 18 burn/NBO, silversulfadiazine: 18 burn/HBO, silversulfadiazine: 18	5	PT	silver sulfadiazine

Table 1. *Cont.*

Author/Year	Species	Nr. Individuals	Study Design	% TBSA	Depth of Burn	Local Treatment
Akin/2002	Rats	54	7 arm; no burn/liquids: 6 no burn/liquids, HBO (short): 8 no burn/liquids, HBO (long): 8 burn/liquids: 16 burn/liquids, HBO (short): 8 burn/liquids, HBO long): 8	30	PT	
Bilic/2005	Rats	70	2 arm randomized; burn/Hyperbaric normoxia: 35 burn/HBO: 35	20	PT	silver sulfadiazine
Türkaslan/2010	Rats	20	4 arm; burn/untreated (evaluation at 24 h): 5 burn/HBO (evaluation at 24 h): 5 burn/untreated (evaluation on day 5): 5 burn/HBO (evaluation on day 5): 5	5	PT	
Selcuk/2013	Rats	32	4 arm; burn/Nicotine, HBO: 8, burn/Nicotine: 8; burn/no nicotine/HBO: 8; burn/no Nicotine: 8	12	PT, FT	
Wu/2018	Rats	36	6 arm; *sham*-burn/sham HBO: 6 sham burn/HBO: 6 burn/1 week sham HBO: 6 burn/2 week sham HBO:6 burn/1 week HBO: 6 burn/2 weeks HBO: 6	1	FT	silver sulfadiazine
Wu/2019	Rats	30	5 arm; Sham-burn/Sham HBO: 6; sham burn/HBO: 6; burn/1 week sham HBO:6; burn/1 week HBO: 6; burn/2 weeks HBO: 6	1	FT	silver sulfadiazine
Hatibie/2019	Rabbits	36	2 arm; burn/untreated; 18 burn/HBO: 18	1	PT	vaseline
Ikeda/1967	Patients	43	case series	>50	PT, FT	silver nitrate 0,5%
Lamy/1970	Patients	27	case series, historical comparator	20 to >80	PT, FT	
Hart/1974	Patients	191	2 arm double blind randomized; (included in observational 138 burn/HBO: 138 and burn/sham HBO: 53)	10 to 50	PT, FT	silver sulfadiazine

Table 1. Cont.

Author/Year	Species	Nr. Individuals	Study Design	% TBSA	Depth of Burn	Local Treatment
			Group I (HBO: 2; sham HBO: 2)	>10 <20		
			Group II (HBO: 2; sham HBO: 2)	>20 <30		
			Group III (HBO: 2; sham HBO: 2)	>30 <40		
			Group IV (HBO: 2; sham HBO: 2)	<40 <50		
Grossmann/1978	Patients	821	2 arm; nonrandomized controls; burn/routine treatment: 419; burn/routine treatment & HBO: 421	>20 <80	PT, FT	silver sulfadiazine
Waisbren/1982	Patients	72	2 arm: matched pairs; burn/routine treatment: 36; burn/routine treatment & HBO: 36	about 50	PT, FT	
Niu/1987	Patients	835	2 arm; nonrandomized comparator; burn/routine treatment: 609; burn/routine treatment & HBO: 226	any; subgroup severe burns	PT, FT	
Cianci/1989	Patients	20	2 arm: nonrandomized controls burn/routine: 12 (had no access to HBO); burn/routine treatment & HBO: 8	18–39	PT, FT	
Cianci/1990	Patients	21	matched pairs burn/routine treatment: 11; burn/routine treatment & HBO: 10,	19–50 (mean: 30)	PT, FT	
Hammarlund/1991	Volunteers	8	2 arm cross-over at 10-day interval burn/untreated: 8 burn/HBO: 8	<1	PT	polyurethane film or hydrocolloid
Brannen/1997	Patients	125	2 arm matched pairs; burn/routine treatment: 62 burn/routine treatment & HBO: 63	20–50 (mean)	PT, FT	
Niezgoda/1997	Volunteers	12	2 arm randomized; burn/NBO: 6 burn/HBO: 6	<1	PT	hydrocolloid
Chong/2013	Patients	17	2 arm randomized; burn/routine treatment: 9 burn/routine treatment & HBO: 8; non-intubated	<35 (mean: 13)	PT, FT	bio-occlusive dressing

Table 1. Cont.

Author/Year	Species	Nr. Individuals	Study Design	% TBSA	Depth of Burn	Local Treatment
Rasmussen/2015	Volunteers	17	2 arm crossover: burn/HBO–NBO: 17 burn/NBO–HBO: 17	1	S	
Chen/2018	Patients	35	2 arm retrospective case control; burn/routine treatment: 17 burn/routine treatment & HBO: 18	<60	PT, FT	
Wahl/2019	Volunteers	21	2 arm crossover; burn/HBO–NBO: 12 burn/NBO–HBO: 9	1	S	

Table 2. HBO treament features; summarized treatment results.

Author/Year	Interval Burn—HBO (hours)	Pressure (ATA)	Duration min	HBO Frequency/Day	Total Number HBO Sessions	Results in Detail
Marchal/1966		3	60	once a day	21	1 rat died, one convulsed; no weight gain during treatment
		3	60	once a day	28	After day 12 better granulation, faster healing, less infection in HBO
		3	60	once a day or every second day	5 to 10	mortality with daily HBO alone higher than in untreated controls. best survival in THAM with HBO every second day
Nelson/1966	0.1	2	60	once	1	hematocrit drops less after HBO
Ketchum/1967		2	60	four times a day with 1 h in between for 23 days	92	healing time reduced by 30%; reduction in positive cultures by 50%, purulent infection reduced
Ketchum/1970		3	60	four times a day with 1 h in between for 28 days	112	angiography: after day 28 extensive capillary proliferation underneath burn in HBO group; Histology: abundant capillary plexus
Benichoux/1968		3	60	once a day	up to 10	positive effect on mortality in THAM and HBO
		3	60	every second day	up to 15	HBO alone has no effect on burn, may even have adverse effect on survival; in THAM improved survival; longest survival in HBO&THAM& antibiotics
Perrins/1969	2	2	60	four times a day	12	burns in HBO group healed slower than in controls
	2	2	60	four times a day	12	no effect of HBO on healing process, no effect on depth of slough.

Table 2. Cont.

Author/Year	Interval Burn—HBO (hours)	Pressure (ATA)	Duration min	HBO Frequency/Day	Total Number HBO Sessions	Results in Detail
Spinadel/1969		2	75			HBO & antibiotics best results concerning healing; HBO alone and antibiotics alone equal but less good; untreated controls do markedly worse.
		3	120			HBO & antibiotics best results concerning healing; HBO alone and antibiotics alone equal but less good; untreated controls do markedly worse.
Gruber/1970	24	3	45	once every week	3	return of pathologically low oxygen tensions to normal achieved by HBO in flaps, grafts or burns; oxygen levels returning to pretreatment values soon after discontinuing HBO
Bleser/1971	0.1	3	60	every second day	4	rapid restoration of total body water; hematocrit, blood volume, plasma volumein HBO; accerlerated recovery in HBO
Bleser/1973	0.1	3	60	once a day	28	first no effect, but soon better granulation, more rapid healing and less infection with HBO.
Härtwig/1974	0.3	2.5	60	three times a day	84	hardly any edema or inflammation in HBO, hardly any loss of fluid; earlier shedding of eschar; microangiography: rapid revascularization in HBO
Korn/1977	0.5	2	90	twice a day	6, 8 or 10	quicker epithelization, no full-thickness conversion in HBO
	0.5	2	90	twice a day	2, 4, 6, or 8	earlier return of vascular patency in HBO
		2	90	twice a day	8	mitotic activity in epithelia of burnt controls not evaluable due to widespread necrosis
Niccole/1977	12	2.5	90	twice a day	(75?)	no difference concerning edema for either FT or PT; no differences in treatement groups for time to epithelization in PT or to eschar separation in FT; less bacterial colonization in FT after HBO& sulfadiazine and in sulfadiazine alone

Table 2. Cont.

Author/Year	Interval Burn—HBO (hours)	Pressure (ATA)	Duration min	HBO Frequency/Day	Total Number HBO Sessions	Results in Detail
Wells/1977	0.5	2	60	once	1	less reduction in plasma volume in HBO
	0.5	3	60	twice	2	less reduction in plasma volume in HBO; less decline in postburn cardiac output in HBO
Arzinger-Jonasch/1978		2	60 or 120	once a day	10	Time until healing of partial or full-thickness burn shortened by 5 days in HBO. Quick reduction of edema, hardly any thromboses, collateral perfusion in HBO. Take of full-thickness skin graft shortened by 2 days in HBO. Positive effect unrelated to time of exposition.
Nylander/1984	<0.1	2.5	45	once a day	1	less local and general edema formation at 2, 6 and 24 h after burn (fluid content of ear post HBO similar to untreated one).
Kaiser/1985	1 in primary HBO; 192 in secondary HBO	3	60	3 times a day	up to 81 (until closure of wounds)	noninfected wounds in controls healed quicker than noninfected HBO treated wound; infected wounds treated with primary HBO healed quicker than infected controls; infected wounds treated with secondary HBO healed somewhat slower.
Kaiser/1988	1	3	60	3 times a day		Extent of burn increased in controls, not in HBO-group; Rapid reduction of wound surface and less edema only in HBO-group
Stewart/1989						
						consistently higher tissue ATP in HBO; 2 HBO/day better than one
	0.5	2.5	60	once a day	1	
	0.5	2.5	60	twice a day	2	
	0.5	2.5	60	once a day	1	
	0.5	2.5	60	twice a day	2 to 10	36 h post injury, with 2 HBO/day more than tenfold increase in tissue ATP compared to 36 h. controls

Table 2. Cont.

Author/Year	Interval Burn—HBO (hours)	Pressure (ATA)	Duration min	HBO Frequency/Day	Total Number HBO Sessions	Results in Detail
Saunders/1989	2	2	60	once a day	up to 4	HBO improved microvascularity in all groups; perfusion of dermal und subdermal vessels beneath burn preserved; less permanent collagen denaturation
Tenenhaus/1994	0.5	2.4	90 or 120	twice a day	2	mesenterial bacterial cultures are postburn sign. HBO: fewer mesenteric bacterial colonies; fewest colonies in fed, HBO treated mice; Villus length in HBO treated, fed mice as long as in nonburnt controls.
			120	twice a day or three times a day	3	fasting produced more bacterial colonies. Three 120 min HBO per 24 h had detrimental effects (seizures);
Espinosa/1995	1	2.8	60	twice a day	8	significant reduction of edema in HBO with or without antibiotic
Hussmann/1996						
		2.5	90	once	1	
		2.5	90	twice a day	up to 14	
	4	2.5	90	once	1	increase of cytotoxic cells unchanged
	4	2.5	90	twice a day	up to 14	increase of cytotoxic cells unchanged
	4	2.5	90	once	1	only regimen to prevent increase of cytotoxic (OX8) T-cells on day 1
	4	2.5	90	twice a day	up to 14	only regimen to downregulate cytotoxic (OX8) T-cells to normal values on days 5 and 15
Germonpré/1996	4	2	60	every 8 h first day, thereafter twice a day	6	Histology day 3: less subepidermal leucocyte infiltration, better preservation of basal membrane * and of skin appendages * after HBO; piracetam has effect only on basal membrane
Shoshani/1998	up to 24	2	90	once within first 24 h, twice a day thereafter	29	epithelization significantly slower with HBO

Table 2. Cont.

Author/Year	Interval Burn—HBO (hours)	Pressure (ATA)	Duration min	HBO Frequency/Day	Total Number HBO Sessions	Results in Detail
Akin/2002		2.5	90	twice a day	4	day 3: HBO prevents intestinal bacterial overgrowth and translocation to lymph nodes, liver and spleen
					14	day 8: HBO prevents bacterial overgrowth and translocation to lymph nodes, liver and spleen
Bilic/2005	2	2.5	60	once a day for up to 21 days	21	Skin samples day 1, 2, 3, 5, 7, 15, 21: less edema, increased neoangiogenesis, higher number of regenatory follicles, earlier epithelization; no significant difference in necrosis staging or margination of leucocytes
Türkaslan/2010	0.5	2.5	90	twice a day	2 or 10	no differences in the 24 h-groups; 5 day group HBO: Vital zones preserved; more cells in proliferative phase, more vital cells; prevents progression from zone of stasis to necrosis, less edema
					10	augmented neovascularization, decreased edema in HBO; no secondary enlargement of burn area
Selcuk/2013	1	2.5	90	once a day	7	After 21 days no difference concerning microbiology; yet best epithlization, lowermost inflammatory cell response, fewest fibrosis in non-nicotine/HBO
Wu/2018	24	2.5	60	once a day	5 or 10	early HBO inhibits Gal-3 dependent TLR-4 pathway; decreases proinflammatory cytokines and proteins in hind horn and paw; suppresses microglia/macrophage activation following burn injury; decreases mechanical withdrawal threshold; promotes wound healing;
Wu/2019	24	2.5	60	once a day	5 or 10	more HBO sessions reduce burn—induced mechanical allodynia (upregulation: melatonin, opioid-receptors, downregulation: brain derived neurotropic factor, substance P, calcitonin gene related peptide)

Table 2. Cont.

Author/Year	Interval Burn—HBO (hours)	Pressure (ATA)	Duration min	HBO Frequency/Day	Total Number HBO Sessions	Results in Detail
Hatibie/2019		2.4	90	once a day	6	day 14: fewer inflammatory cells and more epithelium in HBO; no difference in angiogenesis
Chen/2018		2.5	120	once a day	minimum 20	postburn pain score lower in HBO
Ikeda/1967		3		once or twice a day	5 to 10	6 patients died (those with 90–100% TBSA); no infection during HBO
Lamy/1970		3	60–90	once or twice a day		HBO does not alter mortality in extensive burns; fewer infections, better granulation and healing
Hart/1974	up to 24	2	90	three times on first day, then twice a day until healed	various	healing time, morbidity and mortality decreased in HBO. Healing time related to percentage TBSA
						mean healing time reduced
						mean healing time in relation to %TBSA reduced
Grossmann/1978	up to 4	2	90	every 8 h during first 24 h, twice a day thereafter		fluid requirements, healing time 2nd degree, eschar separation time, donor graft harvesting time, length of hospital stay, complications, mortality all reduced compared to non-HBO group; no paralytic ileus in severe burns and HBO, reduction in cost
Waisbren/1982						worse renal function, lower rate of non-segmented polymorphonuclear leucocytes and higher rate of bacteriemia in HBO; better healing, 75% fewer grafts in HBO
Niu/1987		2.5	90–120	2–3 during 1st 24 h; once a day thereafter		fluid loss reduced, earlier re-epithelization, overall mortality same as controls, less though in high-risk group
Cianci/1989	about 12	2	90	twice a day		duration of hospitalization and number of surgeries reduced in HBO
Cianci/1990	about 12	2	90	twice a day		duration of hospitalization, cost of burn care and number of surgeries reduced in HBO

Table 2. Cont.

Author/Year	Interval Burn—HBO (hours)	Pressure (ATA)	Duration min	HBO Frequency/Day	Total Number HBO Sessions	Results in Detail
Hammarlund/1991	1.5; 10.5; or 21.5	2.8	60	three times a day	3	at day 6: less exsudation, less hyperemia, wound size reduced in HBO; no significant effect on complete epithelization
Brannen/1997	up to 24; mean: 11.5; one third within 8	2	90	twice a day	minimum 10; maximal 1 per % TBSA	no difference in number of surgeries, duration of hospitalization or mortality; less fluid loss (mentioned in discussion); no data provided about the subgroup with early HBO application
Niezgoda/1997	2	2.4	90	twice a day	6	exsudation, hyperemia, wound surface reduced in HBO; no effect on epithelization
Chong/2013	max 15	2.4	90	twice within 22 h	2	no effect of HBO on inflammatory markers IL Beta, 4, 6 and 10; significantly lower rate of positive bacterial cultures (staph aureus, pseudomonas).
Rasmussen/2015	0.1	2.4	90	one (mean crossover interval 37 days)	1	HBO attenuates central sensitation by thermal injury (pin-prick test, thermal threshold, mechanical threshold; seondary hyperalgesia); no peripheral anti-inflammatory effect.
Wahl/2019	0.1	2.4	90	one	1	after one single HBO long-lasting reduction of pain sensitivity surrounding injured area; immediate mitigating effect, long lasting preconditioning effect on hyperalgesia

3.2. Animal Studies

3.2.1. First Decade (1966–1977)

Marchal [37], Nelson [38] and Ketchum [39,40] did the first experimental trials in 1967 [39] followed by Benichoux in 1968 [41], Perrins [42] and Spinadel [43] in 1969, Gruber in 1970 [44], Ketchum again in 1970 [40], and Bleser in 1971 [45] and 1973 [46]. The numbers of animal were impressive amounting up to 520 per study. The investigators focused on both tolerance of HBO at a maximum of 3 ATA in general and influence of HBO on survival following large burns with a total body surface area (TBSA) of 75%. In 25–30% TBSA they studied the effect on healing. Härtwig in 1974 [47], Korn [48], Niccole [49], and Wells [50], all in 1977, investigated burns up to 40% TBSA and applied HBO at a maximum of 2.5 ATA focusing on healing and revascularization. Except Perrins and Wells all researchers did the experiments in rodents, predominantly rats.

Table 3. Animal experiments (*n* = 76), descriptive statistics.

Feature	Number of Experiments (Percentage)/Mean ± SD (Range)
species	
rat	44 (57.9%)
guinea pig	20 (26.3%)
mouse	4 (5.3%)
dog	3 (4.0%)
pig	2 (2.6%)
rabbit	2 (2.6%)
hamster	1 (1.3%)
animals per experiment	19.1 ± 29.4 (2–250)
TBSA (percent)	21.2 ± 22.8 (0–75)
burn thickness	
partial thickness	43 (56.6%)
full thickness	34 (44.7%)
superficial	1 (1.3%)
not provided	3 (3.9%)
hours since injury	8.8 ± 29.6 (0.1–192)
ATA	2.5 ± 0.39 (2.0–3.0)
duration of HBO session	73.2 ± 20.2 (45–120)
HBO sessions per day	1.5 ± 0.9 (0.5–4)
total number of HBO sessions	17.1 ± 26.8 (0–138)

Table 4. Volunteers (*n* = 4) and patients (*n* = 11), descriptive statistics.

Feature	Number of Experiments (Percentage)/Mean ± SD (Range)
patients per clinical experimental group	65.8 ± 111.9 (2–402)
study design	
controlled	10 (66.7%)
randomized	5 (33.3%)
TBSA (percent)	35.2 ± 14.2 (13–65)
burn thickness	
partial thickness	15 (100.0%)
full thickness	15 (100.0%)
hours since injury	18.7 ± 7.4 (4–24)
ATA	2.2 ± 0.4 (2.0–3.0)
duration of HBO session	92.7 ± 8.8 (85–120)
HBO sessions per day	1.8 ± 0.4 (1–2)
total number of HBO sessions	9.8 ± 7.6 (2–20)

Marchal [37] and his co-worker Benichoux [41] found prolonged survival when HBO was given in addition to fluid resuscitation with tris-hydroxymethyl aminomethane (THAM) buffer, in 75% TBSA burns, whereas HBO at 3 ATA without adjunctive treatment proved detrimental. Even unburnt rats tolerated HBO at 3 ATA poorly. Bleser [45,46], from the same group, repeated the experiments in 30% TBSA and documented less fluid loss and reduced fluid requirements as well as higher survival rates following HBO at 3 ATA combined with THAM and antibiotics, thereby also confirming the findings of Nelson [41] who had described a lesser drop of hematocrit following 75% TBSA burn and HBO at 2ATA. In smaller burns (TBSA 20–30%) Marchal was able to demonstrate less fluid loss, better granulation, faster healing, better quality of scars and less infection in the HBO group [37].

Ketchum, after inflicting burns up to 20% TBSA, reported similar results with reduction of both fluid requirements and edema, reduction of bacterial growth on burnt surfaces, lower incidence of sepsis, shortening of healing time by 30% and extensive capillary proliferation beneath the burn injury following HBO at 2 or 3 ATA [39,40].

Spinadel noted enhanced healing of 25% TBSA burns when applying HBO and antibiotics. He noted that guinea pigs seem to be susceptible to HBO at 3 ATA. There was no effect on mortality [43]. Gruber reported a marked increase of tissue-pO2 beneath burnt surfaces following 3 ATA HBO [44].

With HBO at 2.5 ATA in rats following <10% TBSA burns, Härtwig was another investigator to find quicker revascularization, less fluid loss, earlier shedding of scabs with wound healing occurring 6 days earlier than in controls [47]. Similarly, Korn [48] who investigated the effect of 2 ATA HBO in small burns of 5% TBSA in a large series of 211 guinea pigs noticed quicker epithelization, no full-thickness conversion, earlier return of vascular patency, and hardly any edema, loss of fluid or inflammation in HBO, while escars showed earlier shedding. Microangiography revealed rapid revascularization and viable cells beneath burnt areas in the HBO group, whereas mitotic activity in epithelia of controls was not evaluable due to widespread necrosis. Wells, the only one using dogs with 40% TBSA burns, found less reduction in plasma volume and less decline in postburn cardiac output in animals treated with 2 ATA HBO [50].

In contrast, Perrins [42], who was the only investigator using pigs in 12% TBSA experimental burn, documented hardly any local response to HBO treatment at 2 ATA. Of note, he applied HBO four times a day. Likewise, Niccole, when applying 2.5 ATA HBO in rats with 20% TBSA burns found neither difference in edema, time to epithelization nor to eschar separation. Yet, there was less bacterial colonization of burnt surfaces following HBO [49].

3.2.2. Last Two Decades before Turn of the Century (1978–1998)

The investigators in this second phase used only rodents, again predominantly rats. Except Kaiser in 1985 [51] who did HBO at 3 ATA and Espinosa (2.8 ATA) [52], pressures never exceeded 2.5 ATA. While many studies corroborated the findings from earlier ones, new aspects were investigated, such as thrombosis, secondary enlargement of burn, mesenteric bacterial colonies, immunological effects and distinct histological changes within the burnt area.

Arzinger-Jonasch (1978) confirmed previous findings of a reduction in healing time for both full- and partial-thickness 15% TBSA burns and added the evidence that 2 ATA HBO prevented thrombosis beneath burnt areas and entailed a quicker take of full-thickness skin grafts [53]. Nylander (1984) showed a marked reduction of local edema by 2.5 ATA HBO after inflicting a burn on one mouse ear [54]. Kaiser, in 1985, studied the effect of HBO when treating < 10% TBSA burns infected by pseudomonas aeruginosa. He was able to demonstrate that infected wounds following primary HBO healed quicker than infected controls, whereas HBO applied after delay had no positive effect on healing time [51]. In a further study, in 1989, he focused on the secondary enlargement of burn injury. Whereas the phenomenon was reproducible in controls, HBO consistently prevented secondary enlargement of < 10% TBSA burns which in addition showed less edema and a quicker healing [55]. Stewart in 1989 reported consistently higher tissue ATP-levels beneath burnt surfaces when applying HBO [56]. In the same year, Saunders [57] found that 2 ATA HBO improved microvasculature and hence preserved perfusion of dermal und subdermal vessels resulting also in less permanent collagen denaturation subjacent to burnt surfaces. Tenenhaus, in 1994, investigated 30% TBSA burns and found fewer mesenteric bacterial colonies following 2.4 ATA HBO, as villus length in these animals remained normal [58]. Espinosa (1995) same as other investigator reported an HBO (2.8 ATA)—induced reduction of postburn edema following 10% TBSA burn [52]. Hussman, in 1996 was the first to investigate immunologic effects of 2.5 ATA HBO: He described a downregulation of cytotoxic (OX8) T-cells to normal values on days 5 and 15 after 10% TBSA burn [59]. Germonpre, in 1996, studied the influence of 2 ATA HBO on histological features within the burnt area. He documented less subepidermal leucocyte infiltration, better preservation of basal membrane and of skin appendages [60]. The only one reporting negative results in this period was Shoshani (1998) who was unable to find differences in intralesional perfusion between HBO-treated (2 ATA) animals and controls by laser-flowmetry. Besides, he described significantly slower epithelization with HBO [61].

3.2.3. New Millennium (2002–2019)

Again, all studies were done in rodents, and all but one [62] in rats. The investigators set their focuses on intestinal bacteria [63], prevention of inflammation and necrosis as well as on regeneration [62,64–66] and on alleviation of pain [67,68] induced by burn injury. The maximum pressure applied was 2.5 ATA.

Following 2.5 ATA HBO in 30% TBSA burn Akin [34] found lower bacterial colony counts in the distal ileum. Bacterial overgrowth and translocation to lymph nodes, blood liver and spleen were prevented. Bilic (2005) who inflicted 20% TBSA burn injury, confirmed former investigators' results describing reduction of edema, and enhancement of neo-angiogenesis and epithelization. The latter was linked to a higher number of preserved regeneratory follicles [64]. Similarly, Türkaslan in 2010 reported reduced edema as well as preservation of vital cells and cells in the proliferative phase in 5% TBSA burn. Furthermore, HBO prevented progression from zone of stasis to necrosis [65]. Selcuk, in 2013, investigated the effect of HBO on 12% TBSA burn in rats, half of which had undergone pretreatment with nicotine. HBO reduced the degree of necrosis in these animals, while the least degree of necrosis, best epithelization, and lowest inflammatory cell response was present in rats who had HBO treatment and no nicotine [66]. Finally, Hatibie in 2019 was able to show fewer inflammatory cells and better epithelization as well as a trend for enhanced angiogenesis following HBO in 1% TBSA burns [62]. Wu as well inflicted small burns (1% TBSA) when studying wound-healing and postburn pain. Early HBO inhibited the Gal-3 dependent TLR-4 pathway, thus reducing proinflammatory cytokines and proteins both in the affected extremity and in the hind horn. Microglia and macrophage activation following burn injury were suppressed. This resulted in a decrease of the mechanical withdrawal threshold and in a promotion of wound healing (2018) [67]. In a recent study, in 2019, he was able to show, that HBO reduced burn-induced mechanical allodynia, in correlation to the duration of treatment. The effect was accompanied by an upregulation of melatonin and opioid receptors, and by downregulation of brain derived neurotropic factor, substance P and calcitonin gene-related peptide [68].

For detailed baseline data, specifications of HBO and results see Tables 1–4.

3.3. Human Volunteers

The first study in human volunteers was done by Hammarlund in 1991 [26], who used a crossover design inflicting a 5 mm in diameter UV-blister suction wound on the forearm followed by HBO at 2.8 ATA. There was a significant reduction of exsudation and hyperemia as well as of wound size, after HBO but no effect on epithelization. Six years later, Niezgoda used an almost identical setup, yet in a randomized design applying 2.4 ATA HBO. His findings did not differ from those of Hammarlund [13]. In 2015, Rasmussen published another crossover study focused on postburn pain, inflicting a superficial burn with a thermode whereafter HBO at 2.4 ATA was applied. The treatment attenuated the central sensitization by thermal injury. A peripheral inflammatory effect was ruled out [27]. Wahl, from the same group, used an identical setup in 2019. After a single HBO treatment, an immediate mitigating effect on hyperalgesia followed by a long-lasting reduction of pain sensitivity surrounding the injured area was documented [28].

3.4. Clinical Studies

All clinical studies involved full and partial thickness burns. Their extent ranged between 35 and 80%. HBO was administered in addition to routine burn treatment. In contrast to the experimental work, where HBO was almost exclusively administered immediately following burn, this interval varied in the clinical settings: In two studies the patients were treated within 24 h [24,31], in one within 15 [25], in two within 12 [12,30], and in one within four hours after the incident [32]. Brannen stated a mean of 11,5 h with one third of patients treated within 8 h [31]. Five authors did not convey information on this parameter.

Ikeda, in 1967, was the first to report positive effects of 3ATA HBO in 43 extensively burnt (TBSA up to 90%, median 65%) patients after explosion in a mine. They had HBO for additional CO-intoxication and did better than anticipated and better than those who had no HBO treatment. Ikeda underscored the absence of superinfection or sepsis in the HBO collective [36]. In 1979 Lamy published a series of 27 patients with 50% TBSA burns who had 3 ATA HBO with intention to treat. Though mortality was not altered, Lamy noticed better healing and fewer infections [35]. Encouraged by these findings Hart applied 2 ATA HBO both with intention to treat and in a randomized study, published in 1974 [24]. He treated 138 patients with an average TBSA of 35% comparing them to 53 historical controls. Time to healing, morbidity, and mortality decreased beyond the values to be expected in each at risk group. The randomized patients (four with 15%, 25%, 35% or 45% TBSA each) showed reduced mean healing time in relation to %TBSA when compared to the controls. Grossmann administered 2 ATA HBO to patients with an average of 40% TBSA, incorporating the method into routine. He compared 419 patients with routine treatment to 419 who had additional HBO. Fluid requirements, healing time in second-degree burns, eschar separation time in 3rd degree, donor graft harvesting time, length of hospital stay, complications and mortality were all reduced compared to the non-HBO group. In addition, HBO seemed to prevent paralytic ileus in severe burns. In spite the additional treatment Grossman documented a reduction in overall cost [32].

In 1982, Waisbren designed a matched pairs study with 36 patients each, comparing routine treatment to 2.5 ATA HBO in 50% TBSA burn. In contrast to the other investigators, he observed worse renal function, lower rate of non-segmented, polymorphonuclear leucocytes and a higher rate of bacteriemia in the HBO-treated group. Yet, he confirmed former findings of improved healing, resulting in 75% lower requirement of skin grafts in the HBO group [29]. In 1987, Niu published a study comparing 226 patients with 2.5 ATA HBO treatment to 609 historical controls. TBSA was 35%. He added further proof to the evidence of reduced fluid loss and earlier re-epithelization. Yet, the overall mortality was not different from the one of the controls, though it was lower than in controls if only the high-risk group was considered [33].

Cianci and his group in 1989, who similar as Grossman had established HBO as a treatment routine for burn injury, described a small collective of 20 patients with 30% TBSA comparing HBO at 2ATA to historical controls. He found both duration of hospitalization and number of necessary surgical interventions reduced by HBO treatment [12]. A further study in 1990, this time using a matched pairs design in 21 patients, confirmed the former findings. In addition, Cianci stated a reduction of cost in burn care in the HBO-group thereby confirming Grossman´s results [30].

Brannen, in 1997, did a matched-pairs study in 125 patients, 63 of whom had 2 ATA HBO. While renal insufficiency seemed more frequent in the HBO-group, he was unable to document any difference in number of surgeries, length of hospital stay or mortality. On the other hand, Brannen mentioned less fluid loss following HBO. The information about TBSA and details of HBO—application was scant [31]. Chong, in 2013, randomized 8 patients with 13% TBSA burns to 2.4 ATA HBO and 9 to the control group. He found no effect on inflammatory markers IL Beta, 4, 6 and 10, yet a significantly lower rate of positive bacterial cultures of staphylococcus aureus and pseudomonas aeruginosa following HBO [25]. Finally, Chen compared 17 historical controls to 18 patients with 25% TBSA burn who had HBO at 2.5 ATA. Though the post-burn pain scores were better in the HBO group, he noticed no effect on infection or quality of scarring [34].

4. Discussion

We established a comprehensive synopsis of the experimental and clinical work on HBO in burns from its beginning in 1965 to the present, step by step addressing the crucial pathogenetic factors in burns which result from a combination of direct tissue damage by the thermal trauma and initiation of mediator cascades. The latter cause edema, coagulopathy, microvascular stasis and secondary enlargement of the local damage and systemic inflammatory reaction. In large burns, intestinal dysfunction results from both systemic inflammation and imbalance of intestinal microorganisms. Superinfection of burnt surfaces is a further threat [69].

Both experimental and clinical work throughout five decades has yielded unquestionable evidence of beneficial HBO effects the abovementioned factors. Early experiments relied on simple methods of description, whereas later on the evaluation became more sophisticated as insight into underlying molecular mechanisms of HBO developed [8].

Promotion of healing was demonstrable in both partial- and full-thickness burns. It involved quicker epithelization and thus more rapid healing of burnt surfaces based on prevention of secondary enlargement of the injury, preservation and better restoration of the microvasculature and the skin appendages as well as higher levels of intracellular ATP in the burnt area. Earlier shedding of escars was observed in full-thickness burns. Only three out of 32 experimental [42,49,61] and one out of 11 clinical studies [31] did not confirm positive effects of HBO on healing.

An undisputed phenomenon was the marked reduction of post-burn edema and of fluid requirements, respectively [13,26,32,37,38,45,47,48,50,52–55,64,65]. Likewise, inhibition of bacterial growth on both burn wounds and in the intestinum, resulting in fewer cases of sepsis [36] in an absence of bacterial translocation [63] and even in a lower incidence of ileus [32], was confirmed by all investigators focusing on that very issue [25,32,35,36,39,46,49,58,63].

Recent investigations focusing on postburn pain documented marked reduction of sensitation that could be induced by even one single HBO treatment session [27,28,34,67,68].

The findings about the impact of HBO on the prognosis of experimental or clinical burns, respectively, were less consistent: Marchal [37], Benichoux [41] and Bleser [45] reported prolonged survival or less mortality, respectively, in 30 to 75% TBSA burns only when HBO was combined with fluid substitution and buffering or antibiotics, respectively. Spinadel, on the contrary, found no effect on mortality in 25% TBSA experimental burns [43]. From the clinical point of view, Grossmann [32] and Hart [24] reported generally reduced mortality, while Grossmann also noticed fewer complications and fewer surgical interventions in the HBO patients, resulting in shortened hospital stay and lower cost [32]. Cianci confirmed these findings [30]. Niu observed better survival in the high-risk group [33], yet documented an unaltered course in less extensive burns [33]. In contrast, Lamy found prognosis unchanged in extensive burns [35], and Brannen described survival generally unchanged [31].

The reasons for these disparities are most likely based on a variety of factors.

First, the effects of HBO, which basically constitutes a kind of pharmacological treatment, are dose-dependent. The dose of HBO, however, derives from the combination of pressure, duration of exposure, frequency of treatment and total number of treatments—in other words, there is no "HBO" as such. In consequence, all the factors contributing to the HBO dose differed largely between studies and hardly any identical treatment regimens could be identified. What is more, the information about the dose-defining parameters of HBO was incomplete in many clinical studies. The only explicit finding was the gradual use of lower pressure levels. While 3 ATA were applied in the early years of research, there was a general tendency to apply lower pressures as time went by. Evidence of overdose—effects due to high pressure were shown in rats [37,46] and guineapigs [43] at

3 ATA, whereas Tenenhaus noticed negative impact of duration and frequency in mice when applying 2.4 ATA throughout 120 min three times a day [58]. The lack of positive effects of 2 ATA for 60 min used by Perrins may also have been influenced by the fact, that he applied the treatment four times a day [42]. A study on the impact of HBO on bone repair [70] proved that one application per day yielded better results than two and supports this assumption.

In any acute injury HBO has the potential to downregulate mediator cascades if applied within the appropriate time window. In stroke [22] and acute carbon monoxide intoxication [20], this interval seems to last until 6 to 8 h after the acute event. Later on, the inflammatory cascade is less likely to be downregulated by HBO and after 24 h this line of action may be terminated. These limitations probably also apply to HBO in burn injury [18,19,51,54]. The available data from clinical studies are too sparse as to provide an answer to this question.

In summary, though there are recommendations to apply a maximum of 2.5 ATA, there is still no generally established HBO treatment regimen for adjunctive HBO in burns [19].

The delivery of HBO to intensive care patients with precarious fluid balance and requirement for vasopressor treatment and artificial ventilation is a critical issue. The necessary repeated transfer of patients into the chamber for hyperbaric treatment involves further stress and the mere logistics of HBO—delivery may deter therapists from its use. Though HBO can be administered safely and with beneficial effect to severely ill patients, the treatment requires a high degree of experience in hyperbaric medicine and can be demanding for the therapist. Infusion rates, vasopressor doses and ventilation parameters need to be repeatedly adjusted during each HBO session and a meticulous invasive monitoring of cardiorespiratory parameters is mandatory. Thus, in unexperienced hands, HBO treatment may fail to succeed or may even have adverse effects in burn victims [16,32,71,72], a fact that may explain some negative results. The 2018 European Committee for Hyperbaric Medicine (ECHM) consensus paper stresses the point, that HBO treatment in burn should only be administered in burn centers with direct access to highly specialized HBO units [19].

What is more, both experimental and especially clinical studies on burn treatment used different outcome issues or different definitions, respectively, to assess the same outcome issues, while results were evaluated at different time points after the injury [71,73]. In addition, like all reviews of clinical studies in burns, we had to face the heterogeneity of basic parameters including epidemiology, comorbidity, as well as type, degree, TBSA and localization of the burn. Young and colleagues, in a recent systematic review of burn treatment, suggested the development of a core outcome set (COS) enabling the comparison of results of studies on burn treatment [73]. This basic problem when designing trials in burn patients applies also for HBO: Only two clinical studies were randomized including a total of 16 [24] and 15 patients [25], respectively. Other investigators relied on matched pairs [29–31] which allowed for a maximum number of 62 per group. When evaluating the divergent results also the low numbers of patients must be considered.

The main limitation of the study is the lack of comparability of both the various experimental and clinical setups and treatment schedules. In addition, relevant data were not consistently available in all publications.

5. Conclusions

Much experimental and clinical research has been done on the topic of HBO in burn injury, and the authors provide well founded evidence of beneficial interaction with the pathomechanisms of burns and healing processes, albeit focusing on single issues in the various investigations [71]. A comprehensive experimental view on the timeline of patho-molecular events and their interaction with HBO treatment would be desirable. To definitively assess its hitherto disputed clinical value as an adjunctive treatment, however, there is a dire need for well-designed clinical studies. They should involve relevant outcome criteria such as wound-healing time, complications, length of hospital stay, mortality and scar quality, while also defining optimal HBO dose and timing. They will have to be conducted in highly specialized burn treatment units equipped with hyperbaric treatment facilities and expert staff familiar with hyperbaric intensive care. As there is hardly any other single therapeutic measure by which—at least in experimental use—so many aspects of burn can be dealt with, intensified research on this issue is worthwhile.

Author Contributions: Conceptualization, C.S. and J.L.; methodology, C.S.; investigation, C.S. and J.L.; resources, F.-M.S.-J.; writing—Original draft preparation, C.S.; writing—Review and editing, F.-M.S.-J.; supervision, L.K. All authors have read and agreed to the published version of the manuscript.

Funding: This research received no external funding.

Institutional Review Board Statement: Ethical review and approval were waived for this study, due to exclusive use of data from the literature.

Informed Consent Statement: Patient consent was waived due to exclusive use of data from the literature.

Data Availability Statement: Data sharing not applicable. No new data were created or analyzed in this study. Data sharing is not applicable to this article.

Conflicts of Interest: The authors declare no conflict of interest.

References

1. Kindwall, E.P. A History of Hyperbaric Medicine. In *Hyperbaric Medicine Practice*, 2nd ed.; Best Publishing Company: Flagstaff, AZ, USA, 1995; pp. 2–15.
2. Churchill-Davidson, I.; Sanger, C.; Thomlinson, R.H. High-pressure oxygen and radiotherapy. *Lancet* **1955**, *268*, 1091–1095. [CrossRef]
3. Boerema, I. The use of hyperbaric oxygen. *Am. Heart J.* **1965**, *69*, 289–292. [CrossRef]
4. Boerema, I.; Meyne, N.G.; Brummelkamp, W.H.; Bouma, S.; Mensch, M.H.; Kamermans, F.; Stern Hanf, M.; Alderen van, A. Life without blood. *J. Cardiovasc. Surg.* **1960**, *1*, 133–147.
5. Cianci, P. Advances in the treatment of the diabetic foot: Is there a role for adjunctive hyperbaric oxygen therapy? *Wound Repair Regen.* **2004**, *12*, 2–10. [CrossRef]
6. Thom, S.R. Hyperbaric oxygen: Its mechanisms and efficacy. *Plast. Reconstr. Surg.* **2011**, *127*, 131S–141S. [CrossRef]
7. Rothfuss, A.; Speit, G. Investigations on the mechanism of hyperbaric oxygen (HBO)-induced adaptive protection against oxidative stress. *Mutat. Res. Mol. Mech. Mutagen.* **2002**, *508*, 157–165. [CrossRef]
8. Camporesi, E.; Bosco, G. Mechanisms of action of hyperbaric oxygen therapy. *Undersea Hyperb. Med.* **2018**, *41*, 247–252.
9. Domachevsky, L.; Pick, C.G.; Arieli, Y.; Krinsky, N.; Abramovich, A.; Eynan, M. Do hyperbaric oxygen-induced seizures cause brain damage? *Epilepsy Res.* **2012**, *100*, 37–41. [CrossRef]
10. Wada, J.; Ikeda, T.; Kamata, K. Oxygen hyperbaric treatment for carbon monoxide poisoning and severe burn in coal mine gas explosion. *Igakounoaymi* **1965**, *5*, 53–57.
11. Villanueva, E.; Bennett, M.H.; Wasiak, J.; Lehm, J.P. Hyperbaric oxygen therapy for thermal burns. *Cochrane Database Syst. Rev.* **2004**, *2004*, CD004727. [CrossRef]
12. Cianci, P.; Lueders, H.W.; Lee, H.; Shaprio, R.L.; Sexton, J.; Williams, C.; Sato, R. Adjunctive Hyperbaric Oxygen Therapy Reduces Length of Hospitalization in Thermal Burns. *J. Burn Care Rehab.* **1989**, *10*, 432–435. [CrossRef]
13. Niezgoda, J.A.; Cianci, P.; Folden, B.W.; Ortega, R.L.; Slade, J.B.; Storrow, A.B. The effect of hyperbaric oxygen therapy on a burn wound model in human volunteers. *Plast. Reconstr. Surg.* **1997**, *99*, 1620–1625. [CrossRef]
14. Wasiak, J.; Bennett, M.; Cleland, H.J. Hyperbaric oxygen as adjuvant therapy in the management of burns: Can evidence guide clinical practice? *Burns* **2006**, *32*, 650–652. [CrossRef]
15. Weitgasser, L.; Ihra, G.; Schäfer, B.; Markstaller, K.; Radtke, C. Update on hyperbaric oxygen therapy in burn treatment. *Wien. Klin. Wochenschr.* **2019**, 1–7. [CrossRef]
16. Kindwall, E.P.; Gottlieb, L.J.; Larson, D.L. Hyperbaric oxygen therapy in plastic surgery: A review article. *Plast. Reconstr. Surg.* **1991**, *88*, 898–908. [CrossRef] [PubMed]
17. Rogatsky, G.G.; Shifrin, E.G.; Mayevsky, A. Optimal dose as necessary condition for the efficacy of hyperbaric oxygen therapy in is-chemic stroke: A critical review. *Neurol. Res.* **2003**, *25*, 95–98. [CrossRef]
18. Grossmann, A.R.; Grossmann, A.J. Update on hyperbaric oxygen and treatment of burns. *Hyperb. Oxyg. Rev.* **1982**, *3*, 51–59.
19. Mathieu, D.; Marroni, A.; Kot, J. Tenth European Consensus Conference on Hyperbaric Medicine: Recommendations for acepted and non-accepted clinical indications and practic of hyperbaric oxygten treatment. *Diving Hyperb. Med. J.* **2017**, *47*, 24–32. [CrossRef] [PubMed]

20. Weaver, L.K.; Hopkins, R.O.; Chan, K.J.; Churchill, S.; Elliott, G.C.; Clemmer, T.P.; Orme, J.F., Jr.; Thomas, F.O.; Morris, A.H. Hyperbaric oxygen for acute carbon monoxide poisoning. *New Engl. J. Med.* **2002**, *347*, 1057–1067. [CrossRef]
21. Attanasio, G.; Covelli, E.; Cagnoni, L.; Masci, E.; Ferraro, D.; Mancini, P.; Alessandri, E.; Cartocci, G.; Filipo, R.; Rocco, M. Does the addition of a second daily session of hyperbaric oxygen therapy to intratympanic steroid influence the outcomes of sudden hearing loss? *Acta Otorhinolaryngol. Ital.* **2015**, *35*, 272–276.
22. McCormick, J.G.; Houle, T.T.; Saltzman, H.A.; Whaley, R.C.; Roy, R.C. Treatment of acute stroke with hyperbaric oxygen: Time window for efficacy. *Undersea Hyperb. Med.* **2011**, *38*, 321–334.
23. Moher, D.; Liberati, A.; Tezlaff, J.; Altman, D.G.; PRISMA Group. Preferred Reporting Items for Systematic Reviews and Meta-Analyses. The PRISMA Statement. *PLoS Med.* **2009**, *6*, e1000097. [CrossRef]
24. Hart, G.B.; O'Reilly, R.R.; Broussard, N.D.; Cave, R.H.; Goodman, D.B.; Yanda, R.L. Treatment of burns with hyperbaric oxygen. *Surg. Gynecol. Obstet.* **1974**, *139*, 693–696.
25. Chong, S.J.; Kan, E.M.; Song, C.; Soh, C.R.; Lu, J. Characterization of early thermal burns and the effects of hyperbaric oxygen treatment: A pilot study. *Diving Hyperb. Med. J.* **2013**, *43*, 157–161.
26. Hammarlund, C.; Svedman, C.; Svedman, P. Hyperbaric oxygen treatment of healthy volunteers with u.v.-irradiated blister wounds. *Burns* **1991**, *17*, 296–301. [CrossRef]
27. Rasmussen, V.M.; Borgen, A.E.; Jansen, E.C.; Rotboll Nielsen, P.H.; Werner, M.U. Hyperbaric oxygen therapy attenuates central sen-sitization induced by a thermal injury in humans. *Acta Anaesthesiol. Scand.* **2015**, *59*, 749–762. [CrossRef]
28. Wahl, A.M.; Bidstrup, K.; Smidt-Nielsen, I.G.; Werner, M.U.; Hyldegaard, O.; Rotbøll-Nielsen, P. A single session of hyperbaric oxygen therapy demonstrates acute and long-lasting neuroplasticity effects in humans: A replicated, randomized controlled clinical trial. *J. Pain Res.* **2019**, *12*, 2337–2348. [CrossRef]
29. Waisbren, B.A.; Schutz, D.; Collentine, G.; Banaszak, E.; Stern, M. Hyperbaric oxygen in severe burns. *Burns* **1982**, *8*, 176–179. [CrossRef]
30. Cianci, P.; Williams, C.; Lueders, H.W.; Lee, H.; Shapiro, R.L.; Sexton, J.; Sato, R. Adjunctive hyperbaric oxygen in the treatment of thermal burns: An economic analysis. *J. Burn Care Rehabil.* **1990**, *11*, 140–143. [CrossRef]
31. Brannen, A.L.; Still, J.; Haynes, M.; Orlet, H.; Rosenblum, F.; Law, E.; Thompson, W.O. A randomized prospective trial of hyperbaric oxygen in a referral burn center population. *Am. Surg.* **1997**, *63*, 205–208.
32. Wiseman, D.H.; Grossman, A.R. Hyperbaric oxygen in the treatment of burns. *Crit. Care Clin. Plast. Surg.* **1978**, *1*, 163–171. [CrossRef]
33. Niu, A.K.C.; Yang, C.; Lee, H.C. Burns treated with adjunctive hyperbaric oxygen therapy: A comparative study in humans. *J. Hyperb. Med.* **1987**, *2*, 75–85.
34. Chen, K.-L.W.C.-J.; Tseng, W.-S.; Lee, H.-C.; Tsa, T.-P.; Huang, W.-S. Improvement of satisfaction in burn patients recieving adjuvant hyperbaric oxygen therapy. *Formos. J. Surg.* **2018**, *51*, 184–192.
35. Lamy, M.L.; Hanquet, M.M. Application Opportunity for OHP in a General Hospital—A Two Years Experience with a Monoplace Hyperbaric Oxygen Chamber. In *Proceedings of the 4th International Congress on Hyperbaric Medicine Sapporo, Japan, 2–4 September 1969*; Igaku Shoin, Ltd.: Tokyo, Japan, 1970.
36. Ikeda, K.; Ajiki, H.; Nagao, H.; Krino, K.; Sugh, S.; Iwa, T.; Wada, T. Experimental and Clinical Use of Hyperbaric Oxygen in Burns. In *Proceedings of the 4th International Congress on Hyperbaric Medicine Sapporo, Japan, 2–4 September 1969*; Igaku Shoin, Ltd.: Tokyo, Japan, 1970.
37. Marchal, C.; Thibault, G.; Commebias, J.F.; Barlier, J.; Benichoux, R. Effects of OHP and THAM on Experimental Burns of Rats. In *Proceedings of the 3rd International Congress on Hyperbaric Medicine Duke University, Durham, NC, USA, 17–20 November 1965*; National Academy of Sciences Research Council: Washington, DC, USA, 1966.
38. Nelson, B.S.; Stansell, G.B.; Kramer, J.G. Hyperbaric Oxygen in Experimental Burn. In *Proceedings of the 3rd International Congress on Hyper-Baric Medicine Duke University, Durham, NC, USA, 17–20 November 1965*; National Academy of Sciences Research Council: Washington, DC, USA, 1966.
39. Ketchum, S.A.; Thomas, A.N.; Hall, A.D. Effect of hyperbaric oxygen on small first, second, and third degree burns. *Surg. Forum* **1967**, *18*, 65–67.
40. Ketchum, S.A.; Thomas, A.N.; Hall, A.D. Angiographic Studies of the Effect of Hyperbaric Oxygen on Burn Wound Revascularization. In *Proceedings of the 4th International Congress on Hyperbaric Medicine Sapporo, Japan, 2–4 September 1969*; Wada, J., Iwa, T., Eds.; Igaku Shoin, Ltd.: Tokyo, Japan, 1970; pp. 388–394.
41. Benichoux, R.; Marchal, C.; Thibaut, G.; Bertrand, J.P. Hyperbaric oxygen in treatment of severe experimental burns. *J. Chir.* **1968**, *96*, 445–452.
42. Perrins, D.J.D. Failed Attempt to Limit Tissue Destruction in Scalds of Pig´s Skin with Hyperbaric Oxygen. In *Proceedings of the 4th International Congress on Hyperbaric Medicine Sapporo, Japan, 2–4 September 1969*; Igaku Shoin, Ltd.: Tokyo, Japan, 1970.
43. Spinadel, L.; Vymola, F. Influence of hyperbaric oxygenation and antibiotics on burns in animal experiments. *Zent. Chir.* **1969**, *94*, 296–298.
44. Gruber, R.P.; Brinkley, F.B.; Amato, J.J.; Mendelson, J.A. Hyperbaric Oxygen and Pedicle Flaps, Skin Grafts, and Burns. *Plast. Reconstr. Surg.* **1970**, *45*, 24–30. [CrossRef] [PubMed]
45. Bleser, F.; Sztuka, J.C.; Muller, J.-P. Effects of hyperbaric oxygen, THAM and antibiotics on experimental burns in rats. Changes in body fluid compartments, electrolytes and acid-base balance. *Eur. Surg. Res.* **1971**, *3*, 409–420. [CrossRef]

46. Bleser, F.; Benichoux, R. Experimental surgery: The treatment of severe burns with hyperbaric oxygen. *J. Chir.* **1973**, *106*, 281–290.
47. Hartwig, V.J.; Kirste, G. Experimentelle Untersuchungen über die Revaskularisierung von Verbrennungswunden unter Hyperbarer Sauerstofftherapie. *Zent. Chir.* **1974**, *99*, 1112–1117.
48. Korn, H.N.; Wheeler, E.S.; Miller, T.A. Effect of Hyperbaric Oxygen on Second-Degree Burn Wound Healing. *Arch. Surg.* **1977**, *112*, 732–737. [CrossRef] [PubMed]
49. Niccole, M.W.; Thornton, J.W.; Danet, R.T.; Bartlett, R.H.; Tavis, M.J. Hyperbaric oxygen in burn management: A controlled study. *Surg. Gynecol. Obstet.* **1977**, *82*, 727–733.
50. Wells, C.H.; Hilton, J.C. Effects of Hyperbaric Oxygen on Post-Burn Plasma Extravasation. In *Hyperbaric Oxygen Therapy*; Davis, J.C., Hunt, T.K., Eds.; Undersea Medical Society, Inc.: Bethesda, MD, USA, 1977; pp. 259–265.
51. Kaiser, W.; Berger, A.; Von Der Lieth, H.; Heymann, H. Hyperbaric Oxygenation in Burns. *Handchir. Mikrochir. Plast. Chir.* **1985**, *17*, 326–330. [PubMed]
52. Espinosa, C.; Mauvecin, G.; Lopez, C.; Brandon, J.; Ciampagna, H.; Pomar, M.; Lemmi, J. Study of edema regulation by hyperbaric oxygen in an experimental model of thermal burns. *Prensa Med. Argent.* **1995**, *82*, 235–240.
53. Arzinger-Jonasch, H.; Sandner, J.K.; Bittner, H. Effect of hyperbaric oxygen on burns of various depths in anmial experiments. *Z. Exp. Chir.* **1978**, *11*, 6–10.
54. Nylander, G.; Nordström, H.; Eriksson, E. Effects of hyperbaric oxygen on oedema formation after a scald burn. *Burns* **1984**, *10*, 193–196. [CrossRef]
55. Kaiser, W.; Schnaidt, U.; Von Der Lieth, H. Effects of hyperbaric oxygen on fresh burn wounds. *Handchir. Mikrochir. Plast. Chir.* **1989**, *21*, 158–163.
56. Stewart, R.J.; Yamaguchi, K.T.; Mason, S.W.; Rosideh, B.B.; Dabassi, N.I.; Ness, N.T. Tissue ATP levels in burn injured skin treated with hyperbaric oxygen. In Proceedings of the Annual Meeting of the Undersea and Hyperbaric Medical Society, Honolulu, Hawaii, USA, 6–11 June 1989.
57. Saunders, P. Hyperbaric Oxygen Therapy in the Management of Carbon Monoxide Poisoning, Osteoradionecrosis, Burns, Skin Grafts, and Crush Injury. *Int. J. Technol. Assess. Heal. Care* **2003**, *19*, 521–525. [CrossRef]
58. Tenenhaus, M.; Hansbrough, J.F.; Zapata-Sirvent, R.; Neumann, T. Treatment of Burned Mice with Hyperbaric Oxygen Reduces Mesenteric Bacteria but Not Pulmonary Neutrophil Deposition. *Arch. Surg.* **1994**, *129*, 1338–1342. [CrossRef]
59. Hussmann, J.; Hebebrand, D.; Erdmann, D.; Roth, A.; Kucan, J.O.; Moticka, J. Lymphocyte subpopulations in spleen and blood following early burn wound excision and acute/chronic treatment with hyperbaric oxygen. *Handchir. Mikrochir. Plast. Chir.* **1996**, *28*, 103–107.
60. Germonpre, P.; Reper, P.; Vanderkelen, A. Hyperbaric oxygen therapy and piracetam decrease the early extension of deep par-tial-thickness burns. *Burns* **1996**, *22*, 468–473. [CrossRef]
61. Shoshani, O.; Shupak, A.; Barak, A.; Ullman, Y.; Ramon, Y.; Lindenbaum, E.; Peled, Y. Hyperbaric oxygen therapy for deep second degree burns: An experimental study in the guinea pig. *Br. J. Plast. Surg.* **1998**, *51*, 67–73. [CrossRef]
62. Hatibie, M.J.; Islam, A.A.; Hatta, M.; Moenadjat, Y.; Susiolo, R.H.; Rendy, L. Hyperbaric Oxygen Therapy for Second-Degree Burn Healing: An Experimental Study in Rabbits. *Adv. Skin Wound Care.* **2019**, *32*, 1–4. [CrossRef] [PubMed]
63. Akin, M.L.; Gulluoglu, B.M.; Erenoglu, C.; Dundar, K.; Terzi, K.; Erdemoglu, A.; Celenk, T. Hyperbaric oxygen prevents bacterial translo-cation in thermally injured rats. *J. Investig. Surg.* **2002**, *15*, 303–310. [CrossRef]
64. Bilic, I.; Petri, N.M.; Bezic, J.; Alfirevic, D.; Modun, D.; Capkun, V.; Bota, B. Effects of hyperbaric oxygen therapy on experimental burn wound healing in rats: A randomized controlled study. *Undersea Hyperb. Med.* **2005**, *32*, 1–9. [PubMed]
65. Turkaslan, T.; Yogun, N.; Cimsit, M.; Solakoğlu, S.; Ozdemir, C.; Özsoy, Z. Is HBOT treatment effective in recovering zone of stasis? An experimental immunohistochemical study. *Burns* **2010**, *36*, 539–544. [CrossRef] [PubMed]
66. Selçuk, C.T.; Özalp, B.; Durgun, M.; Tekin, A.; Akkoç, M.F.; Alabalik, U.; Ilgezdi, S. The Effect of Hyperbaric Oxygen Treatment on the Healing of Burn Wounds in Nicotinized and Nonnicotinized Rats. *J. Burn Care Res.* **2013**, *34*, e237–e243. [CrossRef]
67. Wu, Z.-S.; Lo, J.-J.; Wu, S.-H.; Wang, C.-Z.; Chen, R.-F.; Lee, S.-S.; Chai, C.-Y.; Huang, S.-H. Early Hyperbaric Oxygen Treatment Attenuates Burn-Induced Neuroinflammation by Inhibiting the Galectin-3-Dependent Toll-Like Receptor-4 Pathway in a Rat Model. *Int. J. Mol. Sci.* **2018**, *19*, 2195. [CrossRef]
68. Wu, Z.-S.; Wu, S.-H.; Lee, S.-S.; Lin, C.-H.; Chang, C.-H.; Lo, J.-J.; Chai, C.-Y.; Wu, C.-S.; Huang, S.-H. Dose-Dependent Effect of Hyperbaric Oxygen Treatment on Burn-Induced Neuropathic Pain in Rats. *Int. J. Mol. Sci.* **2019**, *20*, 1951. [CrossRef]
69. Lang, T.C.; Zhao, R.; Kim, A.; Wijewardena, A.; Vandervord, J.; Xue, M.; Jackson, C.J. A Critical Update of the Assessment and Acute Management of Patients with Severe Burns. *Adv. Wound Care* **2019**, *8*, 607–633. [CrossRef]
70. Barth, E.; Sullivan, T.; Berg, E. Animal Model for Evaluating Bone Repair with and without Adjunctive Hyperbaric Oxygen Therapy (HBO): Comparing Dose Schedules. *J. Investig. Surg.* **1990**, *3*, 387–392. [CrossRef]
71. Cianci, P.; Slade, J.B.; Sato, R.M.; Faulkner, J. Adjunctive hyperbaric oxygen therapy in the treatment of thermal burns. *Undersea Hyperb. Med.* **2013**, *40*, 89–108. [CrossRef]
72. Ratzenhofer-Komenda, B.; Offner, A.; Quehenberger, F.; Klemen, H.; Berger, J.; Fadai, J.H.; Spernbauer, P.; Prause, G.; Smolle-Jüttner, F.M. Hemodynamic and oxygenation profiles in the early period after hyperbaric oxygen therapy: An observational study of intensive-care patients. *Acta Anaesthesiol. Scand.* **2003**, *47*, 554–558. [CrossRef] [PubMed]
73. Young, A.; Davies, A.; Bland, S.; Brookes, S.; Blazeby, J.M. Systematic review of clinical outcome reporting in randomised controlled trials of burn care. *BMJ Open* **2019**, *9*, e025135. [CrossRef]

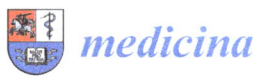

Review
Contemporary Aspects of Burn Care

Arij El Khatib [1,*] and Marc G. Jeschke [2]

1. Unité des Grands Brûlés, University of Montreal Medical Centre Sanguinet, 1051, Rue Sanguinet, Montréal, QC H2X 0C1, Canada
2. Department of Surgery, Division of Plastic Surgery, Department of Immunology, Ross Tilley Burn Centre-Sunnybrook Health Sciences Centre, Sunnybrook Research Institute, University of Toronto, 2075 Bayview Avenue, Rm D704, Toronto, ON M4N 3M5, Canada; marc.jeschke@sunnybrook.ca
* Correspondence: arijabdulhadi@gmail.com

Abstract: The past one hundred years have seen tremendous improvements in burn care, allowing for decreased morbidity and mortality of this pathology. The more prominent advancements occurred in the period spanning 1930–1980; notably burn resuscitation, early tangential excision, and use of topical antibiotic dressings; and are well documented in burn literature. This article explores the advancements of the past 40 years and the areas of burn management that are presently topics of active discussion and research.

Keywords: burn history; burn advancement; burn research

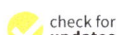

Citation: El Khatib, A.; Jeschke, M.G. Contemporary Aspects of Burn Care. *Medicina* **2021**, *57*, 386. https://doi.org/10.3390/medicina57040386

Academic Editor: Lars P. Kamolz

Received: 8 March 2021
Accepted: 15 April 2021
Published: 16 April 2021

Publisher's Note: MDPI stays neutral with regard to jurisdictional claims in published maps and institutional affiliations.

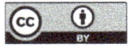

Copyright: © 2021 by the authors. Licensee MDPI, Basel, Switzerland. This article is an open access article distributed under the terms and conditions of the Creative Commons Attribution (CC BY) license (https://creativecommons.org/licenses/by/4.0/).

1. Introduction

Attempts to treat burn injury are as old as man's use of fire. The first depictions of burn injury and treatment have been found in cave drawings [1]. Documentation of treatment recommendations were found in ancient Egyptian writings, the Ebers and Smith papyri, dating over 1500 BC (Before Christ), describing several treatment options including incantations, breast milk, and topical applications of multiple agents including honey, resin, and fabric strips soaked in oil as dressings [1–4]. Chinese medicine in the 6th century BC advocated the use of tea leaf extract on burns [2,3], while Hippocrates in the 4th century BC advocated multiple treatment options for burns including pig fat-soaked dressings, vinegar-soaked dressings, and balms made of oak bark [1–3]. Roman writings in the first century AD (Anno Domini) by Celsus also suggest different topical agents including honey, vinegar, bran, and exposure to air [2,3]. Arabian physicians used ice-cold water as advocated by Rhazes in the ninth century AC [2].

In the 16th century, Ambrose Pare advocated deep burn excision [4]. The first documented classification of burns was coined by Guilhelmus Fabricus Hildanus in the 17th century and was revisited multiple times by different authors including Richter and Dupuytren [3]. The three-degree classification most often used nowadays was coined separately by Petit in 1812 and Boyer in 1814 [3,5]. Reverdin recognized the importance of skin grafting in excised burn wounds, the standard treatment used for most deep burns today, in the 19th century [4]. Scotland is credited with starting the practice of treating burn patients in specialized burn units, with Syme establishing the first burn unit in Edinburgh in 1843 [6].

The 20th century saw a major leap in burn care and major improvements in patient survival. Forty-percent total body surface area burns in adults carried a 50% mortality in the post-World War II era, while in the 1990s, 50% mortality occurred in patients with burns of 80% of total body surface area [4]. This is due to numerous advancements that took place in both burn care, notably burn resuscitation and early excision; and non-burn specific advancements such as discovery of antibiotics and the tremendous improvements in intensive care therapy.

In 1930, Underhill published an article reporting the need for fluid resuscitation in major burn patients after studying blister fluid in patients of the Rialto fire of 1921 [7]. These observations generated further research that culminated in fluid resuscitation formulae utilized to estimate appropriate volume of intravenous fluids to be given to specific body surface area burns. The first resuscitation formula based on body surface area was suggested by Harkins in 1942. Cope and Moore, studying the burn victims of the infamous Coconut Grove Fire in 1942, published their formula based on both extent of burn and patient weight [8]. Other authors followed suit proposing and modifying multiple formulae; culminating in the introduction the formula most widely used nowadays, the Parkland formula, described by Baxter and Shires in 1968 [9].

The World Wars, with unprecedented air warfare that resulted in mass burns contributed to development of burn reconstructive surgery, as these patients were treated in dedicated wards that developed the expertise of the treatment teams. Sir Archibald McIndoe was a pioneer in the field of burn reconstruction for his work on severely burned World War II pilots in the UK [10,11].

Penicillin was discovered in 1929 by Alexander Fleming, but first documented antibiotic use in burn patients was first in the 1940s [12]. Antibiotic therapy, both topical and systemic, became a staple of burn treatment in the 1960s after publication of a series of papers on pseudomonal burn wound sepsis by Mason and Walker, and the reduction of postburn mortality by Pruitt et al. after use of mafenide acetate cream on burns in the 1960s [13–16].

While the tenets of burn surgery, namely the need for deep burn excision, remained the same as described centuries prior; the 20th century saw a paradigm shift to favor early excision as opposed to the earlier recommendations to wait until eschar separation [17,18]. The technique of tangential excision, popularized by Janzekovic in the 1970s, along with improvement in supportive care, made it possible to acutely excise large burns, resulting in decreases in mortality and length of hospital stay [3,18–25].

Most accounts of burn history deal with events up to the consolidation of the method of tangential early excision. Bridging the narrative to contemporary times, this article will discuss the major concepts, developments, and concerns of burn care of the last 40 years. Namely, these are (1) the research on and understanding of hypermetabolism as the pathophysiologic mechanism underlying the corporal response to major burns, (2) description of over-resuscitation for major burns, (3) the continuing battle with burn wound sepsis, (4) tissue bioengineering endeavors to produce an ideal skin substitute, and (5) use of lasers for modulation of burn scars (6) emphasis on mental health (7) rehabilitation, and (8) study of long-term outcomes of burn care.

2. Hypermetabolism

It has long been known that major burns are far from local events, having effects on multiple organ systems and lasting for long periods of time; however, the exact mechanisms of these phenomena have not been well understood. Originally described in the 1930s and supported by studies performed in the 1940s and 50s, the concept of hypermetabolism as the systemic response to burn injury has come into the center-stage of the understanding of burn injury within the last two decades, with intense research on its molecular basis and possible treatments [26–32]. Hypermetabolism is described as a conglomeration of cellular phenomena occurring in response to major trauma, caused by complex hormonal and inflammatory interplays and consisting of changes in glucose, protein, and fat metabolism [27,33–36].

Burn injury initially causes an 'ebb phase' of metabolism characterized by decreased organ function and tissue perfusion which lasts 1–3 days [26]. This is followed by the 'flow phase' which consists of increased inflammatory cytokine secretion, increased tissue perfusion, heightened adrenergic and glucocorticoid responses, and decreased levels of growth hormone [37]. This stage may last up to 2 years after the burn, and as can be inferred, results in increased oxygen and energy expenditure, and caloric requirement [26].

While the evolutionary role of hypermetabolism is to provide the body with substrates to regenerate and fight off insults, it has been recognized that the severity and longevity of this response in burn injury surpasses the bodily needs, becomes deleterious and is in itself a cause of significant morbidity and possibly mortality in burn patients. Glycolysis, proteolysis and lipolysis cause significant catabolism, loss of lean body mass, physiologic exhaustion, delays in wound healing, and immune system dysfunction [37–40].

Traditionally, the two ways of off-setting hypermetabolism in major burn patients is to surgically excise the burn, thereby removing the major source of inflammation; and to provide the patient with adequate nutrition to limit lean body mass wasting and further catabolism [27,39,41].

The most powerful intervention that can be implemented in a major burn patient to curb hypermetabolism and decrease morbidity and mortality is undoubtedly early burn excision and closure of the resulting wounds [27,33]. Historically, this has become possible in the past 4 decades not because of advancement in surgical technique, as excision of burn wounds had been practiced for centuries; but because of advancements in supportive care allowing for the performance of safer surgery. The two fields allowing for this are intensive care which has provided the treatment of infections, blood transfusions, mechanical ventilation, blood pressure support, and enhanced patient monitoring; and the field of bioengineering that has provided skin substitutes allowing options for wound closure.

It is imperative to provide burn patients with adequate nutrition, currently, nutritional support is started enterally as early as possible, usually on the day of injury [27,42]. Nutritional requirements are calculated based on patients' resting energy expenditure; inadequate nutrition is associated with muscle wasting which in turn can lead to immune dysfunction, impaired wound healing, infections, and death; conversely, excess nutrition can lead to hyperglycemia and fatty infiltration of organs [27,42,43]. There is no consensus on the ideal nutrition for burn patients, and while research is actively being conducted to determine the optimal ratios of macro- and micronutrients, it is generally accepted that the majority of calories are to be obtained from carbohydrates with careful control of fatty acids to avoid organ infiltration and dysfunction. It is also standard practice to provide patients with micronutrients including Vitamins A, C, and E; as well as selenium, zinc, copper, and iron to offset oxidative stress, modulate immune function, and promote wound healing [44]. Studies on individual essential amino acids such as glutamine and alanine are also being carried out [27,42,44].

While effective in attenuating the hypermetabolic response, burn excision and adequate nutrition do not completely halt it [26], resulting in attempts to mitigate it using pharmacological agents, including the following:

(a) Insulin: Hyperglycemia has been implicated in multiple detrimental processes in burn patients, including delayed wound healing, infections, and increased mortality. Conversely, keeping a burn patient's glucose controlled around the 130 mg/dL mark has been shown to decrease patient mortality and morbidity associated with sepsis and infections [37,45–48]. Insulin was one of the first agents studied to curb hypermetabolism by controlling hyperglycemia and overcoming insulin resistance that develops in hypermetabolic patients. Insulin has also been shown to downregulate inflammatory cytokines and contribute to improved wound healing [27,37]. A drawback of insulin therapy is that it necessitates rigorous blood glucose measurements to avoid hypoglycemia which may be serious, and potentially fatal in the intensive care setting [37,45].

(b) Metformin: A possible replacement for insulin therapy that is currently being investigated for effectiveness of glucose control and hypermetabolism attenuation is Metformin. Its advantages are the easier dosing and less need for monitoring, as it does not cause hypoglycemia. Metformin may cause lactic acidosis however and renal failure in rare cases [27,37,45].

(c) Propranolol: A non-specific b-adrenergic blocker, propranolol has been shown to decrease the hypermetabolic response due to its ability to block the sympathetic response, thereby decreasing cardiac workload, insulin resistance, and loss of lean body mass, among other beneficial effects [27,49,50].

(d) Recombinant Human Growth Hormone (rHGH): rHGH has been studied as an agent for treatment of hypermetabolism due to the findings that its levels are low in hypermetabolic patients. While it has shown favorable outcomes in pediatric populations, including increase in lean body mass, it is seldom used in adults due to a study that citing high rates of mortality and morbidity in adults with the use of rHGH [27,37,51].

(e) Oxandrolone: A synthetic testosterone analog that possesses only 5% of testos-terone's virilizing effects. Being an anabolic hormone, it helps in maintenance of lean body mass and has been shown to shorten hospital stay in burned children [32,52].

3. Fluid Creep

Fluid resuscitation is a cornerstone of burn treatment; its study and protocolization in the 20th century have led to significant increases in burn patient survival [4]. However, recognition of over-resuscitation, known as fluid creep, and its detrimental effects on patient course and outcomes have dominated the past 2 decades [53]. In 2000, Pruitt famously wrote about the pendulum of resuscitation swinging in the direction of over-resuscitation of acute burns with crystalloid solution and emphasized the need to reverse this phenomenon [54].

There are recognized patient conditions that require higher-than-normal resuscitation volumes. These include very large total body surface area (TBSA) burns, inhalation injury, electrical injury, delayed presentation of burned patient, and polytrauma [55,56]. Recent literature suggests that routine burn patients without the previously mentioned conditions are increasingly receiving volumes of resuscitation fluid in excess of those advocated by resuscitation calculations [55–60]. Adverse effects of fluid creep include increased extremity pressures that may require release in the form of escharotomies or fasciotomies, airway edema potentially requiring intubation, and abdominal compartment syndrome [55–59,61].

While the exact mechanisms of fluid creep have not been delineated, it most probably is a multifactorial phenomenon caused by a combination of the following factors:

(a) Carelessness: patients receiving large volumes as runs by first responders, directly on admission, and reluctance of tapering of high volume infusions for fear of causing renal failure [55,60].

(b) Larger burns: the resuscitation formulae were described when burn survival in patients with very large burns was rare. Therefore, adequacy of the formulas is studied best in moderate-sized burns, whereas fluid requirements for large and very large burns may go beyond what can accurately be predicted by resuscitation formulas [9,55].

(c) Opioid creep: opioid analgesia, which is much more frequently used now than in the past, causes decreases in blood pressure which is then counteracted with larger resuscitation fluid volumes [55,62].

(d) Goal-directed resuscitation: resuscitation to achieve certain urine outputs or base-deficit figures without regard for clinical fluid balances and edema. Studies suggest that certain goals such as base deficit require 24–48 h to normalize even in the setting of adequate resuscitation [55,63]. Interim readings before value normalization may however prompt over-resuscitation [57].

(e) Pure crystalloid: patients resuscitated with crystalloid solution only require higher fluid volumes than those resuscitated with colloid [56,64]. In fact, the earliest version of the Parkland formula included colloid addition in the second day of resuscitation [55,56]. Colloids fell out of favor due to a study by Goodwin et al. in 1983 that showed increased mortality in patients receiving albumin [65]. Newer studies fail to demonstrate increased mortality with the use of colloids but also do not demonstrate a survival benefit with their use [60,66–68].

4. Sepsis in Burns

Sepsis is described as organ damage in the context of a dysregulated systemic inflammatory response to an infectious agent [69]. It is a primary cause of mortality in intensive care units worldwide and is presently the leading cause of death in patients with severe burns [70]. Due to this, sepsis has been the topic of much recent study and discussion. Its definition and diagnostic criteria have been revised frequently in the past three decades, leading to some confusion about the interpretation of study results and the appropriateness of comparison of different therapeutic trials due to use of different defining parameters. The need for standardization of the definition of sepsis has been recognized as a step towards clarity in the clinical diagnosis and therapeutic results of the condition.

Traditionally, sepsis was defined as evidence of an infection in addition to a systemic inflammatory response syndrome (SIRS) [71]; whereas SIRS was defined as two or more of the following: temperature > 38 °C or < 36 °C, heart rate > 90 beats per minute, respiratory rate > 20 breaths per minute or maintenance of $PaCO_2$ < 32 mmHg, or white bloodcount > 12,000/mm^3 or 4000/mm^3 or left shift defined as > 10% bands [72]. The latest widely agreed-upon definition is the Sepsis-3 definition developed by the Third International Consensus Definitions for Sepsis and Septic Shock (Sepsis-3) in 2016 [73–75]. Sepsis-3 defines sepsis in terms of Sequential Organ Failure Assessment (SOFA) variables which are: PaO_2/FiO_2 ratio, Glasgow Coma Scale, mean arterial pressure, vasopressor requirements, serum creatinine or urine output, bilirubin, and platelet count; or quick SOFAs (qSOFAs) which are altered mental status (Glasgow Coma Scale GCS < 13), systolic blood pressure $\leq$ 100 mmHg, and respiratory rate $\geq$ 22 [73]. SOFA and qSOFA variables are essentially proxies for organ dysfunction, and sepsis is defined as 2 or more SOFA criteria, or documented infection in addition to 2 or more qSOFA criteria [73–75].

Burn patients are habitually excluded from sepsis trials due to the overlap of traditional systemic inflammatory response syndrome (SIRS) symptoms such as tachycardia, tachypnea, fever, and leukocytosis with the inflammatory and hypermetabolic reactions seen in response to major burn injury [71,76,77]; therefore, sepsis definitions used in the general patient population are not validated in the burn patient population [71,78,79]. The American Burn Association (ABA) has developed a burn-specific definition of sepsis in 2007 in response to this dilemma, with the following criteria: temperature > 39 °C or < 36.5 °C, progressive tachycardia > 110 beats per minute, progressive tachypnea > 25 breaths per minute, thrombocytopenia < 100,000/mcL, hyperglycemia in the absence of pre-existing diabetes mellitus, inability to continue enteral feedings > 24 h [76]. In addition, the ABA definition requires that a documented infection is identified by a positive culture, or pathologic tissue source, or clinical response to antimicrobials [76]. Several trials have compared the Sepsis-3 and ABA criteria for predicting sepsis in the burn population and found Sepsis-3 to be superior to the ABA criteria [78]. It must be noted that Sepsis-3 definition has come under scrutiny for not being sufficiently specific for sepsis in burn patients [80]. Therefore, the pursuit for a satisfactory definition of sepsis in burn patients is still ongoing.

Major burn patients differ from the general patient population in terms of sepsis in that they present with loss of the body's skin barrier function, which predisposes them to sepsis for prolonged periods of time; this is exacerbated by the immune compromise that is frequently observed in the context of major burns [71]. Additionally, major burn patients often require mechanical ventilation, central venous, arterial, and urinary catheterization, all of which further increase infection risk. As a result, rigorous infection prevention and control measures are the norm in modern burn units in an attempt to reduce the likelihood of infection. These measures include screening for resistant organisms upon admission and discharge of patients, individual patient rooms, contact isolation measures, a strong emphasis on hygiene, daily antimicrobial dressings for burn wounds, monitoring of need and status of all invasive catheters, and careful antimicrobial stewardship [70].

Effort has been put into collecting and protocolizing evidence on sepsis management, with the result being the Surviving Sepsis Campaign (SSC) guidelines that have been developed and published periodically since 2004. These guidelines are presented as collections of treatment recommendations, or 'bundles', that should be implemented within specific time frames or in response to certain signs and symptoms [81–83]. Adherence to these 'bundle' interventions has shown a decrease in mortality rates of sepsis in the general population [69]. While the management recommendations indicated in the Surviving Sepsis Campaign are mostly not new, consisting notably of intravenous fluid resuscitation, administration of antimicrobial agents after taking cultures, vasopressor support to maintain a (mean arterial pressure) MAP $\geq$ 65, renal replacement, and glycemic control [83]. It is the timeliness of these interventions that is an important predictor of survival in sepsis, with evidence of increase in mortality for each hour antimicrobial therapy is delayed after the onset of hypotension [84].

Most of the criteria included in any definition of sepsis are clinical. The few laboratory measurements included (platelet count, bilirubin) are non-specific. The development of a sepsis-specific laboratory marker could greatly help in the prompt diagnosis and follow-up of sepsis, especially in major burn patients, where most of the clinical signs and symptoms are common to both conditions and it is difficult to distinguish etiology. Currently, the two markers used as measures of sepsis are C-reactive protein (CRP) and Procalcitonin. While CRP is sensitive for inflammation, it is less specific for infection and is slower to change, with the half-life of several days [85]. The more expensive Procalcitonin is more specific to infection and has a shorter half-life and may therefore be useful as a marker of change in condition. Although it has been shown to be a relatively good marker for sepsis and survival in burn patients, its levels are subject to fluctuations in response to surgery and different types of microbial agents, making interpretations more complicated [77,86–90].

5. Skin Substitutes

Autograft donor sites in the body are limited. This limitation is compounded by the need for wound coverage after early excision, especially in the case of large burns [91]. One solution for this is the use of skin substitutes, which are naturally-occurring or manufactured alternatives to autografts that can be either temporary or permanent and replace the epidermis, the dermis, or both [17,92]. Ideally, a skin substitute should provide wound coverage to limit fluid loss and bacterial growth, reduce pain and allow for wound healing. There is no perfect skin substitute; the past 4 decades saw a boom of biotechnology in an attempt to make an ideal skin replacement. The following is a limited list of skin substitutes used in burn units today.

The earliest skin substitutes used were allografts, or cadaveric skin, first used by Girdner in 1881 [93,94]. Most major burn centers use allografts as a wound bed preparation material in moderate to large burns, to increase the likelihood of subsequent autograft take [93]. The drawbacks of allograft use are the need for resources (skin banks) for its storage, as well as its antigenicity which usually manifests at around 3 weeks after its application, necessitating its replacement with autograft.

One solution to the antigenicity and impermanence of allografts, while avoiding the morbidity and scarcity of traditional autografts is to culture skin from a small skin sample taken from the burn patient. Cultured keratinocytes, or cultured epithelial autografts (CEA), were first reported in 1981 by O'Connor et al. and required 3–5 weeks for the growth in vitro of sheets of epithelial cells from a small biopsy of a patient's normal skin [17,95–97]. Advantages are lack of immunogenicity and negligible donor sites, disadvantages are fragility of the sheets (due to lack of dermal component which is what gives skin its elasticity and strength), high cost, and time for production [95,98–100]. CEA has evolved from culturing cells in sheets which may take up to 5 weeks, to culturing cells in suspension which takes 2–3 weeks [95,97]. Currently, several systems of suspended keratinocyte delivery are available in the market, these are usually applied over a dermal substitute in order to achieve some elasticity and strength [95,97].

Multiple attempts have also been made at producing a skin substitute that would simultaneously replace the epidermal and dermal layers, with the goal of achieving a skin substitute that is stronger, more elastic, and more resistant to wear than a cultured keratinocyte sheet. One such substitute is the self-assembled skin substitute (SASS) that is composed of a collagen-rich extracellular matrix produced by a patient's fibroblasts which is then seeded with keratinocytes thereby producing a substitute that is non-immunogenic and contains both skin layers [91,98]. Limitations include the time needed for production and high cost.

Numerous non-human tissue skin substitutes have also been developed for use in the burn patient to replace the various skin components. While an exhaustive list of synthetic substitutes is beyond the scope of this text, three substitutes that are prevalent in modern burn units and warrant mention are Biobrane®, Integra®, and BTM®.

Biobrane® is an epidermal substitute that is a synthetic bilayer consisting of an inner nylon mesh and an outer silastic membrane. It is most commonly applied to superficial second degree burns to act as a semi-occlusive dressing, thereby diminishing fluid loss and decreasing pain associated with dressing changes while the superficial burn heals spontaneously [101,102]. It has been particularly useful in pediatric patients with superficial second degree burns, but has also found uses in patients with non-burn epithelial defects such as toxic epidermal necrolysis syndrome (TENS) [103].

Integra® is a dermal regeneration template developed in the 1970s by Yannis and Burke. It consists of a chondroitin-collagen dermis covered by a silastic epidermis [3,4]. The dermal matrix allows for migration of fibroblasts and macrophages and becomes vascularized and incorporated into the body, and the silastic epidermis is removed and autografted 3 weeks after application. Integra carries the advantage of easy storage and decreased contracture compared to autograft only [104,105], and of being able to survive on small exposed areas of bone or tendon, on which autograft alone does not survive. Disadvantages include infections and its high cost [17,105]. Biodegradable Temporizing Matrix, or BTM®, is a synthetic polyurethane dermal substitute developed in 2012 by Greenwood that incorporates into the body through ingrowth of blood vessels and fibroblast infiltration [106,107]. Like Integra®, it contains a sealing membrane that is removed 3–4 weeks after application, allowing the dermal matrix to be skin grafted [17,99]. Preliminary data show decreased contracture rates and decreased infections [99,100].

6. Lasers

Burn scars are a well-recognized sequela of major burn injury. In addition to unsightly appearance, these can limit function through contracture formation, and cause neuropathic pain, itching, and repetitive wound breakdown [108–113]. Increased burn patient survival has meant an increased burden of burn scar morbidity and has brought the need for effective scar therapies to the forefront of burn care.

Traditionally, burn scar treatment has included conservative modalities such as compression garments, applications of intralesional steroids, silicone creams; and surgical modalities such as scar release or excision and grafting [108–113]. Laser therapy has emerged as a novel technique of manipulating scar tissue in the past 20 years [114].

Lasers can be classified as non-ablative and ablative, the difference being their mode of action. Non-ablative lasers target pigments within the skin, and may be used for hyperpigmentation, vascular anomalies and tattoo removal; while ablative lasers vaporize tissues, modulating scar tissue [111].

Pulse-dye lasers are an example of non-ablative lasers, they have a wavelength of 585 nm or 595 nm and target oxygenated hemoglobin within capillaries in the dermis causing the coagulation of these vessels resulting in decreased erythema in the scar [110,111,115–118]. Erbium-yttrium aluminium garnet (Erbium-YAG and CO_2 lasers are examples of ablative lasers, they target abnormal collagen, destroying it and promoting formation of new collagen, consequently remodeling scar tissue [110,111,115–118]. Erbium-YAG has a wavelength of 2490 nm enabling it to target dermal matrix components, while the CO_2 laser has a wavelength of 10,600 nm and is therefore able to effectuate more extensive tissue remodeling due to its ability to vaporize scar tissue and coagulate blood vessels in the scar at the same time. This higher energy however, also carries the potential for more complications due to the higher energy dispersal. Complications of laser therapy include erythema, swelling, pain, skin infection, and hyperpigmentation [110,111,115–118].

Extension of previous laser indications include laser therapy prior to definitive reconstructive surgery for contractures in an attempt to soften scar tissue, making it more malleable; as well as the topical application of corticosteroids just prior to laser therapy, the belief being that laser beams will allow enhanced delivery of the steroids into the scar [110,117,119].

7. Mental Health

The first time mental health was acknowledged as a major component of burn patient recovery was in the work of McIndoe on his patients who were mostly WWII soldiers [120]. The Guinea Pig Club was formed by his patients in 1941 to provide burn reconstruction patients with social and psychological support. Research done in the late 1980s and 1990s demonstrated that up to 45% of adult patients hospitalized for burn injury showed signs of post-traumatic stress disorder 1 year after their initial injury [121]. It has also been demonstrated that prevalence rates of psychological distress and anxiety are high in hospitalized patients and that these symptoms tend to persist after discharge [122]. Compounding the problem of psychiatric issues in burn patients is the high incidence of pre-existing psychiatric conditions, alcoholism, and substance abuse [123–126], which in some cases may be the inciting agents of the burn [127]. Patients with pre-existing psychiatric conditions have been found to have higher rates of complications and require longer hospitalizations after a burn injury, as well as more difficulties in rehabilitation and readjustment post-burn [128–132]. Acute stress disorder starts immediately after hospitalization and if left untreated may be a predictor of future post traumatic stress disorder (PTSD) [127,133]. The burn team needs to be attuned to the patient's psychological wellbeing and symptoms of stress, depression, anxiety, and sleep disturbance must be promptly recognized and treated. Mental health professionals such as counselors, psychologists and psychiatrists are an integral part of any burn unit.

Pain is strongly linked with stress, anxiety, and sleep disorders in burn patients; inversely, patients with these psychological symptoms also become less tolerant to pain and may even have decreased wound healing [134,135]. Pain is a strong predictor of both acute and long-term psychological sequelae, and both pain and psychiatric disorders are strong predictors of long-term functioning in burn patients [123,136–139]. Anxiety and depression caused by excessive pain are decreased with adequate pain management [135].

Pain management is of paramount importance to burn care. The ABA has published guidelines for the management of acute pain and the recommendations include the need for frequent burn assessments, pharmacological therapy that includes opioids as well as adjuncts such as acetaminophen and non-steroidal anti-inflammatory drugs (NSAIDs), agents for neurologic pain such as gabapentin and pregabalin, and the use of ketamine for procedural sedation when needed (by trained personnel) [140]. The guidelines also include the recommendation to offer patients nonpharmacological analgesia techniques, such as cognitive behavioral therapy, hypnosis and virtual reality (VR) when available. Hypnosis has been found to significantly reduce affective pain in burn patients as well as flashbacks to the inciting incident [141–144]. There is significant evidence for the use of virtual reality as a nonpharmacological analgesic technique, it has been found to decrease both pain and anxiety associated with dressing changes, procedures, and physiotherapy and is a powerful analgesic adjunct to pharmacological therapy [121,145–152]. Functional magnetic resonance imagine (MRI) imaging has shown decreased pain-related brain activity with the use of VR [153].

Burn patients need to reintegrate back into their lives and communities after discharge from the burn unit, this is a process that goes hand in hand with physical rehabilitation and may require education of the patients and their families as well as social support. Much in the same tradition of the Guinea Pig Club, burn survivor groups provide an understanding and supportive social network that can assist patients in their recovery [154,155]. Variables affecting success of reintegration include physical impairment, pre- and postburn psychological distress, and substance abuse, among others [122]. About 66% of adult patients are found to be working 2 years after their major burns [156], and presence of work correlates with a better subjective quality of life [157,158].

Followup of children who survive major burns reveals that most of them adapt satisfactorily [159]. In adolescents and young adults, 40–50% were found to be well-adjusted, 50–60% were found to have some degree of psychological distress, and 25% were found to have severe symptoms. In fact, the most debilitating long-term effects of childhood burns are psychological and not physical [160]. Social skills programs have been shown to improve psychosocial competence of adolescent burn survivors [159–162].

8. Rehabilitation

Burn treatment does not end with wound coverage or hospital discharge. Rehabilitation is an integral part of burn care, and probably the stage of burn management that lasts the longest. Burn injuries are notorious for function-limiting sequelae, including contractures, hypertrophic scarring, amputations, pruritus, thermoregulatory anomalies, hyperesthesias and paresthesias.

Rehabilitation has come to play a central role in burn management as survival of burn patients has improved, and quality of life and level of function of patients became the focus of recovery. It nowadays starts in the acute phase just after admission and carries on after patient discharge, and comprises of a vast variety of treatments including physiotherapy, ergotherapy, pain management, pressure garments, masks for hypertrophic scarring, and prosthetics [113,163].

The earliest rehabilitation intervention implemented after patient admission to the burn unit is positioning. The patient as well as the burned body part should be held in a position of comfort that nonetheless minimizes the chances of wound and joint contractures, edema, and pressure injury [164,165]. The strategies used for positioning may include techniques such as splinting, orthoses, special mattresses, foam cushions/wedges, and pressure dressings [165]. The particular strategies used are highly individualized and should be frequently reassessed and modified as the need arises.

The intermediate phase of rehabilitation spans the period of wound healing; priorities at this time are stretching of healing skin, grafts, and joints to prevent contractures and keep the tissues supple [166,167]. Long-term burn rehabilitation occurs after discharge and continues until the patient has gleaned the maximal benefit possible [166]. Rehabilitation programs range from inpatient to outpatient with frequent follow-ups, to patients becoming able to independently effectuate their programs with minimal oversight. The goals of long-term rehabilitation is to achieve maximal range of motion and functionality, and to learn to compensate for function that cannot be restored.

An important aspect of rehabilitation is scar management. Facial masks used to attenuate hypertrophic scarring of facial burns, as well as pressure garments used for scars for other body areas usually fall under the supervision of the burn physiotherapist. Evidence on the efficacy of pressure garments is not indisputable, with multiple studies falling on either side of the debate. The use of pressure to modulate scar healing was first mentioned in the medical literature in the late 1800s and was popularized in the 1970s; the supporters of garment use cite studies showing that application of pressure to a raised scar reduced its thickness and helped in its maturation [168–174]. The detractors argue that the garments do not apply adequate pressure, need to be worn for 23 h a day which is difficult to comply with; and that they cause discomfort, skin breakdown, and limitation of motion [175–178].

9. Long-Term Outcomes

Outcomes of burn care had historically been measured in terms of survival or length of stay. As survival rates of major burns increase, longer-term outcomes such as quality of life, psychosocial well-being, and return to work, may provide greater insights into the consequences of major burns. This in turn allows for patient-centric care and anticipation of patient needs not only in the immediate aftermath of a major burn, but also in the long-run [179–181]. Collection of long-term prospective data on multiple aspects of patient care and its results with respect to patient functioning, as well as periodic review of this data and identification of areas for improvement is a hallmark of major burn units. Verification by the American Burn Association stipulates that every verified burn unit collect data on burn admissions and their complications and outcomes, and creates a framework for collaboration of different burn units and teams on research.

10. Conclusions

Despite the impressive evolution that has taken place in burn care over the past century, there is ample room for further growth. The future will entail developments in the avenues discussed above. Dedicated efforts are being made in order to achieve better understanding and control of hypermetabolism, with ongoing trials on pharmacological agents to modulate the hypermetabolic response; glutamine and combination antihyperglycemics are currently being studied [27]. Research is also ongoing for biomarkers of hypermetabolism, with the goal of discovering markers that are easy to test for and that provide information on response to treatment and prognosis [27,182].

Likewise, optimal ways to resuscitate major burn patients with minimal side effects is an ongoing field of study, one notable trial that is currently in progress is the Acute Burn ResUscitation Multicenter Prospective Trial (ABRUPT2), evaluating acute resuscitation of major burns with crystalloid alone versus crystalloid with the addition of 5% albumin at 8 h post burn [183].

In the field of sepsis, active areas of investigation are the testing of sensitive and specific biomarkers of sepsis, with research into leukocyte biomarkers which may replace the currently used CRP and Procalcitonin measurements [184]. Another important field in sepsis research is the development of techniques that allow the detection of bacterial or fungal DNA within the bloodstream within hours, precluding the need to wait for days for antimicrobial culture results [85]. In addition, investigations on ways to develop therapeutic agents/biotechnology to allow the removal of inflammatory factors and cytokines from the bloodstream, therefore curbing the dysregulated reaction to infection in septic patients is underway [85].

Mesenchymal stem cells (MSCs) have been found to enhance wound healing capabilities [185,186]. It has also been discovered that burnt tissue that is excised in the process of burn debridement contains active MSCs. Research is ongoing on extracting these MSCs from burnt tissue, and incorporating them into a 3D-printed skin substitute that will not use healthy skin as a donor, and will not be immunogenic as the MSCs will come from a patient's own burnt, discarded tissue [187,188]. If successful, this may prove revolutionary as a skin substitute option.

Evaluation and refinement of laser techniques and study of scar modulation techniques are also active areas of research, as are mental health interventions, and burn rehabilitation techniques. In the light of the better understanding of the pathophysiology and treatment of burns and the active research being conducted on many aspects of burn care, the future holds hope of improving outcomes and alleviating the suffering of burn patients.

Author Contributions: A.E.K.: Conceptualization, writing original draft, review and editing. M.G.J.: Supervision, data curation, and editing. All authors have read and agreed to the published version of the manuscript.

Funding: This research received no external funding.

Institutional Review Board Statement: Not Applicable.

Informed Consent Statement: Not Applicable.

Data Availability Statement: Data sharing not applicable.

Conflicts of Interest: The authors declare no conflict of interest.

References

1. Hussain, A.; Choukairi, F. To cool or not to cool: Evolution of the treatment of burns in the 18th century. *Int. J. Surg.* **2013**, *11*, 503–506. [CrossRef]
2. Artz, C.P. Historical Aspects of Burn Management. *Surg. Clin. N. Am.* **1970**, *50*, 1193–1200. [CrossRef]
3. Moiemen, N.S.; Lee, K.C.; Joory, K. History of burns: The past, present and the future. *Burn. Trauma* **2014**, *2*, 169–180. [CrossRef]
4. Liu, H.-F.; Zhang, F.; Lineaweaver, W.C. History and Advancement of Burn Treatments. *Ann. Plast. Surg.* **2017**, *78*, S2–S8. [CrossRef] [PubMed]
5. Denkler, K. History of burns. *Plast. Reconstr. Surg.* **1999**, *104*, 308–309. [CrossRef]
6. Wallace, A.F. Recent advances in the treatment of burns—1843–1858. *Br. J. Plast. Surg.* **1987**, *40*, 193–200. [CrossRef]
7. Underhill, F.P. The significance of anhydremia in extensive superficial burns. *JAMA* **1930**, *95*, 852–857. [CrossRef]
8. Alvarado, R.; Chung, K.K.; Cancio, L.C.; Wolf, S.E. Burn resuscitation. *Burns J. Int. Soc. Burn Inj.* **2009**, *35*, 4–14. [CrossRef]
9. Baxter, C.R.; Shires, T. Physiological response to crystalloid resuscitation of severe burns. *Ann. N. Y. Acad. Sci.* **1968**, *150*, 874–894. [CrossRef] [PubMed]
10. Mayhew, E.R. *The Guinea Pig Club: Archibald McIndoe and the RAF in World War II*; Dundurn Press: Toronto, ON, Canada, 2018.
11. McIndoe, S.A. Total Facial Reconstruction Following Burns. *Postgrad. Med.* **1949**, *6*, 187–200. [CrossRef]
12. Lyons, C. Penicillin therapy of surgical infections in the U. S. ARMY. *J. Am. Med Assoc.* **1943**, *123*, 1007. [CrossRef]
13. Teplitz, C.; Davis, D.; Mason, A.D.; Moncrief, J.A. Pseudomonas burn wound sepsis. I Pathogenesis of experimental pseudomonas burn wound sepsis. *J. Surg. Res.* **1964**, *4*, 200–216. [CrossRef]
14. Teplitz, C.; Davis, D.; Walker, H.L.; Raulston, G.L.; Mason, A.D.; A Moncrief, J. Pseudomonas burn wound sepsis. II Hematogenous infection at the junction of the burn wound and the unburned hypodermis. *J. Surg. Res.* **1964**, *4*, 217–222. [CrossRef]
15. Walker, H.L.; Mason, A.D.; Raulston, L.C.G.L. Surface Infection with Pseudomonas Aeruginosa. *Ann. Surg.* **1964**, *160*, 297–305. [CrossRef]
16. Pruitt, B.A.; O'Neill, J.A.; Moncrief, J.A.; Lindberg, R.B. Successful Control of Burn-Wound Sepsis. *JAMA* **1968**, *203*, 1054–1056. [CrossRef]
17. Kearney, L.; Francis, E.C.; Clover, A.J. New technologies in global burn care—A review of recent advances. *Int. J. Burn. Trauma* **2018**, *8*, 77–87.
18. Herndon, D.N.; Barrow, R.E.; Rutan, R.L.; Rutan, T.C.; Desai, M.H.; Abston, S. A Comparison of Conservative versus Early Excision. *Ann. Surg.* **1989**, *209*, 547–553. [CrossRef]
19. Barret, J.P.; Herndon, D.N. Effects of Burn Wound Excision on Bacterial Colonization and Invasion. *Plast. Reconstr. Surg.* **2003**, *111*, 744–750. [CrossRef] [PubMed]
20. Thompson, P.; Herndon, D.N.; Abston, S.; Rutan, T. Effect of Early Excision on Patients with Major Thermal Injury. *J. Trauma Inj. Infect. Crit. Care* **1987**, *27*, 205–207. [CrossRef] [PubMed]
21. Janžekovič, Z. A new concept in the early excision and immediate grafting of burns. *J. Trauma Inj. Infect. Crit. Care* **1970**, *10*, 1103–1108. [CrossRef]
22. Tompkins, R.G.; Remensnyder, J.P.; Burke, J.F.; Tompkins, D.M.; Hilton, J.F.; Schoenfeld, D.A.; Behringer, G.E.; Bondoc, C.C.; Briggs, S.E.; Quinby, W.C. Significant Reductions in Mortality for Children With Burn Injuries Through the Use of Prompt Eschar Excision. *Ann. Surg.* **1988**, *208*, 577–585. [CrossRef] [PubMed]
23. Pietsch, J.B.; Netscher, D.T.; Nagaraj, H.S.; Groff, D.B. Early excision of major burns in children: Effect on morbidity and mortality. *J. Pediatr. Surg.* **1985**, *20*, 754–757. [CrossRef]
24. Janzekovic, Z. Once upon a time. How west discovered east. *J. Plast. Reconstr. Aesthetic Surg.* **2008**, *61*, 240–244. [CrossRef]
25. Engrav, L.H.; Heimbach, D.M.; Reus, J.L.; Harnar, T.J.; Marvin, J.A. Early excision and grafting vs. nonoperative treatment of burns of indeterminant depth: A randomized prospective study. *J. Trauma* **1983**, *23*, 1001–1004. [CrossRef] [PubMed]
26. Sommerhalder, C.; Blears, E.; Murton, A.J.; Porter, C.; Finnerty, C.; Herndon, D.N. Current problems in burn hypermetabolism. *Curr. Probl. Surg.* **2020**, *57*, 100709. [CrossRef] [PubMed]
27. Jeschke, M.G. Postburn Hypermetabolism: Past, Present, and Future. *J. Burn Care Res.* **2016**, *37*, 86–96. [CrossRef] [PubMed]
28. Wilmore, D.W. Hormonal Responses and Their Effect on Metabolism. *Surg. Clin. N. Am.* **1976**, *56*, 999–1018. [CrossRef]
29. Wilmore, D.W.; Long, J.M.; Mason, A.D.; Skreen, R.W.; Pruitt, B.A. Catecholamines: Mediator of the hypermetabolic response to thermal injury. *Ann. Surg.* **1974**, *180*, 653–669. [CrossRef]
30. Wolfe, R.R.; Herndon, D.N.; Jahoor, F.; Miyoshi, H.; Wolfe, M. Effect of Severe Burn Injury on Substrate Cycling by Glucose and Fatty Acids. *N. Engl. J. Med.* **1987**, *317*, 403–408. [CrossRef]
31. Wolfe, R.R.; Herndon, D.N.; Peters, E.J.; Jahoor, F.; Desai, M.H.; Holland, O.B. Regulation of Lipolysis in Severely Burned Children. *Ann. Surg.* **1987**, *206*, 214–221. [CrossRef]
32. Hart, D.W.; Wolf, S.E.; Ramzy, P.I.; Chinkes, D.L.; Beauford, R.B.; Ferrando, A.A.; Wolfe, R.R.; Herndon, D.N. Anabolic Effects of Oxandrolone After Severe Burn. *Ann. Surg.* **2001**, *233*, 556–564. [CrossRef]
33. Herndon, D.N.; Tompkins, R.G. Support of the metabolic response to burn injury. *Lancet* **2004**, *363*, 1895–1902. [CrossRef]

34. Jeschke, M.G.; Chinkes, D.L.; Finnerty, C.C.; Kulp, G.; Suman, O.E.; Norbury, W.B.; Branski, L.K.; Gauglitz, G.G.; Mlcak, R.P.; Herndon, D.N. Pathophysiologic Response to Severe Burn Injury. *Ann. Surg.* **2008**, *248*, 387–401. [CrossRef] [PubMed]
35. Jeschke, M.G.; Gauglitz, G.G.; Kulp, G.A.; Finnerty, C.C.; Williams, F.N.; Kraft, R.; Suman, O.E.; Mlcak, R.P.; Herndon, D.N. Long-Term Persistance of the Pathophysiologic Response to Severe Burn Injury. *PLoS ONE* **2011**, *6*, e21245. [CrossRef]
36. McCowen, K.C.; Malhotra, A.; Bistrian, B.R. Stress-Induced Hyperglycemia. *Crit. Care Clin.* **2001**, *17*, 107–124. [CrossRef]
37. Auger, C.; Samadi, O.; Jeschke, M.G. The biochemical alterations underlying post-burn hypermetabolism. *Biochim. Biophys. Acta (BBA) Mol. Basis Dis.* **2017**, *1863*, 2633–2644. [CrossRef]
38. Hart, D.W.; Wolf, S.E.; Chinkes, D.L.; Gore, D.C.; Mlcak, R.P.; Beauford, R.B.; Obeng, M.K.; Lal, S.; Gold, W.F.; Wolfe, R.R.; et al. Determinants of Skeletal Muscle Catabolism After Severe Burn. *Ann. Surg.* **2000**, *232*, 455–465. [CrossRef] [PubMed]
39. Orgill, D.P. Excision and Skin Grafting of Thermal Burns. *N. Engl. J. Med.* **2009**, *360*, 893–901. [CrossRef] [PubMed]
40. Porter, C.; Tompkins, R.G.; Finnerty, C.C.; Sidossis, L.S.; E Suman, O.; Herndon, D.N. The metabolic stress response to burn trauma: Current understanding and therapies. *Lancet* **2016**, *388*, 1417–1426. [CrossRef]
41. Gore, D.C.; Chinkes, D.; Sanford, A.; Hart, D.W.; Wolf, S.E.; Herndon, D.N. Influence of Fever on the Hypermetabolic Response in Burn-Injured Children. *Arch. Surg.* **2003**, *138*, 169–174. [CrossRef] [PubMed]
42. Rodriguez, N.; Jeschke, M.; Williams, F.; Kamolz, L.-P.; Herndon, D. Nutrition in Burns: Galveston Contributions. *J. Parenter Enter. Nutr.* **2011**, *35*, 704–714. [CrossRef]
43. Chang, D.W.; DeSanti, L.; Demling, R.H. Anticatabolic and anabolic strategies in critical illness: A review of current treatment modalities. *Shock* **1998**, *10*, 155–160. [CrossRef] [PubMed]
44. Jeschke, M.G.; Shahrokhi, S.; Hall, K.L. Enteral Nutrition Support in Burn Care: A Review of Current Recommendations as In-stituted in the Ross Tilley Burn Centre. *Nutrients* **2012**, *4*, 1554–1565.
45. Jeschke, M.G. Clinical review: Glucose control in severely burned patients—Current best practice. *Crit. Care* **2013**, *17*, 232. [CrossRef] [PubMed]
46. Gore, D.C.; Chinkes, D.; Heggers, J.; Herndon, D.N.; Wolf, S.E.; Desai, M. Association of Hyperglycemia with Increased Mortality after Severe Burn Injury. *J. Trauma Inj. Infect. Crit. Care* **2001**, *51*, 540–544. [CrossRef]
47. Jeschke, M.G.; Kulp, G.A.; Kraft, R.; Finnerty, C.C.; Mlcak, R.; Lee, J.O.; Herndon, D.N. Intensive insulin therapy in severely burned pediatric patients: A prospective random-ized trial. *Am. J. Respir. Crit. Care Med.* **2010**, *182*, 351–359. [CrossRef] [PubMed]
48. Van den Berghe, G.; Wilmer, A.; Hermans, G.; Meersseman, W.; Wouters, P.J.; Milants, I.; Van Wijngaerden, E.; Bobbaers, H.; Bouillon, R. Intensive insulin therapy in the medical ICU. *N. Engl. J. Med.* **2006**, *354*, 449–461. [CrossRef] [PubMed]
49. Flores, O.; Stockton, K.; Roberts, J.A.; Muller, M.J.; Paratz, J.D. The efficacy and safety of adrenergic blockade after burn injury: A systematic review and meta-analysis. *J. Trauma Acute Care Surg.* **2016**, *80*, 146–155. [CrossRef]
50. Brooks, N.C.; Song, J.; Boehning, D.; Kraft, R.; Finnerty, C.C.; Herndon, D.N.; Jeschke, M.G. Propranolol Improves Impaired Hepatic Phosphatidylinositol 3-Kinase/Akt Signaling after Burn Injury. *Mol. Med.* **2012**, *18*, 707–711. [CrossRef]
51. Takala, J.; Ruokonen, E.; Webster, N.R.; Nielsen, M.S.; Zandstra, D.F.; Vundelinckx, G.; Hinds, C.J. Increased Mortality Associated with Growth Hormone Treatment in Critically Ill Adults. *N. Engl. J. Med.* **1999**, *341*, 785–792. [CrossRef] [PubMed]
52. Jeschke, M.G.; Finnerty, C.C.; Suman, O.E.; Kulp, G.; Mlcak, R.P.; Herndon, D.N. The Effect of Oxandrolone on the Endocrinologic, Inflammatory, and Hypermetabolic Responses during the Acute Phase Postburn. *Ann. Surg.* **2007**, *246*, 351–362. [CrossRef]
53. Klein, M.B.; Hayden, D.; Elson, C.; Nathens, A.B.; Gamelli, R.L.; Gibran, N.S.; Herndon, D.N.; Arnoldo, B.; Silver, G.; Schoenfeld, D.; et al. The Association Between Fluid Administration and Outcome Following Major Burn. *Ann. Surg.* **2007**, *245*, 622–628. [CrossRef]
54. Pruitt, B.A. Protection from excessive resuscitation: "Pushing the pendulum back". *J. Trauma* **2000**, *49*, 567–568. [CrossRef] [PubMed]
55. Saffle, J.I.L. The phenomenon of "fluid creep" in acute burn resuscitation. *J. Burn Care Res.* **2007**, *28*, 382–395. [CrossRef] [PubMed]
56. Cartotto, R.; Zhou, A. Fluid creep: The pendulum hasn't swung back yet! *J. Burn Care Res.* **2010**, *31*, 551–558. [CrossRef] [PubMed]
57. Friedrich, J.B.; Sullivan, S.R.; Engrav, L.H.; Round, K.A.; Blayney, C.B.; Carrougher, G.J.; Heimbach, D.M.; Honari, S.; Klein, M.B.; Gibran, N.S. Is supra-Baxter resuscitation in burn patients a new phenomenon? *Burns* **2004**, *30*, 464–466. [CrossRef]
58. Engrav, L.H.; Colescott, P.L.; Kemalyan, N.; Heimbach, D.M.; Gibran, N.S.; Solem, L.D.; Dimick, A.R.; Gamelli, R.L.; Lentz, C.W. A Biopsy of the Use of the Baxter Formula to Resuscitate Burns or Do We Do It Like Charlie Did It? *J. Burn. Care Rehabil.* **2000**, *21*, 91–95. [CrossRef]
59. Cartotto, R.C.; Innes, M.; Musgrave, M.A.; Gomez, M.; Cooper, A.B. How Well Does The Parkland Formula Estimate Actual Fluid Resuscitation Volumes? *J. Burn. Care Rehabil.* **2002**, *23*, 258–265. [CrossRef]
60. Cancio, L.C.; Chávez, S.; Alvarado-Ortega, M.; Barillo, D.J.; Walker, S.C.; McManus, A.T.; Goodwin, C.W. Predicting increased fluid requirements during the resuscitation of thermally injured patients. *J. Trauma* **2004**, *56*, 404–413. [CrossRef]
61. Ivy, M.E.; Atweh, N.A.; Palmer, J.; Possenti, P.P.; Pineau, M.; D'Aiuto, M. Intra-abdominal hypertension and abdominal compart-ment syndrome in burn patients. *J. Trauma* **2000**, *49*, 387–391. [CrossRef]
62. Sullivan, S.R.; Friedrich, J.B.; Engrav, L.H.; Round, K.A.; Heimbach, D.M.; Heckbert, S.R.; Carrougher, G.J.; Lezotte, D.C.; Wiechman, S.A.; Honari, S.; et al. "Opioid creep" is real and may be the cause of "fluid creep". *Burns* **2004**, *30*, 583–590. [CrossRef] [PubMed]
63. Pruitt, B.A.; Mason, A.D.; Moncrief, J.A. Hemodynamic changes in the early postburn patient: The influence of fluid administra-tion and of a vasodilator (hydralazine). *J. Trauma* **1971**, *11*, 36–46. [CrossRef]

64. O'Mara, M.S.; Slater, H.; Goldfarb, I.W.; Caushaj, P.F. A Prospective, Randomized Evaluation of Intra-abdominal Pressures with Crystalloid and Colloid Resuscitation in Burn Patients. *J. Trauma Inj. Infect. Crit. Care* **2005**, *58*, 1011–1018. [CrossRef]
65. Goodwin, C.W.; Dorethy, J.; Lam, V.; Pruitt, B.A. Randomized trial of efficacy of crystalloid and colloid resuscitation on hemo-dynamic response and lung water following thermal injury. *Ann. Surg.* **1983**, *197*, 520–531. [CrossRef]
66. Herndon, D.; Barrow, R.; Linares, H.; Rutan, R.; Prien, T.; Traber, L.D.; Traber, D. Inhalation injury in burned patients: Effects and treatment. *Burns* **1988**, *14*, 349–356. [CrossRef]
67. Dai, N.-T.; Chen, T.-M.; Cheng, T.-Y.; Chen, S.-L.; Chen, S.-G.; Chou, G.-H.; Chou, T.-D.; Wang, H.-J. The comparison of early fluid therapy in extensive flame burns between inhalation and noninhalation injuries. *Burns* **1998**, *24*, 671–675. [CrossRef]
68. Perel, P.; Roberts, I.; Ker, K. Colloids versus crystalloids for fluid resuscitation in critically ill patients. *Cochrane Database Syst. Rev.* **2013**, CD000567. [CrossRef]
69. Laupland, K.B.; Fisman, D.N. Surviving Sepsis? *Can. J. Infect. Dis. Med. Microbiol.* **2011**, *22*, 129–131. [CrossRef] [PubMed]
70. Merchant, N.; Smith, K.; Jeschke, M.G. An Ounce of Prevention Saves Tons of Lives: Infection in Burns. *Surg. Infect.* **2015**, *16*, 380–387. [CrossRef]
71. Greenhalgh, D.G. Sepsis in the burn patient: A different problem than sepsis in the general population. *Burn. Trauma* **2017**, *5*, 23. [CrossRef] [PubMed]
72. Bone, R.C.; Balk, R.A.; Cerra, F.B.; Dellinger, R.P.; Fein, A.M.; Knaus, W.A.; Schein, R.M.; Sibbald, W.J. Definitions for sepsis and organ failure and guidelines for the use of innovative therapies in sepsis. *Chest* **1992**, *101*, 1644–1655. [CrossRef]
73. Singer, M.; Deutschman, C.S.; Seymour, C.W.; Shankar-Hari, M.; Annane, D.; Bauer, M.; Bellomo, R.; Bernard, G.R.; Chiche, J.-D.; Coopersmith, C.M.; et al. The Third International Consensus Definitions for Sepsis and Septic Shock (Sepsis-3). *JAMA* **2016**, *315*, 801–810. [CrossRef]
74. Shankar-Hari, M.; Phillips, G.S.; Levy, M.L.; Seymour, C.W.; Liu, V.X.; Deutschman, C.S.; Angus, D.C.; Rubenfeld, G.D.; Singer, M. Developing a New Definition and Assessing New Clinical Criteria for Septic Shock: For the Third International Consensus Definitions for Sepsis and Septic Shock (Sepsis-3). *JAMA* **2016**, *315*, 775–787. [CrossRef] [PubMed]
75. Seymour, C.W.; Liu, V.X.; Iwashyna, T.J.; Brunkhorst, F.M.; Rea, T.D.; Scherag, A.; Rubenfeld, G.; Kahn, J.M.; Shankar-Hari, M.; Singer, M.; et al. Assessment of Clinical Criteria for Sepsis: For the Third International Consensus Definitions for Sepsis and Septic Shock (Sepsis-3). *JAMA* **2016**, *315*, 762–774. [CrossRef] [PubMed]
76. Greenhalgh, D.G.; Saffle, J.R.; Holmes, J.H.; Gamelli, R.L.; Palmieri, T.L.; Horton, J.W.; Tompkins, R.G.; Traber, D.L.; Mozingo, D.W.; Deitch, E.A.; et al. American Burn Association Consensus Conference to Define Sepsis and Infection in Burns. *J. Burn Care Res.* **2007**, *28*, 776–790. [CrossRef] [PubMed]
77. Chipp, E.; Milner, C.S.; Blackburn, A.V. Sepsis in burns: A review of current practice and future therapies. *Ann. Plast. Surg.* **2010**, *65*, 228–236. [CrossRef]
78. Yan, J.; Hill, W.F.; Rehou, S.; Pinto, R.; Shahrokhi, S.; Jeschke, M.G. Sepsis criteria versus clinical diagnosis of sepsis in burn pa-tients: A validation of current sepsis scores. *Surgery* **2018**, *164*, 1241–1245. [CrossRef]
79. Rech, M.A.; Mosier, M.J.; Zelisko, S.; Netzer, G.; Kovacs, E.J.; Afshar, M. Comparison of Automated Methods Versus the American Burn Association Sepsis Definition to Identify Sepsis and Sepsis With Organ Dysfunction/Septic Shock in Burn-Injured Adults. *J. Burn Care Res.* **2017**, *38*, 312–318. [CrossRef]
80. Yoon, J.; Kym, D.; Hur, J.; Kim, Y.; Yang, H.-T.; Yim, H.; Cho, Y.S.; Chun, W. Comparative Usefulness of Sepsis-3, Burn Sepsis, and Conventional Sepsis Criteria in Patients With Major Burns. *Crit. Care Med.* **2018**, *46*, e656–e662. [CrossRef]
81. Dellinger, R.P.; Carlet, J.M.; Masur, H.; Gerlach, H.; Calandra, T.; Cohen, J.; Gea-Banacloche, J.; Keh, D.; Marshall, J.C.; Parker, M.M.; et al. Surviving Sepsis Campaign guidelines for management of severe sepsis and septic shock. *Crit. Care Med.* **2004**, *32*, 858–873. [CrossRef]
82. Dellinger, R.P.; The Surviving Sepsis Campaign Guidelines Committee including The Pediatric Subgroup*; Levy, M.M.; Rhodes, A.; Annane, D.; Gerlach, H.; Opal, S.M.; Sevransky, J.E.; Sprung, C.L.; Douglas, I.S.; et al. Surviving Sepsis Campaign: International Guidelines for Management of Severe Sepsis and Septic Shock, 2012. *Intensiv. Care Med.* **2013**, *39*, 165–228. [CrossRef] [PubMed]
83. Rhodes, A.A.; Evans, L.E.; Alhazzani, W.; Levy, M.M.; Antonelli, M.; Ferrer, R.; Kumar, A.; Sevransky, J.E.; Sprung, C.L.; Nunnally, M.E.; et al. Surviving Sepsis Campaign: International Guidelines for Management of Sepsis and Septic Shock: 2016. *Intensiv. Care Med.* **2017**, *43*, 304–377. [CrossRef]
84. Kumar, A.; Roberts, D.; Wood, K.E.; Light, B.; Parrillo, J.E.; Sharma, S.; Suppes, R.; Feinstein, D.; Zanotti, S.; Taiberg, L.; et al. Duration of hypotension before initiation of effective antimicrobial therapy is the critical determinant of survival in human septic shock*. *Crit. Care Med.* **2006**, *34*, 1589–1596. [CrossRef]
85. László, I.; Trásy, D.; Molnár, Z.; Fazakas, J. Sepsis: From Pathophysiology to Individualized Patient Care. *J. Immunol. Res.* **2015**, *2015*, 1–13. [CrossRef]
86. von Heimburg, D.; Stieghorst, W.; Khorram-Sefat, R.; Pallua, N. Procalcitonin—A sepsis parameter in severe burn injuries. *Burns* **1998**, *24*, 745–750. [CrossRef]
87. Bargues, L.; Chancerelle, Y.; Catineau, J.; Jault, P.; Carsin, H. Evaluation of serum procalcitonin concentration in the ICU follow-ing severe burn. *Burns* **2007**, *33*, 860–864. [CrossRef] [PubMed]
88. Cabral, L.; Afreixo, V.; Meireles, R.; Vaz, M.; Marques, M.; Tourais, I.; Chaves, C.; Almeida, L.; Paiva, J.A. Procalcitonin kinetics after burn injury and burn surgery in septic and non-septic patients—A retrospective observational study. *BMC Anesthesiol.* **2018**, *18*, 1–10. [CrossRef]

89. Cabral, L.; Afreixo, V.; Meireles, R.; Vaz, M.; Chaves, C.; Caetano, M.; Almeida, L.; Paiva, J.A. Checking procalcitonin suitability for prognosis and antimicrobial therapy monitor-ing in burn patients. *Burns Trauma* **2018**, *6*, 10. [CrossRef]
90. Cabral, L.; Afreixo, V.; Santos, F.; Almeida, L.; Paiva, J.A. Procalcitonin for the early diagnosis of sepsis in burn patients: A retro-spective study. *Burns* **2017**, *43*, 1427–1434. [CrossRef]
91. Germain, L.; Laval, L.C.D.Q.-U.; Larouche, D.; Nedelec, B.; Perreault, I.; Duranceau, L.; Bortoluzzi, P.; Cloutier, C.B.; Genest, H.; Caouette-Laberge, L.; et al. Autologous bilayered self-assembled skin substitutes (SASSs) as permanent grafts: A case series of 14 severely burned patients indicating clinical effectiveness. *Eur. Cells Mater.* **2018**, *36*, 128–141. [CrossRef]
92. Kumar, P. Classification of skin substitutes. *Burns* **2008**, *34*, 148–149. [CrossRef]
93. Paggiaro, A.O.; Bastianelli, R.; Carvalho, V.F.; Isaac, C.; Gemperli, R. Is allograft skin, the gold-standard for burn skin substitute? A systematic literature review and meta-analysis. *J. Plast. Reconstr. Aesthetic Surg.* **2019**, *72*, 1245–1253. [CrossRef]
94. Saffle, J.R. Closure of the excised burn wound: Temporary skin substitutes. *Clin. Plast. Surg.* **2009**, *36*, 627–641. [CrossRef] [PubMed]
95. Ter Horst, B.; Chouhan, G.; Moiemen, N.S.; Grover, L.M. Advances in keratinocyte delivery in burn wound care. *Adv. Drug Deliv. Rev.* **2018**, *123*, 18–32. [CrossRef]
96. O'Connor, N.; Mulliken, J.; Banks-Schlegel, S.; Kehinde, O.; Green, H. Grafting of burns with cultured epithelium prepared from autologous epidermal cells. *Lancet* **1981**, *317*, 75–78. [CrossRef]
97. Wood, F.; Kolybaba, M.; Allen, P. The use of cultured epithelial autograft in the treatment of major burn wounds: Eleven years of clinical experience. *Burns* **2006**, *32*, 538–544. [CrossRef] [PubMed]
98. Beaudoin Cloutier, C.; Goyer, B.; Perron, C.; Guignard, R.; Larouche, D.; Moulin, V.J.; Germain, L.; Gauvin, R.; Auger, F.A. In Vivo Evaluation and Imaging of a Bilayered Self-Assembled Skin Substitute Using a Decellularized Dermal Matrix Grafted on Mice. *Tissue Eng. Part A* **2017**, *23*, 313–322. [CrossRef]
99. Larson, K.W.; Austin, C.L.; Thompson, S.J. Treatment of a Full-Thickness Burn Injury with NovoSorb Biodegradable Temporiz-ing Matrix and RECELL Autologous Skin Cell Suspension: A Case Series. *J. Burn Care Res.* **2020**, *41*, 215–219. [CrossRef]
100. Greenwood, J.E.; Dearman, B.L. Comparison of a Sealed, Polymer Foam Biodegradable Temporizing Matrix against Integra® Dermal Regeneration Template in a Porcine Wound Model. *J. Burn Care Res.* **2012**, *33*, 163–173. [CrossRef] [PubMed]
101. Farroha, A.; Frew, Q.; El-Muttardi, N.; Philp, B.; Dziewulski, P. The use of Biobrane® to dress split-thickness skin graft in paedi-atric burns. *Ann. Burns Fire Disasters* **2013**, *26*, 94–97. [PubMed]
102. Whitaker, I.S.; Prowse, S.; Potokar, T.S. A critical evaluation of the use of Biobrane as a biologic skin substitute: A versatile tool for the plastic and reconstructive surgeon. *Ann. Plast. Surg.* **2008**, *60*, 333–337. [CrossRef]
103. Rogers, A.D.; Blackport, E.; Cartotto, R. The use of Biobrane® for wound coverage in Stevens–Johnson Syndrome and Toxic Epidermal Necrolysis. *Burns* **2017**, *43*, 1464–1472. [CrossRef]
104. Hunt, J.A.; Moisidis, E.; Haertsch, P. Initial experience of Integra in the treatment of post-burn anterior cervical neck contrac-ture. *Br. J. Plast. Surg.* **2000**, *53*, 652–658. [CrossRef] [PubMed]
105. Hicks, K.E.; Huynh, M.N.; Jeschke, M.; Malic, C. Dermal regenerative matrix use in burn patients: A systematic review. *J. Plast. Reconstr. Aesthetic Surg.* **2019**, *72*, 1741–1751. [CrossRef]
106. Li, A.; Dearman, B.L.; Crompton, K.E.; Moore, T.G.; Greenwood, J.E. Evaluation of a novel biodegradable polymer for the genera-tion of a dermal matrix. *J Burn. Care Res.* **2009**, *30*, 717–728. [CrossRef] [PubMed]
107. Wagstaff, M.J.; Salna, I.M.; Caplash, Y.; Greenwood, J.E. Biodegradable Temporising Matrix (BTM) for the reconstruction of defects following serial debridement for necrotising fasciitis: A case series. *Burn. Open* **2019**, *3*, 12–30. [CrossRef]
108. Issler-Fisher, A.C.; Fisher, O.M.; Haertsch, P.; Li, Z.; Maitz, P.K. Ablative fractional resurfacing with laser-facilitated steroid delivery for burn scar management: Does the depth of laser penetration matter? *Lasers Surg. Med.* **2019**, *52*, 149–158. [CrossRef]
109. Issler-Fisher, A.C.; Fisher, O.M.; Smialkowski, A.O.; Li, F.; van Schalkwyk, C.P.; Haertsch, P.; Maitz, P.K. Ablative fractional CO_2 laser for burn scar reconstruction: An exten-sive subjective and objective short-term outcome analysis of a prospective treatment cohort. *Burns* **2017**, *43*, 573–582. [CrossRef] [PubMed]
110. Hultman, C.S.; Friedstat, J.S.; Edkins, R.E.; Cairns, B.A.; Meyer, A.A. Laser resurfacing and remodeling of hypertrophic burn scars: The results of a large, prospective, before-after cohort study, with long-term follow-up. *Ann. Surg.* **2014**, *260*, 519–529. [PubMed]
111. Hultman, C.S.; Edkins, R.E.; Lee, C.N.; Calvert, C.T.; Cairns, B.A. Shine on: Review of Laser- and Light-Based Therapies for the Treatment of Burn Scars. *Dermatol. Res. Pract.* **2012**, *2012*, 1–9. [CrossRef] [PubMed]
112. Taudorf, E.H.; Danielsen, P.L.; Paulsen, I.F.; Togsverd-Bo, K.; Dierickx, C.; Paasch, U.; Haedersdal, M. Non-ablative fractional laser provides long-term improvement of mature burn scars-A randomized controlled trial with histological assessment. *Lasers Surg. Med.* **2015**, *47*, 141–147. [CrossRef]
113. Esselman, P.C.; Thombs, B.D.; Magyar-Russell, G.; Fauerbach, J.A. Burn rehabilitation: State of the science. *Am. J. Phys. Med. Rehabil.* **2006**, *85*, 383–413. [CrossRef] [PubMed]
114. Willows, B.M.; Ilyas, M.; Sharma, A. Laser in the management of burn scars. *Burns* **2017**, *43*, 1379–1389. [CrossRef]
115. Lee, S.J.; Yeo, I.K.; Kang, J.M.; Chung, W.S.; Kim, Y.K.; Kim, B.J.; Park, K.Y. Treatment of hypertrophic burn scars by combination laser-cision and pinhole method us-ing a carbon dioxide laser. *Lasers Surg. Med.* **2014**, *46*, 380–384. [CrossRef] [PubMed]
116. Alster, T.S.; Nanni, C.A. Pulsed Dye Laser Treatment of Hypertrophic Burn Scars. *Plast. Reconstr. Surg.* **1998**, *102*, 2190–2195. [CrossRef]

117. Donelan, M.B.; Parrett, B.M.; Sheridan, R.L. Pulsed dye laser therapy and z-plasty for facial burn scars: The alternative to exci-sion. *Ann. Plast. Surg.* **2008**, *60*, 480–486. [CrossRef] [PubMed]
118. Kawecki, M.; Bernad-Wiśniewska, T.; Sakiel, S.; Nowak, M.; Andriessen, A. Laser in the treatment of hypertrophic burn scars. *Int. Wound J.* **2008**, *5*, 87–97. [CrossRef] [PubMed]
119. Waibel, J.; Wulkan, A.J.; Lupo, M.; Beer, K.; Anderson, R.R. Treatment of burn scars with the 1550 nm nonablative fractional Erbium Laser. *Lasers Surg. Med.* **2012**, *44*, 441–446. [CrossRef] [PubMed]
120. Geomelas, M.; Ghods, M.; Ring, A.; Ottomann, C. "The Maestro": A Pioneering Plastic Surgeon—Sir Archibald McIndoe and His Innovating Work on Patients With Burn Injury During World War II. *J. Burn Care Res.* **2011**, *32*, 363–368. [CrossRef]
121. Faber, A.W.; Klasen, H.J.; Sauer, E.W.; Vuister, F.M. Psychological and social problems in burn patients after discharge. *Scand. J. Plast. Reconstr. Surg.* **1987**, *21*, 307–309. [CrossRef]
122. Fauerbach, J.A.; McKibben, J.; Bienvenu, O.J.; Magyar-Russell, G.; Smith, M.T.; Holavanahalli, R.; Patterson, D.R.; Wiechman, S.A.; Blakeney, P.; Lezotte, D. Psychological Distress After Major Burn Injury. *Psychosom. Med.* **2007**, *69*, 473–482. [CrossRef] [PubMed]
123. Cleary, M.; Visentin, D.C.; West, S.; Kornhaber, R. The importance of mental health considerations for critical care burns patients. *J. Adv. Nurs.* **2018**, *74*, 1233–1235. [CrossRef]
124. Logsetty, S.; Shamlou, A.; Gawaziuk, J.P.; March, J.; Doupe, M.; Chateau, D.; Hoppensack, M.; Khan, S.; Medved, M.; Leslie, W.D.; et al. Mental health outcomes of burn: A longitudinal population-based study of adults hospitalized for burns. *Burns* **2016**, *42*, 738–744. [CrossRef]
125. Öster, C.; Sveen, J. The psychiatric sequelae of burn injury. *Gen. Hosp. Psychiatry* **2014**, *36*, 516–522. [CrossRef] [PubMed]
126. Holmes, W.J.; Hold, P.; James, M.I. The increasing trend in alcohol-related burns: It's impact on a tertiary burn centre. *Burns* **2010**, *36*, 938–943. [CrossRef]
127. McKibben, J.B.A.; Ekselius, L.; Girasek, D.C.; Gould, N.F.; Holzer, C.; Rosenberg, M.; Dissanaike, S.; Gielen, A.C. Epidemiology of burn injuries II: Psychiatric and behavioural perspectives. *Int. Rev. Psychiatry* **2009**, *21*, 512–521. [CrossRef] [PubMed]
128. Dyster-Aas, J.; Willebrand, M.; Wikehult, B.; Gerdin, B.; Ekselius, L. Major depression and posttraumatic stress disorder symp-toms following severe burn injury in relation to lifetime psychiatric morbidity. *J. Trauma* **2008**, *64*, 1349–1356.
129. Low, A.J.; Dyster-Aas, J.; Willebrand, M.; Ekselius, L.; Gerdin, B. Psychiatric morbidity predicts perceived burn-specific health 1 year after a burn. *Gen. Hosp. Psychiatry* **2012**, *34*, 146–152. [CrossRef] [PubMed]
130. Davydow, D.S.; Katon, W.J.; Zatzick, D.F. Psychiatric morbidity and functional impairments in survivors of burns, traumatic injuries, and ICU stays for other critical illnesses: A review of the literature. *Int. Rev. Psychiatry* **2009**, *21*, 531–538. [CrossRef] [PubMed]
131. Van der Does, A.J.; Hinderink, E.M.; Vloemans, A.F.; Spinhoven, P. Burn injuries, psychiatric disorders and length of hospitaliza-tion. *J. Psychosom. Res.* **1997**, *43*, 431–435. [CrossRef]
132. Tarrier, N.; Gregg, L.; Edwards, J.; Dunn, K. The influence of pre-existing psychiatric illness on recovery in burn injury patients: The impact of psychosis and depression. *Burns* **2005**, *31*, 45–49. [CrossRef] [PubMed]
133. Difede, J.; Barocas, D. Acute intrusive and avoidant PTSD symptoms as predictors of chronic PTSD following burn injury. *J. Trauma Stress* **1999**, *12*, 363–369. [CrossRef] [PubMed]
134. Corry, N.H.; Klick, B.; Fauerbach, J.A. Posttraumatic Stress Disorder and Pain Impact Functioning and Disability after Major Burn Injury. *J. Burn Care Res.* **2010**, *31*, 13–25. [CrossRef]
135. Wiechman Askay, S.; Patterson, D.R. What are the psychiatric sequelae of burn pain? *Curr. Pain Headache Rep.* **2008**, *12*, 94–97. [CrossRef]
136. Costa, B.A.; Engrav, L.H.; Holavanahalli, R.; Lezotte, D.C.; Patterson, D.R.; Kowalske, K.J.; Esselman, P.C. Impairment after burns: A two-center, prospective report. *Burns* **2003**, *29*, 671–675. [CrossRef]
137. Patterson, D.R.; Tininenko, J.; Ptacek, J.T. Pain during Burn Hospitalization Predicts Long-term Outcome. *J. Burn Care Res.* **2006**, *27*, 719–726. [CrossRef]
138. Malenfant, A.; Forget, R.; Papillon, J.; Amsel, R.; Frigon, J.-Y.; Choiniere, M. Prevalence and characteristics of chronic sensory problems in burn patients. *Pain* **1996**, *67*, 493–500. [CrossRef]
139. Dalal, P.K.; Saha, R.; Agarwal, M. Psychiatric aspects of burn. *Indian J. Plast. Surg.* **2010**, *43*, S136–S142. [CrossRef]
140. Romanowski, K.S.; Carson, J.; Pape, K.; Bernal, E.; Sharar, S.; Wiechman, S.; Carter, D.; Liu, Y.M.; Nitzschke, S.; Bhalla, P.; et al. American Burn Association Guidelines on the Management of Acute Pain in the Adult Burn Patient: A Review of the Literature, a Compilation of Expert Opinion, and Next Steps. *J. Burn Care Res.* **2020**, *41*, 1129–1151. [CrossRef]
141. Shakibaei, F.; Harandi, A.A.; Gholamrezaei, A.; Samoei, R.; Salehi, P. Hypnotherapy in Management of Pain and Reexperiencing of Trauma in Burn Patients. *Int. J. Clin. Exp. Hypn.* **2008**, *56*, 185–197. [CrossRef]
142. Patterson, D.R.; Questad, K.A.; De Lateur, B.J. Hypnotherapy as an Adjunct to Narcotic Analgesia for the Treatment of Pain for Burn Debridement. *Am. J. Clin. Hypn.* **1989**, *31*, 156–163. [CrossRef]
143. Patterson, D.R.; Everett, J.J.; Burns, G.L.; Marvin, J.A. Hypnosis for the treatment of burn pain. *J. Consult. Clin. Psychol.* **1992**, *60*, 713–717. [CrossRef] [PubMed]
144. Askay, S.W.; Patterson, D.R.; Jensen, M.P.; Sharar, S.R. A randomized controlled trial of hypnosis for burn wound care. *Rehabil. Psychol.* **2007**, *52*, 247–253. [CrossRef]
145. Morris, L.D.; Louw, Q.A.; Grimmer-Somers, K. The effectiveness of virtual reality on reducing pain and anxiety in burn injury patients: A systematic review. *Clin. J. Pain* **2009**, *25*, 815–826. [CrossRef] [PubMed]

146. Arane, K.; Behboudi, A.; Goldman, R.D. Virtual reality for pain and anxiety management in children. *Can. Fam. Physician Med. Fam. Can.* **2017**, *63*, 932–934.
147. Hoffman, H.G.; Rodriguez, R.A.; Gonzalez, M.; Bernardy, M.; Peña, R.; Beck, W.; Patterson, D.R.; Meyer, W.J. Immersive Virtual Reality as an Adjunctive Non-opioid Analgesic for Pre-dominantly Latin American Children With Large Severe Burn Wounds During Burn Wound Cleaning in the Intensive Care Unit: A Pilot Study. *Front. Hum. Neurosci.* **2019**, *13*, 262. [CrossRef] [PubMed]
148. Hoffman, H.G.; Patterson, D.R.; Seibel, E.; Soltani, M.; Jewett-Leahy, L.; Sharar, S.R. Virtual reality pain control during burn wound debridement in the hydrotank. *Clin. J. Pain* **2008**, *24*, 299–304. [CrossRef]
149. Hoffman, H.G.; Doctor, J.N.; Patterson, D.R.; Carrougher, G.J.; Furness, T.A. Virtual reality as an adjunctive pain control during burn wound care in adolescent patients. *Pain* **2000**, *85*, 305–309. [CrossRef]
150. Ahmadpour, N.; Randall, H.; Choksi, H.; Gao, A.; Vaughan, C.; Poronnik, P. Virtual Reality interventions for acute and chronic pain management. *Int. J. Biochem. Cell Biol.* **2019**, *114*, 105568. [CrossRef]
151. Pourmand, A.; Davis, S.; Marchak, A.; Whiteside, T.; Sikka, N. Virtual Reality as a Clinical Tool for Pain Management. *Curr. Pain Headache Rep.* **2018**, *22*, 53. [CrossRef]
152. Eijlers, R.; Utens, E.M.; Staals, L.M.; de Nijs, P.F.; Berghmans, J.M.; Wijnen, R.M.; Hillegers, M.H.; Dierckx, B.; Legerstee, J.S. Systematic Review and Meta-analysis of Virtual Reality in Pediatrics: Effects on Pain and Anxiety. *Anesth. Analg.* **2019**, *129*, 1344–1353. [CrossRef]
153. Li, A.; Montaño, Z.; Chen, V.J.; I Gold, J. Virtual reality and pain management: Current trends and future directions. *Pain Manag.* **2011**, *1*, 147–157. [CrossRef] [PubMed]
154. Esselman, P.C.; Ptacek, J.T.; Kowalske, K.; Cromes, G.F.; DeLateur, B.J.; Engrav, L.H. Community Integration after Burn Injuries. *J. Burn. Care Rehabil.* **2001**, *22*, 221–227. [CrossRef]
155. Blakeney, P.; Partridge, J.; Rumsey, N. Community Integration. *J. Burn Care Res.* **2007**, *28*, 598–601. [CrossRef]
156. Quinn, T.; Wasiak, J.; Cleland, H. An examination of factors that affect return to work following burns: A systematic review of the literature. *Burns* **2010**, *36*, 1021–1026. [CrossRef] [PubMed]
157. Oster, C.; Kildal, M.; Ekselius, L. Return to work after burn injury: Burn-injured individuals' perception of barriers and facili-tators. *J. Burn Care Res.* **2010**, *31*, 540–550. [CrossRef]
158. Mackey, S.; Diba, R.; McKeown, D.; Wallace, C.G.; Booth, S.; Gilbert, P.; Dheansa, B. Return to work after burns: A qualitative research study. *Burns* **2009**, *35*, 338–342. [CrossRef] [PubMed]
159. Blakeney, P.; Meyer, W.; Robert, R.; Desai, M.; Wolf, S.; Herndon, D. Long-Term Psychosocial Adaptation of Children Who Survive Burns Involving 80% or Greater Total Body Surface Area. *J. Trauma Inj. Infect. Crit. Care* **1998**, *44*, 625–634. [CrossRef]
160. Blakeney, P.; Meyer, W.; Moore, P.; Murphy, L.; Broemeling, L.; Robson, M.; Herndon, D. Psychosocial Sequelae of Pediatric Burns Involving 80% or Greater Total Body Surface Area. *J. Burn. Care Rehabil.* **1993**, *14*, 684–689. [CrossRef] [PubMed]
161. Blakeney, P.; Thomas, C.; Holzer, C.; Rose, M.; Berniger, F.; Meyer, W.J. Efficacy of a Short-Term, Intensive Social Skills Training Program for Burned Adolescents. *J. Burn. Care Rehabil.* **2005**, *26*, 546–555. [CrossRef]
162. Meyer, W.J.; Blakeney, P.; Russell, W.; Thomas, C.; Robert, R.; Berniger, F.; Holzer, C. Psychological Problems Reported by Young Adults Who Were Burned as Children. *J. Burn. Care Rehabil.* **2004**, *25*, 98–106. [CrossRef]
163. Esselman, P.C. Burn Rehabilitation: An Overview. *Arch. Phys. Med. Rehabil.* **2007**, *88*, S3–S6. [CrossRef]
164. Richard, R.; Baryza, M.J.; Carr, J.A.; Dewey, W.S.; Dougherty, M.E.; Forbes-Duchart, L.; Franzen, B.J.; Healey, T.; Lester, M.E.; Li, S.K.; et al. Burn Rehabilitation and Research: Proceedings of a Consensus Summit. *J. Burn Care Res.* **2009**, *30*, 543–573. [CrossRef]
165. Moore, M.L.; Dewey, W.S.; Richard, R.L. Rehabilitation of the Burned Hand. *Hand Clin.* **2009**, *25*, 529–541. [CrossRef] [PubMed]
166. Richard, R.L.; Hedman, T.L.; Quick, C.D.; Barillo, D.J.; Cancio, L.C.; Renz, E.M.; Chapman, T.T.; Dewey, W.S.; Dougherty, M.E.; Esselman, P.C.; et al. A Clarion to Recommit and Reaffirm Burn Rehabilitation. *J. Burn Care Res.* **2008**, *29*, 425–432. [CrossRef]
167. Kottke, F.J.; Pauley, D.L.; Ptak, R.A. The rationale for prolonged stretching for correction of shortening of connective tissue. *Arch. Phys. Med. Rehabil.* **1966**, *47*, 345–352. [PubMed]
168. Larson, D.L.; Abston, S.; Evans, E.B.; Dobrkovský, M.; Linares, H.A. Techniques for decreasing scar formation and contractures in the burned patient. *J. Trauma Inj. Infect. Crit. Care* **1971**, *11*, 807–823. [CrossRef] [PubMed]
169. Baur, P.S.; Parks, D.H.; Larson, D.L. The Healing of Burn Wounds. *Clin. Plast. Surg.* **1977**, *4*, 389–407. [CrossRef]
170. Baur, P.S.; Larson, D.L.; Stacey, T.R.; Barratt, G.F.; Dobrkovský, M. Ultrastructural analysis of pressure-treated human hypertrophic scars. *J. Trauma Inj. Infect. Crit. Care* **1976**, *16*, 958–967. [CrossRef]
171. Linares, H.; Larson, D.; Willis-Galstaun, B. Historical notes on the use of pressure in the treatment of hypertrophic scars or keloids. *Burns* **1993**, *19*, 17–21. [CrossRef]
172. Van den Kerckhove, E.; Stappaerts, K.; Fieuws, S.; Laperre, J.; Massage, P.; Flour, M.; Boeckx, W. The assessment of erythema and thickness on burn related scars during pressure garment therapy as a preventive measure for hypertrophic scarring. *Burns* **2005**, *31*, 696–702. [CrossRef]
173. Perkins, K.; Davey, R.B.; Wallis, K. Current materials and techniques used in a burn scar management programme. *Burns* **1987**, *13*, 406–410. [CrossRef]
174. Staley, M.J.; Richard, R.L. Use of pressure to treat hypertrophic burn scars. *Adv. Wound Care J. Prev. Health* **1997**, *10*, 44–46.
175. Macintyre, L.; Baird, M. Pressure garments for use in the treatment of hypertrophic scars–a review of the problems associ-ated with their use. *Burns* **2006**, *32*, 10–15. [CrossRef]

176. Mann, R.; Yeong, E.K.; Moore, M.; Colescott, D.; Engrav, L.H. Do Custom-Fitted Pressure Garments Provide Adequate Pressure? *J. Burn. Care Rehabil.* **1997**, *18*, 247–249. [CrossRef] [PubMed]
177. Cheng, J.; Evans, J.; Leung, K.; Clark, J.; Choy, T.; Leung, P. Pressure therapy in the treatment of post-burn hypertrophic scar—A critical look into its usefulness and fallacies by pressure monitoring. *Burns* **1984**, *10*, 154–163. [CrossRef]
178. Kealey, G.P.; Jensen, K.L.; Laubenthal, K.N.; Lewis, R.W. Prospective Randomized Comparison of Two Types of Pressure Therapy Garments. *J. Burn. Care Rehabil.* **1990**, *11*, 334–336. [CrossRef] [PubMed]
179. Palmieri, T.L.; Molitor, F.; Chan, G.; Phelan, E.; Shier, B.J.; Sen, S.; Greenhalgh, D.G. Long-Term Functional Outcomes in the Elderly After Burn Injury. *J. Burn Care Res.* **2012**, *33*, 497–503. [CrossRef] [PubMed]
180. Holavanahalli, R.K.; Helm, P.A.; Kowalske, K.J. Long-Term Outcomes in Patients Surviving Large Burns: The Musculoskeletal System. *J. Burn Care Res.* **2016**, *37*, 243–254. [CrossRef] [PubMed]
181. Wiechman, S.; Hoyt, M.A.; Patterson, D.R. Using a Biopsychosocial Model to Understand Long-Term Outcomes in Persons with Burn Injuries. *Arch. Phys. Med. Rehabil.* **2020**, *101*, S55–S62. [CrossRef] [PubMed]
182. Bakhtyar, T.S.N. Therapeutic Approaches to Combatting Hypermetabolism in Severe Burn Injuries. *J. Intensiv. Crit. Care* **2015**, *1*. [CrossRef]
183. American Burn Association. The Acute Burn ResUscitation Multicenter Prospective Trial (ABRUPT2). 2020. Available online: https://clinicaltrials.gov/ct2/show/NCT04356859 (accessed on 3 March 2021).
184. Datta, D.; Morris, A.C.; Antonelli, J.; Warner, N.; Brown, K.A.; Wright, J.; Simpson, A.J.; Rennie, J.; Hulme, G.; Lewis, S.M.; et al. Early PREdiction of Severe Sepsis (ExPRES-Sepsis) study: Protocol for an ob-servational derivation study to discover potential leucocyte cell surface biomarkers. *BMJ Open* **2016**, *6*, e011335. [CrossRef]
185. Hassanshahi, A.; Hassanshahi, M.; Khabbazi, S.; Hosseini-Khah, Z.; Peymanfar, Y.; Ghalamkari, S.; Su, Y.W.; Xian, C.J. Adipose-derived stem cells for wound healing. *J. Cell. Physiol.* **2019**, *234*, 7903–7914. [CrossRef]
186. Kosaric, N.; Kiwanuka, H.; Gurtner, G.C. Stem cell therapies for wound healing. *Expert Opin. Biol. Ther.* **2019**, *19*, 575–585. [CrossRef] [PubMed]
187. Amini-Nik, S.; Dolp, R.; Eylert, G.; Datu, A.-K.; Parousis, A.; Blakeley, C.; Jeschke, M.G. Stem cells derived from burned skin—The future of burn care. *EBioMedicine* **2018**, *37*, 509–520. [CrossRef] [PubMed]
188. Martin-Piedra, M.Á.; Alfonso-Rodríguez, C.A.; Zapater Latorre, A.; Durand-Herrera, D.; Chato-Astrain, J.; Campos, F.; Sánchez Quevedo, M.d.C.; Alaminos Mingorance, M.; Garzón Bello, I.J. Effective use of mesenchymal stem cells in human skin sub-stitutes generated by tissue engineering. *Eur. Cell Mater.* **2019**, *37*, 233–249. [CrossRef] [PubMed]

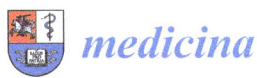

Review

Made in Germany: A Quality Indicator Not Only in the Automobile Industry But Also When It Comes to Skin Replacement: How an Automobile Textile Research Institute Developed a New Skin Substitute

Herbert Leopold Haller [1,*,†], Matthias Rapp [2], Daniel Popp [3], Sebastian Philipp Nischwitz [3] and Lars Peter Kamolz [3]

1. UKH Linz der AUVA, HLMedConsult, Zehetlandweg 7, A-4060 Leonding, Austria
2. Klinik für Orthopädie, Unfallchirurgie und Sporttraumatologie, Zentrum für Schwerbrandverletzte, Marienhospital Stuttgart, Böheimstraße 37, 70199 Stuttgart, Germany; matthias.rapp@vinzenz.de
3. Division of Hand, Plastic and Reconstructive Surgery, Department of Surgery, Medical University of Graz, A-8036 Graz, Austria; daniel.popp@medunigraz.at (D.P.); sebastian.nischwitz@medunigraz.at (S.P.N.); lars.kamolz@medunigraz.at (L.P.K.)
* Correspondence: herberthaller@gmail.com; Tel.: +43-6766393012
† Retired.

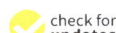

Citation: Haller, H.L.; Rapp, M.; Popp, D.; Nischwitz, S.P.; Kamolz, L.P. Made in Germany: A Quality Indicator Not Only in the Automobile Industry But Also When It Comes to Skin Replacement: How an Automobile Textile Research Institute Developed a New Skin Substitute. *Medicina* **2021**, *57*, 143. https://doi.org/10.3390/medicina57020143

Academic Editor: Edgaras Stankevičius
Received: 10 January 2021
Accepted: 27 January 2021
Published: 5 February 2021

Publisher's Note: MDPI stays neutral with regard to jurisdictional claims in published maps and institutional affiliations.

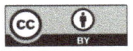

Copyright: © 2021 by the authors. Licensee MDPI, Basel, Switzerland. This article is an open access article distributed under the terms and conditions of the Creative Commons Attribution (CC BY) license (https://creativecommons.org/licenses/by/4.0/).

Abstract: Successful research and development cooperation between a textile research institute, the German Federal Ministry of Education and Research via the Center for Biomaterials and Organ Substitutes, the University of Tübingen, and the Burn Center of Marienhospital, Stuttgart, Germany, led to the development of a fully synthetic resorbable temporary epidermal skin substitute for the treatment of burns, burn-like syndromes, donor areas, and chronic wounds. This article describes the demands of the product and the steps that were taken to meet these requirements. The material choice was based on the degradation and full resorption of polylactides to lactic acid and its salts. The structure and morphology of the physical, biological, and degradation properties were selected to increase the angiogenetic abilities, fibroblasts, and extracellular matrix generation. Water vapor permeability and plasticity were adapted for clinical use. The available scientific literature was screened for the use of this product. A clinical application demonstrated pain relief paired with a reduced workload, fast wound healing with a low infection rate, and good cosmetic results. A better understanding of the product's degradation process explained the reduction in systemic oxidative stress shown in clinical investigations compared to other dressings, positively affecting wound healing time and reducing the total area requiring skin grafts. Today, the product is in clinical use in 37 countries. This article describes its development, the indications for product growth over time, and the scientific foundation of treatments.

Keywords: burn; donor area; wounds; polylactide; lactormone; oxidative stress reduction; analgesia; stabilization; reduced infection

1. Introduction

Stuttgart is one of Germany's most innovative areas, as the location of the headquarters and development centers of several multinational automobile companies, including Daimler AG (Mercedes) and Porsche. Alongside a university and a technology university of applied sciences, many research companies are located there.

Among these is the German Institutes for Textile and Fiber Research Denkendorf (DITF), the largest textile research center in Europe with more than 300 scientific employees. The company's objective is to conduct research projects that ultimately lead to developing degradable materials that do not cause any harm to the environment. The idea of using such a product as a medical wound dressing was the underlying idea behind Suprathel®.

Developing a degradable synthetic skin substitute is a convincing approach to tackling the shortcomings of burn care and biological skin substitutes.

A joint venture between the Institute of Textile Research and Chemical Engineering Denkendorf and Stuttgart Burn Center at the Clinic for Orthopedics, Trauma Surgery and Sports Traumatology of Marienhospital, Stuttgart, Germany, was formed within the scope of the BMOZ (German Center for Biomaterials and Organ Substitute Stuttgart–Tübingen), supported by the German Federal Ministry of Education and Research, the Federal Country of Baden-Württemberg, and the University of Tübingen to develop a material "combining the advantages of biological and synthetic substitutes" [1,2].

This material was needed to advance skin substitution processes to improve burn and wound care. A transparent, permanent wound dressing was to be developed, allowing the proper assessment of the treated wound. It needed to serve as an epithelial replacement until the wound had healed completely, enabling both analgesia and the undisturbed regeneration of the damaged epithelium. The durability also had to prevent infection or iatrogenic compromise when changing the dressing. Dressing changes, if necessary, had to be as painless and straightforward as possible.

Later on, a spin-off of the institute was founded (PolyMedics Innovations GmbH) to further investigate said medical dressing and to promote its development.

This article explains the requirements of this product and reviews the developmental steps and published literature on the use of Suprathel® (Polymedics Innovations GmbH. Denkendorf, Germany).

2. Technical Features in the Development of a Skin Substitute

2.1. The Choice of Materials

It was an obvious choice to use materials from components already available in the healthy human metabolism. Hydrocarbons are common and usually present in a cyclic form. As the material needs some stability over a specific time, which should reduce during degradation and resorption, polymers of lactic acid seemed to be suitable as an essential product. Polymers with a higher molecular weight degrade in a humid environment into monomers of lactic acid, buffered physiologically. It has been demonstrated that externally applied lactic acid at a lower concentration positively influences keratinocyte-derived growth factors such as VEGF (Vascular Endothelial Growth Factor [3,4]. Lactates, the salts of lactic acid, are known to scavenge superoxide radicals and to inhibit lipid peroxidation. When lactate oxidizes to pyruvate, this molecule can scavenge hydrogen peroxide and superoxide radicals as well [5,6]. Both lactic acid and lactate can enter the cells. Lactic acid, due to its small molecules and lack of polarity, being small enough to permeate through the lipid membrane, can enter cells via the monocarboxylate transporter (MCT) protein shuttle system [7]. Once inside the cell, lactate can serve as an energy source via the Cori cycle, wherein it is converted into glucose. Lactate does not cause acidosis within a physiological range [8].

Lactate dehydrogenase can alternatively convert lactate into pyruvate, which is oxidized to acetyl Co-A, producing water, carbon dioxide, and NADH (nicotinamide adenine dinucleotide plus hydrogen) in the mitochondria [9]. It can serve as an energy source and as an energy transport system [10,11].

2.1.1. The Chemical Structure

The chemical structure influences the degradation time, potential toxicity, and foreign body reactions in a wound environment. The initial molecular weight and structure, as well as the chirality of polylactides, influence the speed of degradation and the degree of formation of crystalline products [12]. Schakenraad showed, in 1991, that the initial hydrolysis of amorphous poly-L-lactide might increase crystallinity and can lead to a long degradation time [13]. Therefore, the challenge was to develop a chemical compound without developing crystallinity and a foreign body reaction with a shorter resorption time.

2.1.2. The Material Structure

The material had to provide a certain degree of stability, as it was intended primarily for temporary use in the place of human biological skin. This was combined with other human skin qualities such as water vapor permeability and mechanical strength, flexibility, and adherence to the wound bed.

The impact of morphology on the degradation and resorption speed was described by Taylor et al. [12]. Different structures, resulting in a different porosity, showed a different impact on angiogenesis [14–17]. Many materials with different structures and thicknesses, such as foams, fleeces, and hot melt blows, were analyzed. The angiogenic response, structural stability, and degradation had to be balanced in order to not create hypertrophic granulation tissue, to provide sufficient water vapor permeability and stability, and to preserve a moist wound environment. A balance of these properties would allow the product to be used for partial-thickness burns, supporting wound healing and the regeneration of the epithelium without generating granulation tissue. These considerations finally resulted in the pore size and structure used in Suprathel® (Polymedics Innovations GmbH, Denkendorf, Germany).

3. Results of the Development Process
3.1. Material Properties

This development process resulted in a specific microporous structure for Suprathel®. This microporous structure provides an increased moisture vapor permeability at the beginning of the treatment. Induced by fibrine and the outer dressing, the water vapor permeability of Suprathel® is reduced over the time to that of healthy human skin.

Suprathel® consists of DL-lactide (>70%), trimethylene carbonate, and ε-caprolactone. A unique processing technique creates a porous membrane with a nearly symmetrical cross-section, with an interconnected pore structure and varying pore sizes between 2 and 50 μm. The initial porosity of the material is >80%. Due to its plasticity, it adapts to the wound bed at body temperature. It promptly adheres to a fresh wound. The membrane has a thickness of 70–150 μm and an elongation potential between 100% and 250% [18]. Storage at room temperature is possible for three years without the loss of quality. Degradation and loss of stability occur within four weeks in vitro; in vivo, it is stabilized by fibrin, and the separation layer and remnants are removed after wound healing. Examples for the use of Suprathel® are shown in Figures 1 and 2a,b.

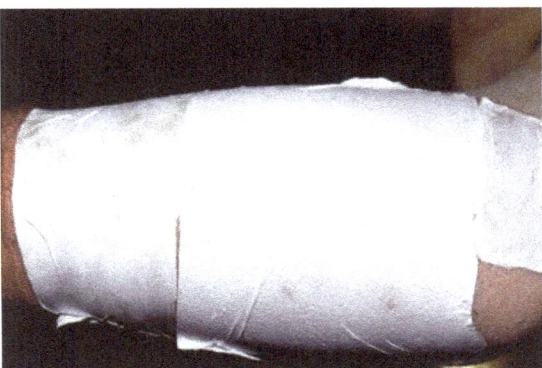

Figure 1. Shows the first application of Suprathel® in 1999 in a donor site (courtesy of Dr. Rapp).

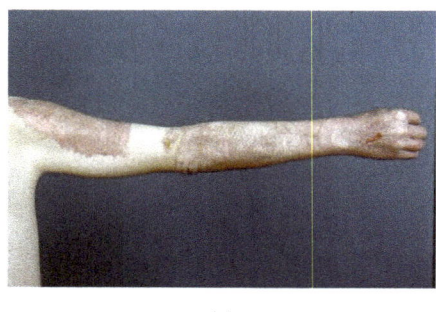 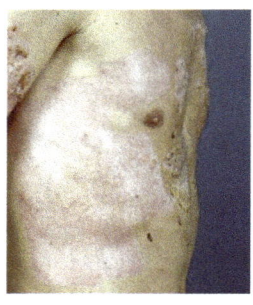

(a) (b)

Figure 2. (a) Shows healed areas after the application of Suprathel on a mesh-grafted area; and (b) shows a healed donor area after Suprathel application on day 13 post op. (courtesy of Dr. Rapp).

3.2. Medical Aims of Suprathel Development

Table 1 gives an overview on the medical key points of the development of Suprathel®. The effects are described in detail in the following paragraphs.

Table 1. Medical and handling key points of the development of Suprathel®.

- Pain reduction;
- Reduction in oxidative stress and the systemic inflammatory response;
- Reduction in the need for skin transplantations and consecutive donor wounds;
- Support for wound healing and more efficient healing;
- Low infection rate;
- Good cosmetic results and scar quality;
- Reduction in workload;
- Economic efficiency.

3.3. Detailed Results of Development

3.3.1. Basic Mechanism

Suprathel® offers positive effects on wound healing. These include the barrier effect, the effect on dermal tissue, the effect on epidermal tissue, and systemic effects. The barrier effect provides bacterial tightness and reduces fluid and energy loss [1,19]. The effect of lactate has been described above. It works as a radical scavenger and energy source for cells. Lactate simulates hypoxic conditions for cells, while oxygen tension is normal [11], supporting the metabolism and wound healing in dermal tissue. It increases VEGF [20], the number of vessel sprouts and functional vessel density, red blood cell velocity, as well as interconnections in capillaries. It supports fibroblast migration and extracellular matrix generation [21] and collagen synthesis [22]. Lactate's effect on TGF-β (Transforming Growth Factor β) generation is limited to two weeks, preventing myofibroblast generation but supporting early wound healing [23–25]. In epidermal tissue, it supports keratinocyte activation by redifferentiation and forming filopodia, enabling keratinocyte migration and wound closure under lactate-induced TGF-β [26]. Cleavage during wound closure by decorin limits this effect [27]. Systemic effects support burn wound healing by influencing the inflammatory response, as demonstrated in children with a mean TBSA (total burned surface area) burn of 39.95% [28].

3.3.2. Pain Reduction

Suprathel® has been shown to significantly reduce pain when applied to fresh wounds. This effect is nearly unique to Suprathel® and is only comparable to dressings with an incorporated analgesic and antiphlogistic medication such as Ibuprofen [29]. One reason for this might be the radical scavenging ability of the free radicals released after trauma by keratinocytes and other cells [28]. ROS (reactive oxygen species) induces the synthesis of PGE2 (Prostaglandin E2) [30]. A specific PGE2 receptor, EP1, is responsible for pain perception. EP1-knockout mice only show 50% of the pain perception of wild-type mice. The reduction in free radicals results in reduced pain triggers, as demonstrated by Stock et al. [31]. Reduced PGE2 also influences local edema formation as a component of inflammation [31], as demonstrated by Kaartinen et al. [32]. The reduction in oxidative stress and pro-inflammatory cytokines might significantly influence the reduction in pain [28,33].

Another reason might be the protective effect on wound desiccation, known from other materials [34], hindering pain from free nerve endings [35]. This effect alone is not sufficient to explain the degree of pain reduction in Suprathel®. When compared directly to other products, Suprathel® shows superiority in hindering desiccation [32]. Suprathel® can significantly reduce resting and procedural pain due to its structure, as well as to inner dressing changes being omitted [36–38]. As the Suprathel® skin template covered with the separation layer remains adherent until the wound is healed, it protects the wound from irritation and disruption during dressing changes. The degradation of the absorbent layer does not trigger additional pain.

The Practical Meaning of Pain Reduction

Based on its physiological effect, several randomized controlled trials have demonstrated the excellence of Suprathel® in pain reduction. Significant superiority was found when compared to Jelonet [39], Mepilex [29,32], and Omiderm [40]. Pain reduction, which was in the range of 30–63%, was statistically significant in all of these studies. Biatain Ibu showed a faster but weaker effect than Suprathel® but had to be changed after three days to preserve the pain-reducing ability [29]. To date, more than 20 studies, including prospective, retrospective, and case reports, have confirmed the excellent effect on pain reduction in partial-thickness burns [38,41–45] and donor sites, radiation injuries [46], and burn-like syndromes [47–49], as well as successful use in high-risk and complicated patients [50,51] and cauterizations [52]. Some publications have even demonstrated a significant reduction in opioids [37,45,51,53,54].

The other positive side effects include pain reduction, which has several positive side effects. This enables the early return of function and early mobilization, as well as a lower need for sedation, preparation, and surveillance before, during, and after procedures. Furthermore, it reduces the side effects of opioid use, such as obstipation, dizziness, loss of appetite, and hypotension, which might be compensated for by more fluid application linked with edema and fluid-creep, triggering dependency on opioids [55,56]. Short et al. [52] and others [44] have reported that it also enables outpatient care.

The reduction in opioids means less of a sedation effect, which facilitates early extubating and prevents the complications that come with longer periods of artificial ventilation, as demonstrated in the Burn Repository 2017 of the ABA (American Burn Association) [57] by reductions in fluid retention and acute kidney injury [58–61]. The goal of opioid reduction is to prevent long-term opioid use (opioid dependency) [62].

3.3.3. The Effect of Treatment with Suprathel® on Workload and Stress to Both Patients and Medical Staff

The basic principle for Suprathel® treatment is the initial application of Suprathel® to the wound. The outer dressing typically consists of a separation layer (i.e., fatty gauze), followed by an absorbent dressing and a compression layer. Only the outer dressing is replaced during dressing changes.

This results in a reduced frequency of dressing changes and a reduced overall time necessary for each dressing change, since the inner dressing remains attached to the wound bed. Kukko et al. found a reduction in dressing changes to 42% compared to SSD silver sulfa diazine (SSD) [63], while Markl et al. found a reduction from a mean of 4.0 in Mepitel to 0.3 in Suprathel (7.5%). The time needed for dressing changes was Ø2.25 min for Suprathel® and Ø10.58 min for Mepitel®.

3.3.4. Effects of Suprathel® on Water Vapor Permeability and Fluid Management on the Patient

Suprathel® reduces bleeding and is permeable for water and serum during the initial treatment and causes less fluid secretion than other products [32]. It works well on donor sites as it does not form a "cement-like clot" like other products (e.g., Biobrane) [64]. Hence, donor sites are an excellent indication for Suprathel®.

As several case reports show, in products such as Biobrane® [65,66], Integra® [67], and Opsite® [68], or even skin grafts [69], toxic shock syndrome can be a severe side effect that is likely related to fluid retention underneath the dressing. There are no reports of toxic shock syndrome with the use of Suprathel®. This might be due to the increased water vapor permeability.

Suprathel® does not support hematoma formation or fluid retention at the beginning of treatment, and therefore observation is less frequently necessary. This is in contrast to several other materials, which have to be closely observed for these complications [70]. The water vapor permeability of Suprathel® at the beginning of the treatment is below 50% of a partial thickness burn in vitro. This reduces even further to below 25% within 20 days [71]. In vivo, it links with fibrin and cells from the wound, such as red blood cells, thrombocytes, and leukocytes, reducing permeability within four to five days to nearly 0%. After this time, the dressing stays dry, and further dressing changes are only necessary for on-demand or hygienic reasons.

3.3.5. Effects of Suprathel® on the Energy Balance

Water vapor permeability is an essential component of energy balance. Loss of water and serum over the wound causes a wet surface, resulting in cooling by evaporation. This results in a drop in body temperature, and energy is lost in an attempt to maintain body temperature. Occlusive dressings can substantially reduce energy requirements [72,73]. The semi-occlusive properties of Suprathel® at the beginning of treatment, turning into a nearly occlusive treatment over the early treatment course, might reduce energy requirements and the inflammatory response and therefore improve the metabolic situation in favor of a better wound healing situation [74,75]. Demircan demonstrated a substantial reduction in healing time after Suprathel® treatment, possibly reducing oxidative stress and attenuating energy loss. This attenuation of energy balance might also lead to a reduction in areas that require skin grafts, as demonstrated by Uhlig et al. [76], Schriek et al. [77], and Blome-Eberwein et al. [78].

3.3.6. Reduction in the Oxidative Stress and the Systemic Inflammatory Response

Gürünlüoglu et al. investigated the effect of Suprathel® on the systemic inflammatory response. They found a positive impact on the total antioxidant and reduced total oxidant capacity compared to hydrofiber (HF) Ag at a highly statistically significant level [28]. Wound healing was also significantly faster in the Suprathel® group. They were the first to demonstrate the systemic effects of wound dressings on oxidative stress in humans.

The same group also investigated the impact of Suprathel® on cytokine levels. IL-6 (Interleukin 6) and TNF-α (Tumor Necrosis Factor α) were significantly lower in the Suprathel® group than in HF Ag, and TGF-β was significantly higher throughout the two weeks and reduced to nearly normal levels after the third week [25].

Gürünlüoglu et al. also demonstrated the impact of oxidative stress reduction on skin quality using Suprathel® by measuring telomerase activity in healed skin after Suprathel® treatment compared to HF Ag. This study demonstrated higher telomerase activity and a higher cell count, with higher skin viscoelasticity, in the Suprathel® group, concluding a better result in regard to skin quality after Suprathel® treatment [79].

3.3.7. The Practical Meaning of the Reduction in Oxidative Stress

Severe thermal injury induces a pathophysiological response that affects most of the body's organs, including the liver, heart, lungs, and skeletal muscle, and leads to inflammation and hypermetabolism as a hallmark of post-burn damage. Oxidative stress has been implicated as a critical component in developing an inflammatory and hypermetabolic response after a burn [80]. Mitochondria are a primary site of free oxygen radical metabolism. In burn victims, it has been found that a burn-related cardiac dysfunction involves mitochondria under oxidative stress [81]. Hypermetabolism and Hyperkatabolism have been found to accompany mitochondrial stress. Burn trauma alters mitochondrial defenses against free oxygen radicals, which can be positively influenced by antioxidants [81]. Suprathel® applied topically systemically reduces oxidative stress and might decrease organ damage as a consequence [28].

The semi-occlusive properties and a lower inflammatory response by reducing oxidative stress can explain the reduced need for fluid and the patient's early stabilization with Suprathel® treatment [30,74,82]. Free radicals cause a "shedding" of the mostly hyaluronic acid-based glycocalyx of the capillaries and vessels, causing a higher permeability for fluids and the formation of edema, which can be reduced by the radical scavenging abilities of Suprathel®. Systemic stabilization under Suprathel® treatment can occur, as Rubenbauer et al. described in a case of epidermal necrolysis treated with a silver product prior to Suprathel®. The patient developed fluid retention with massive potassium needs and required intubation and ventilation. After changing the treatment to Suprathel®, the patient stabilized quickly, could be extubated on day one after Suprathel® treatment, and was shortly thereafter able to be discharged from the ICU (intensive care unit) [74]. Short described similar cases [51].

A significant reduction in the need for fluids with Suprathel® was reported by Hentschel et al. when comparing Suprathel® to the standard of care (SOC) [81]. The reduced need for fluids with less edema formation might aid in reducing complications such as compartment syndrome, organ failure, and reduced graft take.

Burn wound conversion is the progression of tissue damage over the first days after a burn, resulting in the deepening of the burn. Clinically, areas primarily evaluated as healing spontaneously convert to areas that need skin grafts.

In two retrospective studies, a reduction in the need for grafting in Suprathel®-treated cases versus SOC indicated a reduction in burn wound conversion. The degree of reduction ranged from 27% (historical SOC) to 7% and 2.1% [36,77]. Prospective studies have shown reduced systemic oxidative stress [28] and inflammatory responses [25], possibly as critical causes for reducing burn wound conversion. Additionally, Suprathel® positively affects telomeric kinetics, a significant event in oxidative stress regulation [79]. Apoptosis, combined with connexin's upregulation, seems to be part of burn wound progression [83]. Anti-apoptotic measures such as reducing connexin by addition of poly-L-lactide, as a component of Suprathel®, reduces apoptosis and supports faster wound healing [84]. All of these components support the positive effect of Suprathel® on burn wound conversion.

As there are many influencing components of burn wound conversion, Suprathel® has been shown to potentially reduce some of them. It hinders desiccation, reduces free oxygen radicals and lipid peroxidation, reduces the inflammatory response, and undergoes sympathetic activation by pain, followed by minder perfusion. It supports cells with energy by the lactate shuttle [85], and releases wound healing cytokines [33]. Reduced burn wound conversion means a reduction in areas to be grafted and reduces donor areas, meaning a faster reduction in the total wound area and positively influencing the course of healing. As demonstrated by Blome-Eberwein et al., Suprathel® can reduce the number of patients with partial-thickness burns to be grafted from 20% previously to 0% of all cases, compared to historical SOC, after three weeks. Schriek et al. showed that this reduced from 30% in the historical group to 7–9% after 11 days [77,78].

3.4. Studies and Reports on the Use of Suprathel® for Different Indications

Suprathel® is a versatile dressing in burns treatment and can be used for most indications during treatment. More than 160 reports, studies, and abstracts have been published for various indications.

3.4.1. Donor Areas

Donor areas are often neglected in the treatment of skin defects. Particularly in older people, non-healing donor sites can cause long-lasting morbidity and burden [86]. Suprathel® has been successfully used for donor areas, and many studies have shown excellent results. Pain reduction, reduced workload, very low infection rates, and fast healing times are the main advantages [32,54,71,87]. Berg presented a case with repetitive harvesting 12 times from the scalp without causing alopecia [88]. Healing time can be expected in the range of seven and eight days in children [42,87,88] and from nine days (clinical experience) to 13 days in adults [29].

3.4.2. Superficial and Partial-Thickness Burns

Superficial and partial-thickness burns covered with Suprathel®, especially in more extensive burns, provide a comfortable and nearly painless treatment, with reduced stress for patients and reduced stress and workload for medical staff [89]. It can be combined with the tangential excision or enzymatic debridement in partial-thickness burns, and given the presence of a sufficient number of epidermal remnants, healing without complications can be expected in deeper partial-thickness burns, it can reduce the need for grafting [90–93] and can provide better cosmetic results than in mesh-grafted areas. This has been confirmed by validated scar scales (i.e., POSAS (Patient and Observer Scar Assessment Scale) and VSS (Vancouver Scar Scale) six months after the burn. The cosmetic result measured on a five-point scale was significantly better after one month with Suprathel®, and patients were more satisfied than with Mepilex® [32].

3.4.3. Partial-Thickness and Small Third-Degree Burns

In burns that are mostly partial thickness with small areas of only third-degree burns, treatment with Suprathel® is particularly useful. The whole wound can be treated with Suprathel®. The majority of the wound will heal spontaneously, and only the remaining small areas that do not heal spontaneously within a defined range of time will have to be excised and grafted. This leads to an overall better cosmetic outcome with fewer surgical procedures [76,93,94]. This technique can also be applied in more extensive mixed burns. In areas that will not heal spontaneously, Suprathel® will not be adherent, and the need for grafting will be clear after 10–14 days [76]. During this time, the patient can be stabilized and/or transported. Thus, Suprathel® is the ideal dressing for burn treatment for mass casualties at a lower level of care or under combat conditions. After incomplete debridement and disinfection and covering with Suprathel®, the patient can be transported, and excision of necrotic tissue can be done in a delayed manner under controlled infection conditions [95]. As mentioned above, the main advantages are pain reduction, attenuated fluid balance, and protection from infection.

3.4.4. Full-Thickness Burns

After the complete excision of a burn wound, Suprathel® can be used as a temporary dressing, reducing pain and workload with the advantage of avoiding skin staples, as only the external dressing needs to be changed, which reduces blood and fluid loss [76,96,97].

3.4.5. Suprathel® and Cells

Suprathel® has shown excellent adhesion over and proliferation of keratinocytes and fibroblasts [98,99]. The results of covering sprayed keratinocytes were first published in 2012 [100–102]. The healing time of Suprathel®-covered sprayed cultured and non-cultured keratinocytes was better or equivalent to the results with other dressings published in the literature [101,103]. After application to deep partial-thickness burns, the mean healing time was, on average, eight days after the clinical evaluation of the wound depth and 10 days after laser doppler imaging (LDI). In comparison, the wounds healed, on average, three days faster than in other studies. Furthermore, Suprathel® also protected these wounds with applied cells from infection [104,105].

3.4.6. Suprathel® and the Meek Technique

After removing a Meek nylon pleated wound coverage after 10–14 days, Suprathel® is a good option for covering the incompletely healed wound areas. Suprathel® can be left on the confluent Meek Islands until the wound is fully healed, allowing for more secure epithelialization. This procedure leads to faster healing and a reduction in the rate of wound infections [106].

3.4.7. Suprathel® after Enzymatic Debridement

Suprathel® has been suggested as a dressing after enzymatic debridement (ED) in several consensus meetings, mainly because of the reduced need for dressing changes and its wound-healing abilities. In the European consensus update, it was declared as appropriate, and in the Spanish consensus [107–109], it was declared as a most appropriate dressing material after E.D. in different publications [107–112]. Due to the increased effusion after E.D., a prolonged after soaking period of 5–8 h is indicated [112]. In a retrospective study assessing healing time after E.D., Suprathel® showed a shorter healing time overall than polyurethane foam and cream application, especially in burns with a higher Baux Index, offering all the known advantages of Suprathel® [113,114].

3.4.8. Suprathel® in Burn-Like Syndromes

Excellent results, especially in high-risk toxic epidermal necrolysis (TEN) cases, have been described, including the youngest case ever published before 2006 [115]. The main factors might be reducing the overall mortality due to insufficient wound care, linked with pain reduction, reduced stress, the prevention of life-threatening infections, and the stabilization of the patient [115–120]. It has been shown to be superior to an allograft. Successful case reports have been published as well on staphylococcal scalded skin syndrome [49], phototoxic plant burns [121–123], frostbites [124,125], cotton wool babies [126], and aplasia cutis [127].

3.4.9. Suprathel® in Radiation Injuries

Rothenberger et al. described its successful use in exfoliative dermatitis [46]. Radiation therapy could be continued from 40 Grey to 64 Grey while the wound was able to heal. Immediate pain relief was a positive side effect. Similar cases are currently being peer reviewed.

3.4.10. Suprathel® in Ulcus Cruris

Sari et al. described the positive effect of Suprathel^{CW} in treating chronic wounds in venous, arterial, diabetic, and mixed ulcers. The use of Suprathel^{CW} resulted in a reduction in size or healing of the ulcer. Pain levels were significantly reduced, the skin's inflammatory reaction was significantly reduced, and the wound secretion decreased [128].

3.5. Cost-Effectiveness

When describing costs, material costs and total treatment costs must be taken into account. For Suprathel®, the lower total costs were described by Schwarze et al. [40], Everett et al. [37], and Fischer et al. [50].

4. Limitations

In practical use, instructions have to be followed. It is necessary to overlap Suprathel® over the wound margins and to overlap between sheets. A separation layer and some compression must be applied to prevent adherence to the external absorbent layers and the dislocation of the Suprathel®.

In dressing changes, Suprathel® stays in place, as does the separation layer. Only the absorbent layer and the compressions are changed. Not to do so, causes complications, as described by Rashaan et al. [43]. Experience in the use of Suprathel® in full-thickness burns and ulcers is limited and must be expanded. Costs are sometimes described as a limiting aspect. Although the material may be more expensive than other treatment modalities, different authors have described its cost-effectiveness when considering the total treatment costs.

5. Conclusions

The positive cooperation of a tech company with research institutes and clinical departments, with public funding support and a spin-off, proven to be the source of success for developing and further improving a medical product, which was primarily not in the company's scope.

A fully synthetic and fully resorbable epidermal template based on lactic acid, a physiological and essential product of the human metabolism, opened a new product line and eliminated complicated and laborious production steps. Biocompatibility has been achieved before in other products by the genetic modification of animal-derived tissue [129], which remains limiting in terms of viral, bacterial, and prion safety. By using physiological components only in Suprathel® (i.e., lactic acid), these safety limitations could be eliminated [130].

After the initial regulatory studies, scientific curiosity expanded and later helped find essential wound healing mechanisms relevant to the product. Physical properties such as the adaptation of water vapor permeability over time supported by the body wound healing interactions made a new dressing and treatment scheme possible, reducing complications and the need for inner dressing changes, in contrast to other products [32,130]. A new understanding of lactate and its mechanism positively impacted the local and systemic inflammatory response and (hyper-) metabolism and cell regeneration compared to other products [28,78]. Lactate's effects on particular pain-related receptors could explain the strong pain-reducing effect [131].

Author Contributions: H.L.H. and M.R. contributed substantially to conceptualization, data acquisition, and paper writing. D.P. and S.P.N. contributed essentially to structuring and writing the paper. L.P.K. contributed to the contents and the structure of the article. All authors have read and agreed to the published version of the manuscript.

Funding: Polymedics GmbH Germany paid the publishing fee. No further external funding was received.

Institutional Review Board Statement: Ethical review and approval were waived for this study, due to the nature of a literature review.

Informed Consent Statement: Patient consent was waived due to giving no information on individual patients.

Data Availability Statement: No new data were created or analyzed in this study. Data sharing is not applicable to this article.

Acknowledgments: The article was text edited by MDPI editing service.

Conflicts of Interest: Herbert L. Haller and Matthias Rapp are consultants for training and teaching for Polymedics Innovations GmbH. The other authors declare no conflict of interest. Polymedics GmbH had no role in the design of the study; in the collection, analyses, or interpretation of data; in the writing of the manuscript, or in the decision to publish the results.

References

1. Uhlig, C.; Uhlik, C. Suprathel: The Facts Suprathel. 2004. Available online: https://www.yumpu.com/de/document/view/21238041/suprathel-fakten-stapleline (accessed on 22 December 2020).
2. Hierlemann, H.; Uhlig, C.; Rapp, M. Entwicklung eines resorbierbaren Epithelersatzes für die Verbrennungsmedizin. *Z. Für Wundheilung* **2002**, *4*, 150–151.
3. Rendl, M.; Mayer, C.; Weninger, W.; Tschachler, E. Topically applied lactic acid increases spontaneous secretion of vascular endothelial growth factor by human reconstructed epidermis. *Br. J. Dermatol.* **2001**, *145*, 3–9. [CrossRef] [PubMed]
4. Hunt, T.K.; Aslam, R.; Hussain, Z.; Beckert, S. Lactate, with oxygen, incites angiogenesis. *Adv. Exp. Med. Biol.* **2008**, *614*, 73–80.
5. Herz, H.; Blake, D.R.; Grootveld, M. Multicomponent investigations of the hydrogen peroxide- and hydroxyl radical-scavenging antioxidant capacities of biofluids: The roles of endogenous pyruvate and lactate. *Free Radic. Res.* **1997**, *26*, 19–35. [CrossRef]
6. Yanagida, S.; Luo, C.S.; Doyle, M.; Pohost, G.M.; Pike, M.M. Nuclear magnetic resonance studies of cationic and energetic alterations with oxidant stress in the perfused heart. Modulation with pyruvate and lactate. *Circ. Res.* **1995**, *77*, 773–783. [CrossRef] [PubMed]
7. Philp, A.; Macdonald, A.L.; Watt, P.W. Lactate—A signal coordinating cell and systemic function. *J. Exp. Biol.* **2005**, *208*, 4561–4575. [CrossRef] [PubMed]
8. Robergs, R.A.; Ghiasvand, F.; Parke, D.; Parker, D. Biochemistry of exercise-induced metabolic acidosis. *Am. J. Physiol. Regul. Integr. Comp. Physiol.* **2004**, *287*, 2005–2007. [CrossRef] [PubMed]
9. Lampe, K.J.; Namba, R.M.; Silverman, T.R.; Bjugstad, K.B.; Mahoney, M.J. Impact of lactic acid on cell proliferation and free radical-induced cell death in monolayer cultures of neural precursor cells. *Biotechnol. Bioeng.* **2009**, *103*, 1214–1223. [CrossRef] [PubMed]
10. Gladden, L.B.; Gladden, L.B. Lactate metabolism: A new paradigm for the third millennium. *J. Physiol.* **2004**, *558*, 5–30. [CrossRef] [PubMed]
11. Gladden, L.B. Current Trends in Lactate Metabolism: Introduction. *Med. Sci. Sports Exerc.* **2008**, *40*, 475–476. [CrossRef] [PubMed]
12. Taylor, M.S.; Daniels, A.U.; Andriano, K.P.; Heller, J. Six bioabsorbable polymers: In vitro acute toxicity of accumulated degradation products. *J. Appl. Biomater.* **1994**, *5*, 151–157. [CrossRef]
13. Schakenraad, J.M.; Dijkstra, P.J. Biocompatibility of poly (DL-lactic acid/glycine) copolymers. *Clin. Mater.* **1991**, *7*, 253–269. [CrossRef]
14. Wake, M.C.; Patrick, C.W.; Mikos, A.G. Pore morphology effects on the fibrovascular tissue growth in porous polymer substrates. *Cell Transplant.* **1994**, *3*, 339–343. [CrossRef]
15. Malda, J.; Woodfield, T.B.F.; Van Der Vloodt, F.; Kooy, F.K.; Martens, D.E.; Tramper, J.; Van Blitterswijk, C.A.; Riesle, J. The effect of PEGT/PBT scaffold architecture on oxygen gradients in tissue engineered cartilaginous constructs. *Biomaterials* **2004**, *25*, 5773–5780. [CrossRef]
16. Yannas, I.V.; Burke, J.F. Design of an artificial skin. I. Basic design principles. *J. Biomed. Mater. Res.* **1980**, *14*, 65–81. [CrossRef]
17. Chiu, Y.C.; Cheng, M.H.; Engel, H.; Kao, S.W.; Larson, J.C.; Gupta, S.; Brey, E.M. The role of pore size on vascularization and tissue remodeling in PEG hydrogels. *Biomaterials* **2011**, *32*, 6045–6051. [CrossRef]
18. Rapp, M.; Uhlig, C.; Hierlemann, H.; Planck, H.; Dittel, K.-K. A New Permanent Wound Dressing in the Treatment of Superficial Burns and Donor Sites. In *Proceedings of the Skin Substitutes: Quality and Standards*; European Burns Association—State of the Art Symposium, Ed.; European Burns Association: Brünn, Czech Republic, 2000; pp. 37–38.
19. Haller, H.; Held-Föhn, E. Investigation of Germ Patency of a Polylactic Acid-based Membrane for the Treatment of Burns, Abstract. *J. Burn Care Res.* **2020**, *41*, S173. [CrossRef]
20. Pinney, E.; Liu, K.; Sheeman, B.; Mansbridge, J. Human three-dimensional fibroblast cultures express angiogenic activity. *J. Cell. Physiol.* **2000**, *183*, 74–82. [CrossRef]
21. Stern, R.; Shuster, S.; Neudecker, B.A.; Formby, B. Lactate stimulates fibroblast expression of hyaluronan and CD44: The Warburg effect revisited. *Exp. Cell Res.* **2002**, *276*, 24–31. [CrossRef] [PubMed]
22. Green, H.; Goldberg, B. Collagen and cell protein synthesis by an established mammalian fibroblast line. *Nature* **1964**, *204*, 347–349. [CrossRef] [PubMed]
23. Kottmann, R.M.; Kulkarni, A.A.; Smolnycki, K.A.; Lyda, E.; Dahanayake, T.; Salibi, R.; Honnons, S.; Jones, C.; Isern, N.G.; Hu, J.Z.; et al. Lactic acid is elevated in idiopathic pulmonary fibrosis and induces myofibroblast differentiation via pH-dependent activation of transforming growth factor-β. *Am. J. Respir. Crit. Care Med.* **2012**, *186*, 740–751. [CrossRef] [PubMed]
24. Kwan, P.O.; Ding, J.; Tredget, E.E. Serum Decorin, IL-1beta, and TGF-beta Predict Hypertrophic Scarring Postburn. *J. Burn Care Res.* **2015**, *37*, 1–11.
25. Demircan, M.; Gurunluoglu, K. 354 The IL-6, TNF-alpha, and TGF-ß Levels in Serum and Tissue in Children with Treated by Different Burn Dressings. *J. Burn Care Res. Abstr.* **2019**, *40*, S154. [CrossRef]
26. Rousselle, P.; Braye, F.; Dayan, G. Re-epithelialization of adult skin wounds: Cellular mechanisms and therapeutic strategies. *Adv. Drug Deliv. Rev.* **2019**, *146*, 344–365. [CrossRef] [PubMed]
27. Zhang, Z.; Garron, T.M.; Li, X.J.; Liu, Y.; Zhang, X.; Li, Y.Y.; Xu, W.S. Recombinant human decorin inhibits TGF-β1-induced contraction of collagen lattice by hypertrophic scar fibroblasts. *Burns* **2009**, *35*, 527–537. [CrossRef] [PubMed]

28. Gürünlüoğlu, K.; Demircan, M.; Taşçı, A.; Üremiş, M.M.; Türköz, Y.; Bağ, H.G.; Akıncı, A.; Bayrakçı, E. The effects of two different burn dressings on serum oxidative stress indicators in children with partial burn. *J. Burn Care Res.* **2019**, *40*, 444–450. [CrossRef] [PubMed]
29. Markl, P.; Prantl, L.; Schreml, S.; Babilas, P.; Landthaler, M.; Schwarze, H. Management of split-thickness donor sites with synthetic wound dressings: Results of a comparative clinical study. *Ann. Plast. Surg.* **2010**, *65*, 490–496. [CrossRef] [PubMed]
30. Hu, Y.P.; Peng, Y.B.; Zhang, Y.F.; Wang, Y.; Yu, W.R.; Yao, M.; Fu, X.J. Reactive Oxygen Species Mediated Prostaglandin E2 Contributes to Acute Response of Epithelial Injury. *Oxid. Med. Cell. Longev.* **2017**. [CrossRef]
31. Stock, J.L.; Shinjo, K.; Burkhardt, J.; Roach, M.; Taniguchi, K.; Ishikawa, T.; Kim, H.S.; Flannery, P.J.; Coffman, T.M.; McNeish, J.D.; et al. The prostaglandin E2 EP1 receptor mediates pain perception and regulates blood pressure. *J. Clin. Investig.* **2001**, *107*, 325–331. [CrossRef]
32. Kaartinen, I.S.; Kuokkanen, H.O. Suprathel® causes less bleeding and scarring than Mepilex® transfer in the treatment of donor sites of split-thickness skin grafts. *J. Plast. Surg. Hand Surg.* **2011**, *45*, 200–203. [CrossRef]
33. Mehmet Demircan, M.D.; Kubilay Gürünlüoğlu, M. The IL6, TNF-α, and TGF-β Levels in Serum in Children with Treated by Different Burn Dressings Searching of the ideal burn wound dressing continues. *JBCR* **2019**, *40*, 354.
34. Wei, L. The application of moist dressing in treating burn wound. *Open Med.* **2015**, *10*, 452–456. [CrossRef]
35. Dubin, A.E.; Patapoutian, A. Nociceptors: The sensors of the pain pathway. *J. Clin. Investig.* **2010**, *120*, 3760–3772. [CrossRef]
36. Blome-Eberwein, S.A.; Amani, H.; Lozano, D.D.; Gogal, C.; Boorse, D.; Pagella, P. A bio-degradable synthetic membrane to treat superficial and deep second degree burn wounds in adults and children—4 year experience. *Burns* **2020**, in press. [CrossRef]
37. Everett, M.; Massand, S.; Davis, W.; Burkey, B.; Glat, P.M. Use of a copolymer dressing on superficial and partial-thickness burns in a paediatric population. *J. Wound Care* **2015**, *24*, S4–S8. [CrossRef]
38. Highton, L.; Wallace, C.; Shah, M. Use of Suprathel for partial thickness burns in children. *Burns* **2012**, *39*, 2–7. [CrossRef] [PubMed]
39. Schwarze, H.; Ku, M.; Uhlig, C.; Hierlemann, H.; Prantl, L.; Küntscher, M.; Uhlig, C.; Hierlemann, H.; Prantl, L.; Noack, N.; et al. Suprathel, a new skin substitute, in the management of donor sites of split-thickness skin grafts: Results of a clinical study. *Burns* **2007**, *33*, 850–854. [CrossRef] [PubMed]
40. Schwarze, H.; Küntscher, M.; Uhlig, C.; Hierlemann, H.; Prantl, L.; Ottomann, C.; Hartmann, B. Suprathel, a new skin substitute, in the management of partial-thickness burn wounds: Results of a clinical study. *Ann. Plast. Surg.* **2008**, *60*, 181–185. [CrossRef] [PubMed]
41. Eberwein, S.B.; Pagella, P. Results from Application of an Absorbable Synthetic Membrane to Superficial and Deep Second Degree Burn Wounds. 2014. Available online: http://www.silon.com/wp-content/uploads/2014/09/ECPB2014-Results-from-Application-of-an-Absorbable-Synthetic-Membrane.pdf (accessed on 20 December 2020).
42. Glat, P.M.; Burkey, B.; Davis, W. The use of Suprathel® in the treatment of pediatric burns: Retrospective review of first pilot trial in a burn unit in the United States. *J. Burn Care Res.* **2014**, *35*, S159.
43. Rashaan, Z.M.; Krijnen, P.; Allema, J.H.; Vloemans, A.F.; Schipper, I.B.; Breederveld, R.S. Usability and effectiveness of Suprathel in partial thickness burns in children. *Eur. J. Trauma Emerg. Surg.* **2016**, *43*, 549–556. [CrossRef] [PubMed]
44. Hundeshagen, G.; Collins, V.N.; Wurzer, P.; Sherman, W.; Voigt, C.D.; Cambiaso-Daniel, J.; Nunez Lopez, O.; Sheaffer, J.; Herndon, D.N.; Finnerty, C.C.; et al. A prospective, randomized, controlled trial comparing the outpatient treatment of pediatric and adult partial-thickness burns with suprathel or Mepilex Ag. *J. Burn Care Res.* **2018**, *39*, 261–267. [CrossRef] [PubMed]
45. Merz, K.M.; Sievers, B.R. Suprathel® bei zweitgradig oberflächlichen Verbrennungen im Gesicht Material und Methoden. *GMS Verbrennungsmedizin* **2011**, *4*. [CrossRef]
46. Rothenberger, J.; Held, M.; Stolz, A.; Tschumi, C.; Olariu, R.; Pdf, D.; Constantinescu, M.A.; Held, M.; Aebersold, D.M.; Stolz, A.; et al. Use of a Polylactide—Based Copolymer as a Temporary Skin Substitute for a Patient With Moist Desquamation Due to Radiation. *Wounds* **2016**, *7*, E26–E30.
47. Mueller, E.; Haim, M.; Petnehazy, T.; Acham-Roschitz, B.; Trop, M. An innovative local treatment for staphylococcal scalded skin syndrome. *Eur. J. Clin. Microbiol. Infect. Dis.* **2010**, *29*, 893–897. [CrossRef]
48. Lindford, A.J.; Kaartinen, I.S.; Virolainen, S.; Vuola, J. Comparison of Suprathel® and allograft skin in the treatment of a severe case of toxic epidermal necrolysis. *Burns* **2011**, *37*, 6–11. [CrossRef]
49. Baartmans, M.G.A.; Dokter, J.; Den Hollander, J.C.; Kroon, A.A.; Oranje, A.P. Use of Skin Substitute Dressings in the Treatment of Staphylococcal Scalded Skin Syndrome in Neonates and Young Infants. *Neonatology* **2011**, *100*, 9–13. [CrossRef] [PubMed]
50. Fischer, S.; Kremer, T.; Horter, J.; Schaefer, A.; Ziegler, B.; Kneser, U.; Hirche, C. Suprathel® for severe burns in the elderly: Case report and review of the literature. *Burns* **2016**, *42*, e86–e92. [CrossRef] [PubMed]
51. Short, T.; Johnson, D.; Bennett, D. An Evaluation of Patients that Failed Outpatient Management but Rescued by the Use of Synthetic Lactic Acid Polymer Referenten. *J. Burn. Care Res.* **2018**, *39*, S193–S194. [CrossRef]
52. Liodaki, E.; Schopp, B.E.E.; Lindert, J.; Krämer, R.; Kisch, T.; Mailänder, P.; Stang, F. Kombination von universellem Antidot und temporärem Hautersatz bei VerätzungenCombination of a universal antidote and temporary skin substitute for chemical burns. *Unfallchirurg* **2015**, *118*, 804–807. [CrossRef] [PubMed]
53. Grigg, M.; Brown, J. Donor site dressings: How much do they affect pain? *Ejcb* **2020**, *1*, 88.

54. Grigg, M.; Clenwen, T.; Jason, B. Donor Site Dressings: How Much Do They Affect Pain? 2018. Available online: https://www.mendeley.com/reference-manager/reader/8ea85f41-059c-3096-ab92-ee76df2b04e4/1e556e1f-5932-1173-6f10-287641fb2542/ (accessed on 15 May 2020).
55. Mahinda, T.B.; Lovell, B.M.; Taylor, B.K. Morphine-induced analgesia, hypotension, and bradycardia are enhanced in hypertensive rats. *Anesth. Analg.* **2004**, *98*, 1698–1704. [CrossRef]
56. Stoicea, N.; Costa, A.; Periel, L.; Uribe, A.; Weaver, T.; Bergese, S.D. Current perspectives on the opioid crisis in the US healthcare system: A comprehensive literature review. *Med. Baltim.* **2019**, *98*, e15425. [CrossRef]
57. American Burn Association NBR Advisory Committee; American Burn Association; Committee NBRA; American Burn Association NBR Advisory Committee. National Burn Repository 2017. *Am. Burn. Assoc.* **2017**, *60606*, 1–141.
58. Mackie, D.P. Inhalation injury or mechanical ventilation: Which is the true killer in burn patients? *Burns* **2013**, *39*, 1329–1330. [CrossRef] [PubMed]
59. Mackie, D.P.; Spoelder, E.J.; Paauw, R.J.; Knape, P.; Boer, C. Mechanical ventilation and fluid retention in burn patients. *J. Trauma Inj. Infect. Crit. Care* **2009**, *67*, 1233–1238. [CrossRef] [PubMed]
60. Cancio, L.C.; Chávez, S.; Alvarado-Ortega, M.; Barillo, D.J.; Walker, S.C.; McManus, A.T.; Goodwin, C.W. Predicting Increased Fluid Requirements During the Resuscitation of Thermally Injured Patients. *J. Trauma Inj. Infect. Crit. Care* **2004**, *56*, 404–414. [CrossRef] [PubMed]
61. van den Akker, J.P.; Egal, M.; Groeneveld, A.J. Invasive mechanical ventilation as a risk factor for acute kidney injury in the critically ill: A systematic review and meta-analysis. *Crit. Care* **2013**, *17*, R98. [CrossRef]
62. Peluso, H.; Georgi, M.S.; Caffrey, J. The Opioid Dependence Paradox in Among Patients with Burn Injury. *J. Burn Care Res.* **2020**, *41*, S81. [CrossRef]
63. Kukko, H.; Kosola, S.; Pyörälä, S.; Vuola, J. Suprathel® in treatment of children's scald injuries. *Burns* **2009**, *35*, S22. [CrossRef]
64. Greenwood, J.E.; Clausen, J.; Kavanagh, S. Experience with biobrane: Uses and caveats for success. *Eplasty* **2009**, *9*, e25. [PubMed]
65. Weinzweig, J.; Gottlieb, L.J.; Krizek, T.J. Toxic shock syndrome associated with use of biobrane in a scald burn victim. *Burns* **1994**, *20*, 180–181. [CrossRef]
66. Egan, W.C.; Clark, W.R. The toxic shock syndrome in a burn victim. *Burns* **1988**, *14*, 135–138. [CrossRef]
67. Shirley, R.; Teare, L.; Dziewulski, P.; Frame, J.; Navsaria, H.; Myers, S. A fatal case of toxic shock syndrome associated with skin substitute. *Burns* **2010**, *36*, 2009–2011. [CrossRef] [PubMed]
68. Blomqvist, L. Toxic shock syndrome after burn injuries in children. Case report. *Scand. J. Plast. Reconstr. Surg. Hand Surg.* **1997**, *31*, 77–81. [CrossRef]
69. Withey, S.J.; Carver, N.; Frame, J.D.; Walker, C.C. Toxic shock syndrome in adult burns. *Burns* **1999**, *25*, 659–662. [CrossRef]
70. Vig, K.; Chaudhari, A.; Tripathi, S.; Dixit, S.; Sahu, R.; Pillai, S.; Dennis, V.A.; Singh, S.R. Advances in skin regeneration using tissue engineering. *Int. J. Mol. Sci.* **2017**, *18*, 789. [CrossRef]
71. Uhlig, C.; Rapp, M.; Hartmann, B.; Hierlemann, H.; Planck, H.; Dittel, K.K. Suprathel-an innovative, resorbable skin substitute for the treatment of burn victims. *Burns* **2007**, *33*, 221–229. [CrossRef] [PubMed]
72. Caldwell, F.T.J.; Bowser, B.H.; Crabtree, J.H. The effect of occlusive dressings on the energy metabolism of severely burned children. *Ann. Surg.* **1981**, *193*, 579–591. [CrossRef] [PubMed]
73. Caldwell, F.T.; Wallace, B.H.; Cone, J.B.; Manuel, L. Control of the hypermetabolic response to burn injury using environmental factors. *Ann. Surg.* **1992**, *215*, 485–490, discussion 490–491. [CrossRef] [PubMed]
74. Rubenbauer, J. Erfolgreiche Behandlung eines Lyellpatienten mit Suprathel. Available online: https://www.egms.de/static/en/meetings/dav2018/18dav54.shtml (accessed on 4 January 2021).
75. Kloeters, O.; Schierle, C.; Tandara, A.; Mustoe, T.A. The use of a semiocclusive dressing reduces epidermal inflammatory cytokine expression and mitigates dermal proliferation and inflammation in a rat incisional model. *Wound Repair Regen.* **2008**, *16*, 568–575. [CrossRef]
76. Uhlig, C.; Rapp, M.; Dittel, K.-K. New strategies for the treatment of thermally injured hands with regard to the epithelial substitute Suprathel. *Handchir. Mikrochir. Plast. Chir.* **2007**, *39*, 314–319. [CrossRef]
77. Blome-Eberwein, S.A.; Amani, H.; Lozano, D.; Gogal, C. 501 Second-Degree Burn Care with a Lactic Acid Based Biodegradable Skin Substitute in 229 Pediatric and Adult Patients. *Proc. J. Burn Care Res.* **2018**, *39*, S223. [CrossRef]
78. Gürünlüoğlu, K.; Demircan, M.; Koç, A.; Koçbıyık, A.; Taşçı, A.; Durmuş, A.; Gürünlüoğlu, S.; Bağ, H.G. The effects of different burn dressings on length of telomere and expression of telomerase in children with thermal burns. *J. Burn Care Res.* **2019**, *40*, 302–311. [CrossRef] [PubMed]
79. Szczesny, B.; Brunyánszki, A.; Ahmad, A.; Oláh, G.; Porter, C.; Toliver-Kinsky, T.; Sidossis, L.; Herndon, D.N.; Szabo, C. Time-dependent and organ-specific changes in mitochondrial function, mitochondrial DNA integrity, oxidative stress and mononuclear cell infiltration in a mouse model of burn injury. *PLoS ONE* **2015**, *10*, e0143730. [CrossRef] [PubMed]
80. Zang, Q.; Maass, D.L.; White, J.; Horton, J.W. Cardiac mitochondrial damage and loss of ROS defense after burn injury: The beneficial effects of antioxidant therapy. *J. Appl. Physiol.* **2007**, *102*, 103–112. [CrossRef] [PubMed]
81. Hentschel, S.; Göbel, P. Anpassung der Infusionstherapie nach Suprathel-Deckung? Nachuntersuchung von Patienten nach Suprathel-Therapie bei Verbrennung/Verbrühung in einem Kra. 2013. Available online: https://www.egms.de/static/de/meetings/dav2013/13dav55.shtml (accessed on 20 December 2020).
82. Schriek, K.; Sinnig, M. The Use of Caprolactone Dressing in Pediatric Burns—A Gold Standard? *JBCR* **2018**, *39*, S209.

83. Feng, J.; Thangaveloo, M.; Siang, Y.; Jack, S.; Joethy, J.; Becker, D.L. Connexin 43 upregulation in burns promotes burn conversion through spread of apoptotic death signals. *Burns* **2020**. [CrossRef] [PubMed]
84. Ahmed, S.; Tsuchiya, T. Novel mechanism of tumorigenesis: Increased transforming growth factor-β1 suppresses the expression of connexin 43 in BALB/cJ mice after implantation of poly-L-lactic acid. *J. Biomed. Mater. Res. Part A* **2004**, *70*, 335–340. [CrossRef] [PubMed]
85. Draoui, N.; Feron, O. Lactate shuttles at a glance: From physiological paradigms to anti-cancer treatments. *DMM Dis. Model. Mech.* **2011**, *4*, 727–732. [CrossRef]
86. Fatah, M.F.; Ward, C.M. The morbidity of split-skin graft donor sites in the elderly: The case for mesh-grafting the donor site. *Br. J. Plast. Surg.* **1984**, *37*, 184–190. [CrossRef]
87. Demidova, O.; Manushin, S. Alloplastic skin substitute (SUPRATHEL®) dressings in treatment of donor sites in children with burns. *Moressier* **2019**, *2019*, 2017.
88. Berg, L. SuprathelTM: Where and How to Use It? Helsinki. 2013. Available online: info@polymedics.comonrequest (accessed on 20 December 2020).
89. Rapp, M.; Al-Shukur, F.; Liener, U.C. Der Einsatz des Alloplastischen Epithelersatzes Suprathel®bei Großflächigen Gemischt 2.-Gradigen Verbrennungen über 25% KOF—Das Stuttgarter Konzept. 2010. Available online: https://www.egms.de/static/en/meetings/dav2010/10dav18.shtml (accessed on 27 November 2020).
90. Selig, H.F.; Keck, M.; Lumenta, D.B.; Mittlböck, M.; Kamolz, L.P. The use of a polylactide-based copolymer as a temporary skin substitute in deep dermal burns: 1-year follow-up results of a prospective clinical noninferiority trial. *Wound Repair Regen.* **2013**, *21*, 402–409. [CrossRef]
91. Keck, M.; Selig, H.F.; Lumenta, D.B.; Kamolz, L.P.; Mittlböck, M.; Frey, M. The use of Suprathel® in deep dermal burns: First results of a prospective study. *Burns* **2012**, *38*, 388–395. [CrossRef]
92. Rapp, M.; Junghart, K.; Liener, U. The Treatment of Mixed Superficial and Deep Dermal Facial Burns of Adults Using the Hydrolytic Epithelial Substitute Suprathel. Available online: http://www.medbc.com/annals/review/vol_28/num_3b/text/vol28n3bp347.pdf (accessed on 4 January 2021).
93. Rapp, M.; Uhlig, C.; Dittel, K.-K.; Rapp, M.; Uhlig, C.; Dittel, K.-K. The Treatment of Mass Burn Casualties Resulting from Mass Disaster. *Osteosynth. Trauma Care* **2007**, *15*, 8–16. [CrossRef]
94. Rapp, M.; Junghardt, K.; Junghardt, U.C. Experiences with the Hydrolytic Epithelial Substitute Suprathel®in Extended Superficial and Deep Dermal Burns over 25% TBSA (097). Available online: http://www.medbc.com/annals/review/vol_28/num_3b/text/vol28n3bp348.htm (accessed on 27 December 2020).
95. Cancio, L.C.; Barillo, D.J.; Kearns, R.D.; Holmes, J.H.; Conlon, K.M.; Matherly, A.F.; Cairns, B.A.; Hickerson, W.L.; Palmieri, T.; Young, A.W.; et al. Guideline for Burn Care Under Austere Conditions Surgical and Nonsurgical Wound Management. *J. Burn Care Res.* **2017**, *38*, 203–214. [CrossRef]
96. Selig, H.F. Suprathel versus autologous split-thickness skin in deep-partial-thickness burns. *Burns* **2011**, *37*, S19. [CrossRef]
97. Hierlemann, H.; Rapp, M. New approach—Synthetic resorbable skin epithelial skin substitute for treatment of deep dermal injuries. *J. Burn Care Res.* **2017**, *38*, 56.
98. Nolte, S.V.; Xu, W.; Rodemann, H.P.; Rennekampff, H.O. Suitability of Biomaterials for cell delivery in vitro. *Trauma Care* **2007**, *15*, 42–47. [CrossRef]
99. Kawecki, M.; Kraut, M.M.; Klama-Baryła, A.; Łabuś, W.; Kitala, D.; Nowak, M.; Glik, J.; Sieroń, A.L.; Utrata-Wesołek, A.; Trzebicka, B.; et al. Transfer of fibroblast sheets cultured on thermoresponsive dishes with membranes. *J. Mater. Sci. Mater. Med.* **2016**, *27*, 111. [CrossRef] [PubMed]
100. Herold, C.; Busche, M.N.; Vogt HOR, P.M. Autologe nichtkultivierte Keratinozytensuspension in der Verbrennungschirurgie—Indikationen und Anwendungstechniken Autologous non-cultivated keratinocytesuspension in burn surgery—Indications and techniques Zusammenfassung Einleitung. *GMS Verbrennungsmedizin* **2011**, *4*, 1–8.
101. Hartmann, B.; Haller, H.L. Use of Polylactic Membranes as Dressing for Sprayed Keratinocytes-Retrospective Review Over103 Cases. *J. Burn Care Res.* **2019**, *40*, S224. [CrossRef]
102. Hartmann, B.; Ekkernkamp, A.; Johnen, C.; Gerlach, J.C.; Belfekroun, C.; Küntscher, M.V. Sprayed cultured epithelial autografts for deep dermal burns of the face and neck. *Ann. Plast. Surg.* **2007**, *58*, 70–73. [CrossRef]
103. Holmes, J.H.; Molnar, J.A.; Shupp, J.W.; Hickerson, W.L.; King, B.T.; Foster, K.N.; Cairns, B.A.; Carter, J.E. Demonstration of the safety and effectiveness of the RECELL® System combined with split-thickness meshed autografts for the reduction of donor skin to treat mixed-depth burn injuries. *Burns* **2019**, *45*, 772–782. [CrossRef]
104. Wood, F.; Martin, L.; Lewis, D.; Rawlins, J.; McWilliams, T.; Burrows, S.; Rea, S. A prospective randomised clinical pilot study to compare the effectiveness of Biobrane® synthetic wound dressing, with or without autologous cell suspension, to the local standard treatment regimen in paediatric scald injuries. *Burns* **2012**, *38*, 830–839. [CrossRef] [PubMed]
105. Wood, F.M.; Kolybaba, M.L.; Allen, P. The use of cultured epithelial autograft in the treatment of major burn wounds: Eleven years of clinical experience. *Burns* **2006**, *32*, 538–544. [CrossRef]
106. Rapp, M.; Schappacher, R.; Liener, C.U. Zweizeitige Deckung von Spalthaut-Meek-Inseln nach 7–10 Tagen mit einer Polylactid-Membran (Suprathel). In Proceedings of the Jahrestagung der Deutschsprachigen Arbeitsgemeinschaft für Verbrennungsbehandlung, Zell am See, Austria, 13 January 2020. [CrossRef]

107. Dos Santos, B.; Serracanta, J.; Aquuilera-Saez, J.; Dos Santos, B.P.; Serracanta Verdaguer, E.; Barret, J. Designing an algorithm for the use of Suprathel® following enzymatic debridement with Nexobrid ®in burn injuries in hands. *EBA 2019 E-Poster* **2017**. [CrossRef]
108. Dadras, M.; Wagner, J.M.; Wallner, C.; Sogorski, A.; Sacher, M.; Harati, K.; Lehnhardt, M.; Behr, B. Enzymatic debridement of hands with deep burns: A single center experience in the treatment of 52 hands. *J. Plast. Surg. Hand Surg.* **2020**, *54*, 220–224. [CrossRef] [PubMed]
109. Schulz, A.; Perbix, W.; Shoham, Y.; Daali, S.; Charalampaki, C.; Fuchs, P.C.; Schiefer, J. Our initial learning curve in the enzymatic debridement of severely burned hands—Management and pit falls of initial treatments and our development of a post debridement wound treatment algorithm. *Burns* **2017**, *43*, 326–336. [CrossRef]
110. Schiefer, J.L.; Daniels, M.; Grigutsch, D.; Fuchs, P.C.; Schulz, A. Feasibility of pure silk for the treatment of large superficial burn wounds covering over 10% of the total body surface. *J. Burn Care Res.* **2020**, *41*, 131–140. [CrossRef]
111. Schulz, A.; Shoham, Y.; Rosenberg, L.; Rothermund, I.; Perbix, W.; Christian Fuchs, P.; Lipensky, A.; Schiefer, J.L. Enzymatic Versus Traditional Surgical Debridement of Severely Burned Hands: A Comparison of Selectivity, Efficacy, Healing Time, and Three-Month Scar Quality. *J. Burn Care Res.* **2017**, *38*, e745–e755. [CrossRef]
112. Ziegler, B.; Hundeshagen, G.; Cordts, T.; Kneser, U.; Hirche, C. State of the art in enzymatic debridement. *Plast. Aesthetic Res.* **2018**, *5*, 33. [CrossRef]
113. Sander, F.; Omankowsky, A.; Radtke, F.; Delmo Walter, E.M.; Haller, H.; Branski, L.; Kamolz, L.P.; Hartmann, B. Do Dressing Materials Influence the Healing Time after Enzymatic Debridement? In Proceedings of the 18th European Burns Association Congress, Helsinki, Finland, 4–7 September 2019.
114. Sander, F.; Haller, H.; Hartmann, B. Factors Influencing Healing Time After Enzymatic Debridement. *J. Burn Care Res.* **2020**, *41*, S193–S194. [CrossRef]
115. Rapp, M.; Uhlig, C.; Dittel, K.-K. Der Einsatz von Suprathel in der Behandlung einer großflächigen toxischen epidermalen Nekrolyse (TEN) im Rahmen eines Lyell-Syndroms über 62% KOF. *DAV 2006 Abstr. B* **2006**, 47–48.
116. Rapp, M.; Lorch, R.L.U. Die Behandlung der Toxisch Epidermalen Nekrolyse (TEN) mit SuprathelTM und Immungobulin-G—Das Stuttgarter Behandlungskonzept. 2015. Available online: https://www.egms.de/static/en/meetings/dav2015/15dav74.shtml (accessed on 28 November 2020).
117. Pfurtscheller, K.; Zobel, G.; Roedl, S.; Trop, M. Use of Suprathel® in Two Paediatric Patients with Toxic Epidermal Necrolysis (Ten). n.d. Use of Suprathel® in Two Paediatric Patients with Toxic Epidermal Necrolysis (Ten). Available online: https://suprathelu.com/wp-content/uploads/2017/05/6.1.TEN_Poster_2007.pdf (accessed on 22 December 2020).
118. Renkert, M.; Schöler, M.; Mockenhaupt, B.; Lange, B. Toxische Epidermale Nekrolyse im Kindesalter: 100%iger Epidermisersatz mit Suprathel- Ein Fallbericht. In Proceedings of the 35th Jahrestagung der Deutschsprachigen Arbeitsgemeinschaft für Verbrennungsbehandlung, Chur, Switzerland, 11–14 January 2017.
119. Polymedics Innovations GmbH. TEN (Toxic Toxic Epidermal Necrolysis)with TBSA 80% 2a with One Operation and Treatment with Suprathel. Available online: https://suprathelu.com/wp-content/uploads/2017/05/Indications_6_Case_Study_3.pdf (accessed on 22 December 2020).
120. Sandner, A. Suprathel als Therapieoption bei Exfoliativ Nekrotisierenden Dermatitiden. 26 Jahrestagung der Deutschsprachigen Arbeitsgemeinschaft für Verbrennungsbehandlung. 2008. Available online: https://www.egms.de/static/de/meetings/dav2008/08dav32.shtml (accessed on 22 December 2020).
121. Rapp, M.; Al-Shukur, F.-F.; Junghardt, K.; Liener, U. Kontaktverbrennung durch Pflanzen. *Hautnah Dermatol.* **2018**, *34*, 30–33. [CrossRef]
122. Pfurtscheller, K.; Trop, M. Phototoxic plant burns: Report of a case and review of topical wound treatment in children. *Pediatr. Dermatol.* **2014**, *31*, e156–e159. [CrossRef]
123. Rapp, M.; Al-Shukur, F.F.; Junghardt, K.; Liener, U. Kontaktverbrennung durch Pflanzen. *MMW-Fortschr. Med.* **2017**, *159*, 42–46. [CrossRef]
124. Mądry, R.; Struzyna, J.; Stachura-kułach, A.; Drozdz, Ł.; Bugaj, M.; Mądry, R.; Strużyna, J.; Stachura-kułach, A.; Drozdz, Ł.; Bugaj, M.; et al. Effectiveness of Suprathel® application in partial thickness burns, frostbites and Lyell syndrome treatment. *Pol. Prz. Chir. Pol. J. Surg.* **2011**, *83*, 541–548. [CrossRef]
125. Strużyna, J.; Mądry, R. Treatment of Frostbites—Six Cases Experience. Effectiveness of Suprathel Application. Polymedics Lunch Symp. 2017. Available online: https://suprathelu.com/wp-content/uploads/2017/05/6.4.Lunchsymposium-DAV-2011_Madry.pdf (accessed on 22 December 2020).
126. Sari, E.; Eryilmaz, T.; Tetik, G.; Ozakpinar, H.R.; Eker, E. Suprathel®-assisted surgical treatment of the hand in a dystrophic epidermolysis bullosa patient. *Int. Wound J.* **2014**, *11*, 472–475. [CrossRef]
127. Krohn, C.; Mihatsch, W.; Grundhuber, H.; Hosie, S. A Step Beside Burn Surgery: Suprathel as Wound Dressing in a Neonate with Aplasia Cutis—A Case Report. In Proceedings of the ECPB 2015 Scientific Program, Lyon, France, 24–26 June 2015; p. 75.
128. Shubitidze, D.; Rapp, M.; Strölin, A.; Beckert, S.; Ghahremani, M.; Kiparski, S. Lokaltherapie des Ulcus cruris mit einer neuen Wundauflage Suprathel®. *Gefäßchirurgie* **2013**, *5*, 462–463.
129. Yamamoto, T.; Iwase, H.; King, T.W.; Hara, H.; Cooper, D.K.C.C. Skin xenotransplantation: Historical review and clinical potential. *Burns* **2018**, *44*, 1738–1749. [CrossRef]

130. Phillips, L.G.; Robson, M.C.; Smith, D.J.; Phillips, W.A.; Gracia, W.D.; McHugh, T.P.; Sullivan, W.G.; Mathoney, K.; Swartz, K.; Meltzer, T. Uses and abuses of a biosynthetic dressing for partial skin thickness burns. *Burns* **1989**, *15*, 254–256. [CrossRef]
131. De La Roche, J.; Walther, I.; Leonow, W.; Hage, A.; Eberhardt, M.; Fischer, M.; Reeh, P.W.; Sauer, S.; Leffler, A. Lactate is a potent inhibitor of the capsaicin receptor TRPV1. *Sci. Rep.* **2016**, *6*, 1–13. [CrossRef] [PubMed]

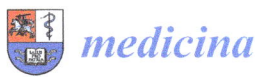

Review

Porcine Xenograft and Epidermal Fully Synthetic Skin Substitutes in the Treatment of Partial-Thickness Burns: A Literature Review

Herbert L. Haller [1,*], Sigrid E. Blome-Eberwein [2], Ludwik K. Branski [3], Joshua S. Carson [4], Roselle E. Crombie [5], William L. Hickerson [6], Lars Peter Kamolz [7], Booker T. King [8], Sebastian P. Nischwitz [7], Daniel Popp [7], Jeffrey W. Shupp [9] and Steven E. Wolf [2]

[1] HLMedConsult, Zehetlandweg 7, 4060 Leonding, Austria
[2] Lehigh Valley Health Network 1200 S. Cedar Crest Blvd. Kasych 3000, Allentown, PA 18103, USA; sibloeb@yahoo.com (S.E.B.-E.); swolf@utmb.edu (S.E.W.)
[3] Department of Surgery—Burn Surgery, The University of Texas Medical Branch and Shriners Hospitals for Children, 301 University BLVD, Galveston, TX 77555, USA; lubransk@UTMB.EDU
[4] Department of Surgery, UF Health Shands Burn Center, University of Florida, 1600 SW Archer Rd, Gainesville, FL 32610, USA; Joshua.Carson@surgery.ufl.edu
[5] Connecticut Burn Center, Yale New Haven Heal System, 267 Grant St, Bridgeport, CT 06610, USA; Roselle.Crombie@bpthosp.org
[6] Memphis Medical Center Burn Center, 890 Madison Avenue, Suite TG032, Memphis, TN 38103, USA; whicker1@uthsc.edu
[7] Division of Plastic, Aesthetic and Reconstructive Surgery, Department of Surgery, Medical University, 8053 Graz, Austria; lars.kamolz@medunigraz.at (L.P.K.); sebastian.nischwitz@medunigraz.at (S.P.N.); daniel.popp@medunigraz.at (D.P.)
[8] Division of Burn Surgery, Department of Surgery, 101 Manning Drive CB #7206, Chapel Hill, NC 27599, USA; bookert@email.unc.edu
[9] The Burn Center, Department of Surgery, MedStar Washington Hospital Center, 110 Irving St NW, Washington, DC 20010, USA; Jeffrey.W.Shupp@medstar.net
* Correspondence: herberthaller@gmail.com

Abstract: *Background and Objectives*: Porcine xenografts have been used successfully in partial thickness burn treatment for many years. Their disappearance from the market led to the search for effective and efficient alternatives. In this article, we examine the synthetic epidermal skin substitute Suprathel® as a substitute in the treatment of partial thickness burns. *Materials and Methods*: A systematic review following the PRISMA guidelines has been performed. Sixteen Suprathel® and 12 porcine xenograft studies could be included. Advantages and disadvantages between the treatments and the studies' primary endpoints have been investigated qualitatively and quantitatively. *Results*: Although Suprathel had a nearly six times larger TBSA in their studies ($p < 0.001$), it showed a significantly lower necessity for skin grafts ($p < 0.001$), and we found a significantly lower infection rate ($p < 0.001$) than in Porcine Xenografts. Nonetheless, no significant differences in the healing time ($p = 0.67$) and the number of dressing changes until complete wound healing ($p = 0.139$) could be found. Both products reduced pain to various degrees with the impression of a better performance of Suprathel® on a qualitative level. Porcine xenograft was not recommended for donor sites or coverage of sheet-transplanted keratinocytes, while Suprathel® was used successfully in both indications. *Conclusion*: The investigated parameters indicate that Suprathel® to be an effective replacement for porcine xenografts with even lower subsequent treatment rates. Suprathel® appears to be usable in an extended range of indications compared to porcine xenograft. Data heterogeneity limited conclusions from the results.

Keywords: dressing changes; epidermal skin substitute; grafting; healing time; infection rate; partial thickness burns; porcine xenograft; resorbable; suprathel; synthetic; workload

1. Introduction

Contemporary burn care aims at rapid closure of open wounds, either temporarily or permanently. Wound closure reduces infectious complications and downregulates inflammation and other detrimental systemic responses. Moreover, it curbs the hypermetabolic response and supports re-establishment of undisturbed energy expenditure in the mitochondria [1,2].

Porcine xenograft (PX) (Mölnlyke, Peachtree Corners, GA, USA) and biosynthetic and synthetic dressings, such as human skin allografts, amniotic membrane, Biobrane® (Dow Hickman/Bertek Pharmaceuticals, Sugarland, TX, USA), Dermagraft™ (Organogenesis, Canton, MA, USA), Appligraf® (Organogenesis, Canton, MA, USA), OrCel® (ORTEC int. Inc., New York, NY, USA), Hyalomatrix® (Medline Industries, Northfield, IL, USA), Transcyte® (Takeda Pharmaceutical Co. Ltd., Tokyo, Japan), and Suprathel® (ST) (Polymedics Innovations GmbH, Denkendorf, Germany) as epidermal skin substitutes, have been used for the closure of partial-thickness wounds. The requirements of these products include safety, ease of application, a short healing time, effectiveness, hypo- allergenicity, and non-oncogenicity, while being able to be stored easily and cost-effective. The PX EZ Derm® was used with numerous indications but is not available on the market anymore, yielding the need for finding the optimal replacement and delivering the motivation for this review.

This paper compares the biological pig skin-derived skin substitute (EZ Derm) to a fully synthetic and biodegradable epidermal substitute (ST) based on the published literature. After describing general product characteristics, we conducted a modified systematic review of the literature to evaluate the suitability or advantages of products other than PX.

2. Materials and Methods

Given the absence of studies directly comparing PX and ST® treatment in burns, we extracted data from studies comparing either PX or ST® to other treatment modalities.

2.1. Data Retrieval

PubMed®, Science Direct®, and Google Scholar® were searched. The primary strategy was to find studies describing the results of the different products in partial thickness burns.

2.2. Study Selection

Studies were selected according to the PRISMA guidelines. We selected articles published in peer-reviewed journals or reviewed and published abstracts of an international meeting on burns.

2.3. Exclusions

Studies on the treatment of mainly or exclusively deep partial-thickness burns were not described. We excluded studies on donor site areas, porcine small intestine submucosa, genetically modified pigskin, and full-thickness burns. We excluded in vitro studies and studies that were not relevant, mentioning one treatment method without numerical data. Non-English articles or articles without full-text have been excluded as well.

2.4. Search Method and Search Results Based on the PRISMA Flow Chart

Figure 1 shows the Prisma procedure.

The following data were retrieved from the studies: study type (prospective, retrospective, randomized, non-randomized, descriptive); study population (pediatric, adult, or mixed); sex distribution (male, female); age; cause of burn (scald, flame, contact, flash); timing of epidermal substitute application; description of use in donor sites (Yes/No); information on detailed burn depth (partial superficial, partial deep, or full-thickness burn); technique of dressing application; wound ground preparation; dressing method and dressing change frequency; healing time; information and percentage of infections;

hypertrophic scarring percentage; product replacement frequency and necessity; hospital length of stay (LOS).

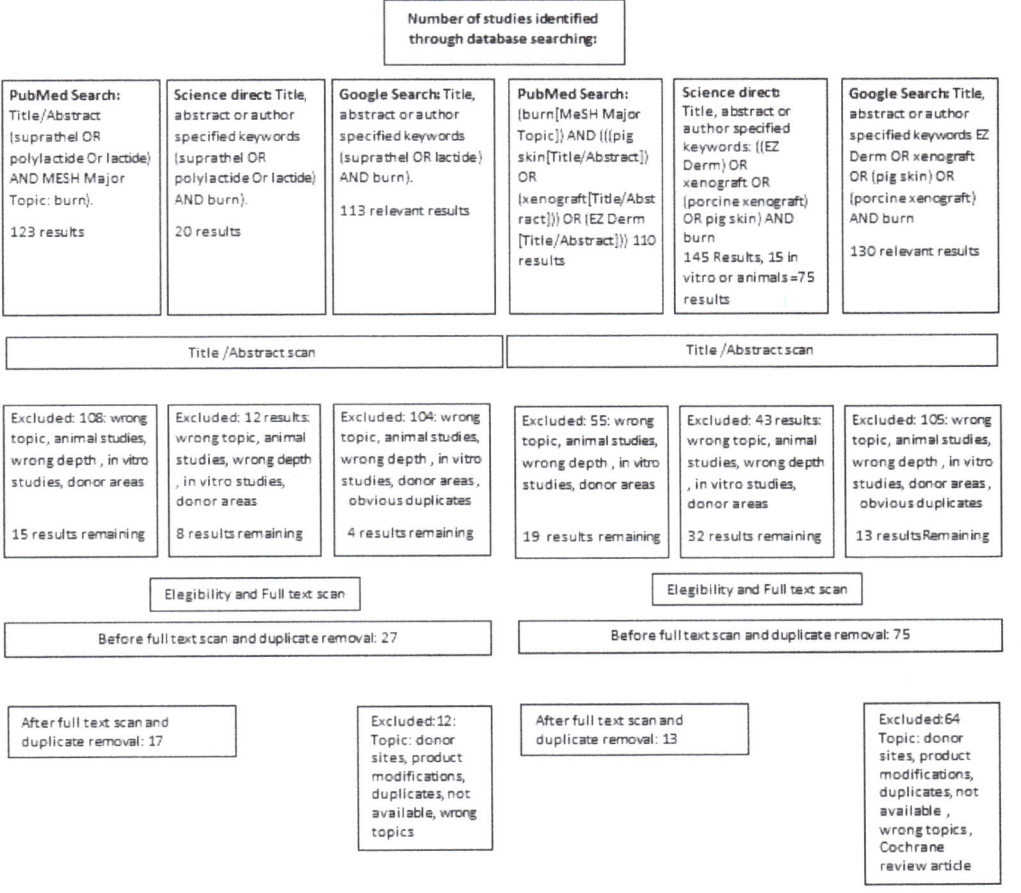

Figure 1. The PRISMA procedure.

2.5. Statistics

In many of the primary studies, the variance was not described. The validity of these studies' statistical output is limited and can only be seen as an approximation. Only studies themselves could have been compared and not individuals treated in the studies. The data were weighted on the number of patients in the studies. Medians were transformed to means as described by Hozo et al. [1] when indicated for comparison. SPSS 20 was used for statistics. The Kolmogorov–Smirnov test was used to identify data for normal distribution and the Levene test for homogeneity of variance. Student T-Test was used for normally distributed data and Kruskal–Wallis and Welch's test for not normally distributed ones. Being well aware of the shortcomings, the statistical efficiency was calculated on pooled data from the studies [2]. A level of $p < 0.05$ was considered statistically significant.

The number of average dressing changes was calculated by dividing healing time by interval of dressing changes in the studies.

2.6. Effect Size of Treatment Modalities

The effect size calculated can only be a rough estimate due to the heterogeneity of studies. The standard effect size was calculated using the SPSS *T*-Test and Two-Sample *T*-Test Calculator from statistics Kingdom for unknown unequal standard deviation [3]. The effect size interpretation was made with no effect when d_{Cohen} was <0.1, a small effect with a d_{Cohen} of 0.2 to 0.4, a medium effect with d_{Cohen} of 0.4–0.6, and a large effect d_{Cohen} of >0.6.

3. Results

In total, 29 studies have been found with two of them describing pediatric and adults separately and where counted separately. There was no special evaluation of mixed populations (pediatric and adult). After exclusion of non-relevant studies (see above), 17 and 16 studies have been included dealing with ST and PX, respectively.

3.1. Quality of Studies

In the ST studies, nine out of 17 studies were done prospectively. Five of the studies were randomized.

In the PX studies, six out of 16 studies were prospective and four of them were randomized. Details are given in Tables 1 and 2.

Table 1. Calculation of the effect size for healing time, percentage of infections, the percentage to be grafted, and dressing changes with weighted data. Stdev = standard deviation.

	Healing Time	Infected %	Grafted %	Dressing Changes
Mean ST	13.59	3.83	2.50	4.38
Mean PX	7.03	7.04	8.36	4.79
Stdev ST	1.86	6.44	4.05	1.83
Stdev PX	2.09	15.62	13.14	4.28
Sample size ST	371	625	681	398
Sample size PX	143	1124	1136	286
Standardized Effectsize at 95% Confidence Intervall	0.19	0.2	0.52	0.13

Table 2. Healing time in ST studies.

Name of the First Study Author	Number of Patients	Study Design	Age	TBSA	Inclusion	Healing Time Days
Blome Eberwein [4]	229	Retro	P (Pediatric): 138, a (adults): 91	Ø 8.6 1–60.5	Superficial and deep second degree	Mean 13.7 d (days) p: 11.9 d A: 14.7 d
Everett [5]	17	Retro	P, Ø 33 m (months)	Ø 5%	Superficial and partial thickness	Mean 9.4 (5–24) d
Fischer [6]	1	Case report	A, 81 a	51%	Partial thickness	14 d
Glat [7]	12	Prospective	Ø 3.6 y (years)	Ø 5.5%	Superficial and mixed	Mean 8.4 d
Glik [8]	24	Retrospective unblinded pair control	Ø 48 y (21–86 y)	Ø 23.8	Burns of both hands to minimize differences	From Figure 1: complete healing d 20
Gürünlüoglu [9]	20	Prospective randomized	4.9 ± 3.8 y	Ø 31.95 ± 4.43%	Acute burns, 1–60 y, 20–50% including deep burns 5–10%	Median 13.5 d (range 9–21 d) Mean 14.25 ±3.46 d

Table 2. Cont.

Name of the First Study Author	Number of Patients	Study Design	Age	TBSA	Inclusion	Healing Time Days
Highton [10]	33	Prospective	P: Ø 29 m (5 m–11 y)	Ø 4 (1–13)%	Superficial partial $n = 24$ mid-dermal: $n = 19$ deep $n = 10$, >21 d and infection	Median 16 (range 9–38) d; Mean 19.5 ± 8.4 d
Hundeshagen [11]	30	Prospective randomized	A: Ø 24.0 ± 23.0	Ø 5.5 ± 4.6%	Partial thickness, FT excl.	Median 12.0 d,
Iqbal [12]	65	Prospective	Ø 4.9 y (4 m–11 y)	Ø 23.6% (8–45)	Superficial dermal 16, mid-dermal 34, deep-dermal 15	Mean 15 (10–35) d
Kukko [13]	8	Retrospective	Ø 18 mo, range 10–39	Ø 7.6 Stdev. missing	Scald injuries	All burns healed by the end of the third week.
Madry [14]	15	Retrospective	1 p, 14 a	Not defined	partial thickness within 96 h after injury	Application: (a) ≤24 hs; (b) 24–48 h; (c) >48 h
Radu [15]	30	Prospective randomized	Median 42 y, (range 18–80 years)	Ø 18% (range 6–36)	Superficial partial thickness burn >3%	Not defined
Rashaan [16]	21	Prospective observational	Median 2.4 y (range 5 m–14 y)	4.0% (range 1–18)	All consecutive partial thickness burns < 48 h after injury and age < 18 years SPTB: 12 DPTB: 9	Median 13 (range 7–29); without bacterial contamination: 13 (7–18); with bacterial contamination 15 (9–29) Mean: 15.5 ± 6.36 d
Schiefer [17]	24	Prospective randomized	Ø 39.8 ± 18 y	0.5 ± 3.0%	All patients with superficial partial thickness burn of the hands	All patients after 7 to 10 days healed completely
Schriek [18]	149 (last year)	Retrospective	Pediatric	Not defined	All partial thickness burns	After 10–12 days, 7–9% grafted
Schwarze [19]	30	Prospective, randomized bicentric	a	1.5%		0

3.2. Inclusion Criteria

Studies showed various inclusion criteria, burn causes, time to admission, total burn surface area (TBSA), TBSA grafted, and data quality. For some topics, data reports were sparse, and therefore these topics are not discussed further.

3.3. Biocompatibility and Systemic Effects

Wound closure with PX reduces pain, fluid, and heat loss [20–22]. Gal and non-Gal antigens are essential pig xenoantigens, causing an endothelial complement-mediated injury, resulting in PX thrombosis [23] which will not be incorporated. A "xenograft reaction" is described anechoically but not published yet by users with an increased leukocytosis and elevated body temperature, even after some days (personal communication from Dr. Joshua Carson).

ST degrades lactate due to its composition (Polylactid). The increase in the ionized lactate level signals hypoxic conditions to cells despite normal oxygen levels without changing the actual pH [24]. It serves as an alternative energy source by the pyruvate and lactate transfer [25], enhances angiogenesis, and generates fibroblasts and extracellular matrix [26,27]. Groussard et al., and, recently, Gürünlüoglu et al., demonstrated lactate's ability to act as a scavenger of free radicals demonstrating the influence on the inflammatory response [9,28]. A positive effect on wound healing was demonstrated compared to Hydrofiber Ag, showing increased keratinocyte generation and faster healing [29,30].

3.4. Wound Preparation

3.4.1. Wound Bed Preparation

Preparation of the wounds before applying the epidermal templates can be considered similar in both products. After cleaning, debridement, and necrectomy [12], both products were usually applied under general anesthesia [20,21,31,32] or moderate-to-deep sedation [22], primarily due to the patient's stress after the injury. The wound bed preparation technique varies among the studies: abrasion was performed using scratchpads or other metallic sponges, brushes, dermabrasion, Versajet, or dermatomes [21,32]. Generally, wound bed preparation was done similarly, depending on the burn depth, and necrosectomy was sometimes performed to induce punctate bleeding [33].

3.4.2. Template Fixation

For template fixation, most authors used staples for mechanical fixation of PX [31,32,34–36] and in some cases fibrin glue [20,22] cyanoacrylate glue [20] topical skin adhesives [36], or sutures [21]. Alternatively, xenograft fixation on superficial partial-thickness burns was achieved by 1-day compression [32] and additional dressing changes on day 1 in PX studies to drain blood or serum retention and control the substitutes' adherence. Frequently, splints were used during the first days to reduce the mobilization of extremities.

However, ST was not mechanically fixated in most studies [10,19,37] with only a secondary dressing holding it in place (see below).

3.4.3. Separation Layer

A separation layer was applied between the product and an absorptive protective dressing in both groups with different dressings, such as antibiotic-loaded agents, silicone, fatty gauze, or nylon dressings being used.

Troy et al. used external dressings with a separation layer until the first dressing change on postoperative day 1, and the PX was exposed to air [32].

3.5. Healing Time

3.5.1. Healing Time in Partial Thickness Burns

The comparison was impeded by a missing or inconsistent description of the healing status.

Effects of grafting or conservative treatment were not specified. Therefore, the healing time was considered in uncomplicated wounds without infections or transplantations.

The two treatment groups had a significantly different TBSA with ST mean $11.36 \pm 7.37\%$ and PXs with 4.79 ± 5.78 (p-value of 0.035) or as weighted data 11.72 ± 7.37 and 1.58 ± 3.44 ($p < 0.001$). Nevertheless, the healing time was not significantly different ($p = 0.067$).

3.5.2. ST Studies

Data were derived from 16 ST studies with 676 patients (See details in Table 2). Eight were excluded as no data at all or no sufficient data on healing time were provided. The remaining nine studies weighted on the number of patients: a mean healing time of 13.59 days with a mean TBSA of $11.73\% \pm 7.37\%$ can be reported. The study populations were composed of children, adults, or both. Rashaan et al. found the healing time range's upper values to be 38 days and 29 days, respectively.

3.5.3. PX Studies

Thirteen PX studies included 1136 patients (see details in Table 3), and seven of them did not provide sufficient data for comparison of healing time and were excluded. After weighting, a mean healing time of 13.22 ± 2.79 days was found in the remaining six studies. The TBSA in studies of patients treated with xenografts had a weighted mean of 1.58 ± 3.44%.

Table 3. Healing time in PX studies.

The Name of the First Study Author	Number of Patients	Study Design	Age	TBSA	Inclusion	Healing Time
Bukovcan [38]	109	Retrospective	Ø 7.6 ± 15.3	Ø 13 ± 8.2%	Superficial and partial thickness burns	Ø 15.1 d ± 11.6 total
Burkey [31]	164	Retrospective	Pediatric	Ø 5.8 ± 4.4%	Superficial partial thickness burns	Not described
Chiu [34]	2	Case reports	Ø 14	Not described	Partial thickness burns of the face, mesh graft pattern	Healed after 10 days
Diegidio [39]	534	Retrospective	Ø 3.41	Ø 8.41%	Scalds from ABA and own registry	Not described
Duteille [35]	20	Prospective	Ø 16.45% range	Ø 27.75%	Intermediary 2nd-degree facial burns	Initial healing time after excision: Ø 13.4 d, 3 grafted
Elmasry [20]	67	Retrospective	Median: 1 y, IQR 1–2	Median 6.2 IQR 4–11	Scalds treated with xenograft (deep and FT)	Not defined
Healy [40]	16	Prospective randomized	Ø 2.6 y ± 7.0	Ø 1.8 ± 0.8%	Partial- thickness burns < 10% BSA	12.9 days in spontaneously healed patients (=47%)
Karlsson [22]	58	Prospective randomized	Ø 21 m (11–59)	Median 5% (3–22)	Partial thickness, <72 h after injury, 6 m–6 y	Median 97% healing 15 d (range 9–29) Ø 17 Median 100% healing: 20.5 range 11–42
Klosova [36]	91	Retrospective	2.5	1–20%	Partial thickness and burn center admission	12–14 d
Klosova	10	Retrospective	42	1–20%	Partial thickness and burn center admission	
Priebe [41]	17	Prospective	15 < 28 m	Not defined	Areas with comparable aspects of 2nd degree	13 of 17 healed in 15 days,
Rodriguez Ferreyra [42]	20	Not defined	Ø 19.2 y	Ø 14.8, no std	Not described	No healing time described.
Troy [32]	133	Retrospective	Ø 17.7, range	Ø 16 ± 37.7%	partial thickness burns, no hands, no pediatric pat	Not described

In the xenograft studies, the maximum healing time was 42 days [22]. Duteille reported excision 7.6 days after injury, and healing occurred after 13.4 days in all but three patients.

3.6. Change of the Templates or Discontinuation of Treatment

Troy et al. described adhesion loss in their PX studies in 6.8% of patients [32]. Klosova et al., using XE Derma, found adhesion loss in 16% of patients and at least partial disintegration of xenografts in an additional 12% of patients [36]. Out of eight xenograft studies describing unexpected or not defined autografting, adhesion loss was found in five studies, and xenograft change was done between daily and every third day in three studies.

Early detachment or poor wound healing was mentioned in three of the ST® studies. In all these wounds, conservative treatment until wound closure was performed due to the residual defects' small size. Two studies described at least a partial removal of ST®. In one study, early detachment occurred in 33% of the patients [16], attributed to the method of debridement or dressing. In the other study, in three of 15 patients, a dressing removal was necessary without a reason given [14] (Table 4).

Table 4. Change or discontinuation of Suprathel or PX treatment.

	ST®			Xenograft	
First Author	ST®	Comment	First Author	Xenografts Change or Diss.	Comment
Blome Eberwein [4]	No change and no autografts.	In 5.2% failure or progression to full thickness, residual defects treated conservatively	Burkey [31]	11% of 164 not anticipated autografting + prolonged topical wound care in 6 pat. (3.7%) not anticipated and 22 (14%) anticipated	14.7% (in a total of not anticipated autografting or prolonged wound care)
Everett [5]	No change		Burleson [43] cited by Chiu [34]	Change every two days	Partial-thickness porcine split skin
Fischer [6]	No change		Duteille [35]	EZ derm in place after surgery for three days, followed by grafting or topical wound care	Grafting in 3 patients,
Gürünüloglu [9]	No change		Elmasry [20]	20% needed an operation	No use in hands
			Klosova [36]	19% (81% no signs of dissolution)	XE derma
Hundeshagen [11]	No change		Priebe [41]	EZ Derm replaced every third day	
Madry [14]	No change	One dressing removal necessary when ST applied at 24–48 h; 2 removals necessary, applied >48 h after injury (reasons nor specified).	Rappaport [44] cited by Chiu [34]	Daily change of xenograft	Deep Frozen pigskin
Rashaan [16]	No change, early detachment in 43% treated conservatively	33% contamination before ST®, detachment is linked to the method of debridement and topical wound care when detached.	Troy [32]	6.8% with premature graft separation, 15% lost for follow-up	After separation, local wound care
Schiefer [17]	No change				
Schwarze [19]	No change				

3.7. Auto-Grafting as Indicator for Burn Wound Conversion

Sufficient data on grafting rates were mentioned in 13 and 17 studies in the PX and ST groups, respectively.

In PX studies, Troy et al. described excision and autografting in 4.5% of patients in a "no variable burn depth group with only partial-thickness burns" [32]. In their retrospective, unselected study, Elmasry et al. [20] had a grafting rate of 30% due to non-closure after two weeks. Details are shown in Table 5. Only clearly defined grafting procedures were included in the table. The time to evaluate the necessity of the use of autografting varied. Blome-Eberwein evaluated skin grafting after three weeks, while Schriek and Sinnig did their evaluation after 11 to 14 days.

Table 5. Grafting rates in partial thickness burns.

	ST®				PX				
Study	n=	% Grafted	n=	Type of Burn	Study	n=	% Grafted	Number of Grafted	Type of Burn
Blome Eberwein [4]	229	0%	0	2nd degree burns superficial and partial	Bukovcan [38]	109	3.7%	4	superficial partial scald burns
Everett [5]	17	0%	0	Partial thickness within 6 h	Burkey [31]	167	5.5% unexpected	3 + 21	Superficial partial-thickness inclusion
Fischer [6]	1	0%	0	Partial thickness	Duteille [35]	20	15%	3	Intermediate face burns
Gürünlüoglu [9]	20	0%	0	Superficial and deep partial thickness burns	Elmasry [20]	67	30%	20	Only superficial partial-thickness burns
Hundeshagen [11]	30	6.6%	1	Partial thickness burns	Healy [40]	32	7 out of 16 EZ Derm 44%	7	Partial, no hands or faces
Iqbal [12]	65	0%	0	Partial-thickness burns	Karlsson [22]	29	13%	6	No palms, soles, or faces
Madry [14]	15	26%	2	Children, Flame and scald burns	Klosova [36]	91 children	30%	27	Partial thickness burns and full thickness
Rashaan [16]	21	14%	3	Superficial. and deep partial, 7% of all patients colonization before ST®	Klosova [36]	10 adults	90%	9	Partial thickness burns and full thickness
Schulz [17]	24	0%	0	Partial thickness	Priebe [41]	15	13%	2	Scald burns, children
Schriek and Sinnig [18]	149	9%	11 last year of table	Superficial and partial deep burns	Rodriguez Ferreyra [42]	20	0%	0	superficial
Schwarze [19]	30	0%		Superficial or mid dermal burns	Troy [32]	157	8.6%	6.8 + 4.5 + 2.2	Partial, no hands, no faces

According to the studies analyzed, treatment resulted in a mean grafted rate of 2.50% ± 4.05% per ST and 8.63% ± 13.14% per PX study ($p < 0.0001$) as weighted values.

The same effect could be verified by evaluating the statistical effect size of 0.58, demonstrating a medium effect of ST to reduce grafting.

3.8. Infection Rates in Partial Thickness Burns

Infection rates were described in 11 studies on PX and 14 on ST. Infection was evaluated only where explicitly described as "infection" (Table 6). Reasons for autografting might overlap these results, as they were not distinguished to prolonged healing time or infection.

Table 6. Infection rates in partial thickness burn studies (p = pediatric, a = adult).

ST					Xenograft				
First Author	N=	Infections	Infect. %	Healing Time	First Author	N=	Infections	Infect. %	Healing Time
Blome Eberwein [4]	138 p 91 a	0 8	0 8.8%	13.9 14.70	Bukovcan [38]	109 p	4	4%	15.10
Everett [5]	17 p	0	0	9.40	Burkey [31]	167 p	4	2%	insuff. Data
Glat [7]	12 p	0	0	8.40	Diegidio [39]	534 p	3	0.01%	Insuff. Data
Hundeshagen [11]	31 a	1	6.45%		Duteille [35]	20 a	3	15%	insuff. Data
Iqbal [12]	65 p	13	20%	15.00	Elmasry [20]	20 p	7	35%	insuff. Data
Rashaan [16]	21 p	1	4.76%	15.56	Healy [40]	16 a	7	43%	insuff. Data
Schwarze [19]	30 a	0	0	10.20	Karlsson [22]	58 p	9	16%	17.00
					Klosova [36]	101 p + a	5	5%	Nd
					Priebe [41]	15 p	Nd (Not defined)		Nd
					Rodriguez Ferreyra [42]	20 p + a	0	0%	insuff. Data
					Troy [32]	15 a	2	13%	insuff. Data
Average per study		3.83%	±6.34		Average per studies		7.039	15.62	

3.8.1. Infection Rate ST

Weighted infection rates in the ST studies were 3.83 ± 6.34 in the ST studies. In 24 of 631 (3.8%) participants, a wound infection was described in the ST studies with no difference between pediatric and adult patients.

3.8.2. Infection Rate PX

Weighted infection rates in the studies was 3.83 ± 6.34 in the ST, and 7.04 ± 15.62 in the PX studies. No difference could be found between pediatric and adult patients ($p = 0.10$).

3.9. Pain Reduction

Both products were found to reduce pain.

In the ST group, Everett et al. demonstrated a significantly reduced need for intravenous narcotics after ST application [5]. A direct comparison was not possible due to the use of different scales used to investigate pain.

VAS with different ranges were used by Schwarze et al. [19], Blome Eberwein et al. [4], and Hundeshagen et al. [11], showing pain reduction by the ST dressings, partly significant in comparison to other dressings. Wong–Baker and Comfort B scores used by Glat et al. [7]

and Rashaan et al. [16] showed values between no pain and minimal pain after ST treatment. Glik et al. [8] showed OASIS superior only on day four without statistical significance.

In the PX group, medication use was evaluated by Burkey et al. [31], finding reduced narcotic doses in 32.4% of the patients and 6.1% needing sedation who did not need it before. Karlsson et al. [22] used Parents Postoperative Pain Measure (PPPM) scores and found no difference in opioid and analgesics use compared to the use of silver foam. Routine use of analgesics was described by Zajicek et al. [45]. Elmasry et al. [20] used the FLACC score, showing a reduction after two days to minimal pain values (3 of 10). Other authors experienced, discussed, or claimed pain reduction without detailed information.

3.10. Frequency of the Secondary Dressing Changes

In the study by Fischer et al., the hospital length-of-stay was 69 days, during which nine dressing changes were performed, even though the wounds were closed after 14 days [6]. In five studies, dressing changes were performed every 1–10 days (Table 7).

Table 7. The frequency of outer dressing changes.

ST Studies, First Author	Outer Dc Every Day	Approx. Healing Time	Total Number of DC	PX Studies, First Author	Outer Dc Every Day	Approx. Healing Time	Total Number of DC
Blome Eberwein [4]	1–4 (2.5)	14.2	5.68	Burkey [31]	Average DC 1.6	Healing time not described	1.6
Everett [5]	5–7 (6)	9.5	1.59	Bukovcan [38]	2	15.1	7.6
Hundeshagen [11]	3–5 (4)	12	3	Elmasry [20] *	1	12.2	12
Iqbal [12]	4–5 (4.5)	15	3.33	Duteille [35]	3 days then moistened gauze	3 *	* excluded
Rashaan [16]	3	15	5	Karlsson [22]	3 regularly, up to three times a week, Number of DC: 5 (−9), time for DC 20 min (10–50)	Time to 95% healing 15 days	5
				Priebe [41]	3	15	5
The average number of dressing changes during Healing time and		13.61	3.43 ± 1.46 Median 3.165 Range 4.09			14.33	7.4 ± 2.86 Median 5 Range 10.4

* The study of Duteille et al. was excluded, as no exact healing time and dressing changes were provided.

Often the frequency was described as an interval of dressing changes. Calculating the number of dressing changes, the weighted healing time given in the respective studies was divided by the interval of dressing changes. The number of dressing changes in the ST group was on average 4.38 ± 1.83 dressing changes during the healing period and 4.79 ± 4.29 in the PX studies ($p = 0.139$).

3.11. Outpatient Visits and Hospital Length of Stay

Hospital length of stay (LOS) was described in 11 and eight of the PXs and ST® studies, respectively, in different non-comparable modalities. The number of outpatient visits and hospital length of stay depends on the frequency of dressing changes, the burn unit's policy, and the study design. Burn severity might also influence hospital LOS, which could not be considered due to insufficient data. In prospective ST and PX studies, hospital LOS ranged from 0 [5] to 23.3 days [9] and 2 to approximately 40 days [8], respectively.

3.12. Results of the Literature Review on Other Indications for Epidermal Templates in Burns Treatment

When covering freshly harvested keratinocytes after seeding and culturing or precultured keratinocytes, PX did not adhere to the keratinocytes and, therefore, did not survive the first week [46].

In a prospective study of 19 patients, ST was successfully used to cover sprayed keratinocytes in deep dermal burns of the face, with excellent cosmetic outcomes [47]. Moreover, similar results were found in a retrospective study of 103 patients with keratinocytes applied to deep partial-thickness burns and covered with ST [48]. The studies mentioned above showed a mean healing time of 8.04 days, which was shorter than that in the literature wherein other dressings were used [49–51]. Neither other wound-associated infections nor patient age influenced the duration of wound healing.

In the sandwich technique, both ST® and PX can be used over a meek graft or a widely meshed autograft to reduce the risk of infection and fluid loss [52].

3.13. Results from the Literature on Oxidative Stress during Burns Treatment

Karlsson et al. compared C-reactive protein (CRP) levels during treatment with a silver foam dressing and found lower levels in the PX group without significant intergroup differences [22]. Feng et al. [53] used PX and found a significantly decreased CRP level than in the use of betadine gauze [53]. Iwase et al. could demonstrate that an IL-6 antagonist could reduce the inflammatory response on pig derived transplants, but not on D-dimer [54].

ST decreases total oxidant capacity, increases total antioxidant capacity [29], restores telomere length [9], reduces IL-6 and TNF α activity, and increases TGF-β generation [55] over two weeks in comparison to a silver-containing Hydrofiber product, possibly mediated by the radical scavenging ability of lactate released during degradation accompanied by a shorter healing time [29,55].

4. Discussion

PX's disappearance from the United States market raises several fundamental challenges for burn treatment and the question of the best available replacement.

4.1. General Aspects
4.1.1. Viral and Prion Safety

Concerns about the safety of biological products are accompanying the use, at least as a theoretical consideration. In Internet-based research by Wurzer et al. [56] with 111 burn specialists over 36 countries in 2016, the participants rated the risk associated with xenografts as essential in only 32%, which may have changed during the current pandemic situation. The approximately hypothetical risk has been well-known over time [34]; however, epidermal skin replacement's urgent need supported the application. Unique methods nowadays even might allow for the use of virus-free animals, at least for transplantation trials with pervasive and expensive means so that they are not in general use.

A fully synthetic and biocompatible epidermal skin substitute makes a biological risk assessment needless, as it poses no viral or prion or (probably) even nowadays unknown pathogens risk.

4.1.2. Biocompatibility

Not decellularized PX's lack of biocompatibility is caused by endothelial membrane-bound Gal and non-Gal antigens. Besides, human monocytes can also recognize porcine endothelial cells [57] causing thrombosis in the template and hindering PX incorporation in the dermal scaffold. The decellularization procedure might reduce thrombosis and increase viral safety to a more theoretical aspect, cross-linking of collagen by aldehyde treatment reduced antigenicity, and rejection and inflammation but could not eliminate it [58–61]. Even when PX does not vascularize, it remains a biological cover, thereby increasing inflammation as described by Salisbury and Vanstraelen [62,63]. Moreover, the lack of vascularization led to frequent dressing changes in many studies [41], a high rate of unexpected autografting [31,36], prolonged topical wound care after dissolution [36], and the generation of granulation tissue in long term use [21].

Biogenetically reengineered PX could avoid these unwanted effects; nonetheless, it is not yet clinically used [64,65]. Troy et al. [32] discussed rejection and stated a "self-limiting effect by host epidermis reconstitution under the dressing" in partial thickness burns.

The observed, but until now unpublished "xenograft reaction" with leukocytosis and fever might be provoked by this.

Although no actual trans-species viral transmissions are reported in the PX, a potential risk remains [66]. Hume et al. described mitigating factors in viral inactivation such as sample volume and protein content and underscored the necessity to evaluate inactivation protocols of BSL-4 pathogens (viruses) using "worst-case scenarios" [67]. Risks are eliminated with the non-availability of PXs are no more available. Other potential risks of biological replacement products like prions were unknown until the first cases with Creutzfeldt Jacobs Disease remain.

Karlsson et al. compared C-reactive protein (CRP) levels during treatment with a silver foam dressing and found lower levels in the PX group without significant intergroup differences [22]. Feng et al. described a lower CRP level to controls in the early and late treatment phases and hypothesized a positive effect on SIRS by PXs [68] but Iwase et al. demonstrated evidence of a sustained systemic inflammatory response [54].

ST® is biocompatible, fully resorbed without a foreign body reaction, and does not cause rejection as tested in CE and FDA 510 k clearance. Shelf-life discussions are irrelevant in a non-available product. Other similar products are not the topic of this paper.

4.1.3. Ethical and Religious Considerations for a Replacement Decision

Non-availability of PXs eliminates, at least in the US, Deliberations linked to the use.

In the areas of the world with pigskin production like XE-Derma [45], the aspects as described by Eriksson et al. [69] are still relevant: Sunni and Shiite Muslims who reject porcine-derived products, whereas, for Hindus and Sikhs, these are acceptable if no alternative product is available and if the treatment is considered life-prolonging. In Iran, lyophilized PX has been legalized [21]. Therefore, PX use requires the patient's informed consent or its legal deputy [70]. For ST®, no ethical, cultural, or religious limitations are described as a fully synthetic product.

4.2. Usability

4.2.1. The Usability in Donor Areas

The safe and effective treatment of donor areas is of concern, as these artificially created wounds are of partial thickness, and nonhealing donor areas may prolong morbidity.

The use in donor areas was seen differently. Although PX is described as indicated for donor site closure, many authors disagreed with this because it might trigger local site inflammation [22,62,63,71]. ST® is widely used to cover donor sites [7,72–74], and many authors described a positive impact on wound healing, pain control, patient comfort, and ease of use [5,7,72,73,75–77].

4.2.2. Covering Keratinocytes

When used as a cover for cultured keratinocytes, PX did not adhere to the wounds, and the keratinocytes did not survive the first week [46] no matter whether precultured or not-precultured keratinocytes were used. In a prospective study of 19 patients, ST was successfully used to cover sprayed keratinocytes in deep dermal burns of the face, with reasonable cosmetic outcomes [47]. Moreover, similar results were found in a retrospective study of 103 patients with keratinocytes applied to deep partial-thickness burns and covered with ST [48]. The studies' results revealed a mean healing time of 7.34 ± 2.84 days after application, which was shorter than that in the literature wherein other dressings were used [49–51]. Neither wound-associated infections nor patient age influenced the duration of wound healing in this case-series.

4.2.3. The Use as a Sandwich Technique

Using a sandwich technique, both PX and ST® have been used successfully over Meek grafts or widely meshed autograft to reduce the risk of infection and fluid loss [52,78]. The potent pain-reducing abilities of ST® and the reduced number of dressing changes may be advantageous in this indication.

4.2.4. The Use for Preparation of the Wound Bed by Xenografts

Xenografts can be used to prepare the wound bed before grafting, thereby creating granulation tissue in deeper parts [21], and ST can be used to prepare the wound bed as well [79] and to induce tissue neoformation and is reported to reduce the sizes of areas to be grafted and therefore donor areas [37].

4.3. The Use of the Products to Provide Undisturbed Wound Healing

Healing time, the frequency of dressing changes, the rate of infections, dissolution of the epidermal skin substitute, grafting rates, and pain during treatment and dressing changes might be indicators for undisturbedness.

4.3.1. Healing Time

Data are presented in Tables 1 and 2. Healing time only seems to be an easy parameter for undisturbed wound healing. The number of dressing changes, infection rates, and grafting rates is other parameters. The healing time evaluated in this paper was the time of uncomplicated healing in wounds without transplantations. When evaluating healing time, the number of patients grafted has to be considered, as must be considered, as the indication for grafting might be a predictable prolonged healing time. It also has to be considered that the wounds covered with ST were nearly six times as large as those covered with PXs.

Healing Time in Partial Thickness Burns

With similar inclusion and exclusion criteria, the healing time in uncomplicated wound healing was in the ST Ø 13.59 ± 1.86 days and the PX group Ø 13.22 ± 2.1 days after weighting the data.

Comparison of weighted data showed a healing time in the ST studies, with a statistically not significant difference of $p = 0.067$. The difference might influence this in weighted TBSA, which was about seven times as high in the ST group (11.36 ± 7.37%, compared to 1.58 ± 344%), a significantly higher infection rate (3.85 ± 6.35 versus 7.03 ± 15.65). Early grafting based on the evaluation that no spontaneous healing was expected within three weeks and early infections may have classified patients as drop-out for wound healing time evaluation and shortened by this the PX average healing time. The impact on the standardized effect size of mean wound healing days was small (0.19).

No study provided data with a healing time without infections and grafting as signs of undisturbed healing in the xenograft group.

In the ST group, undisturbed wound healing was reported in six studies with 218 patients.

In the ST® studies, 96.8% of the patients healed without transplants, while 91.7% in the PX studies. Infections without transplantation prolonged the healing time from about ten days to 16 days; the healing time after transplantations remains unclear.

Mixed and Deep Partial Thickness Burns

The treatment of mixed and deep partial-thickness burns is of high interest, as the standard procedure suggested for this condition is grafting [37]; treatment with an epidermal skin substitute may reduce the area grafted, thereby reducing donor sites. Grafting in partial-thickness burns has cosmetic consequences, especially with mesh grafts [37], where a graft pattern and graft margins may remain visible. Healing time® in mixed burns is an essential parameter for the choice of conservative or operative treatment and ranged from 8.4 [9] to >38 days, indicating the presence of minor full thickness burns or the influence of infections on the healing process.

Healing time in mixed burns in the xenograft group was described by Bukovcan et al., who reported a correlation with TBSA. Patients with a TBSA < 10% and >20% had healing times of 13.6 ± 11.1 days and 24.6 ± 12.7 days, respectively. The mean healing time not regarding TBSA was 13.47 days in PX treated children and in adults, the mean healing time was 15 days in their study. Highton et al. [10] described a median healing time in their superficial and deep dermal wounds of 16 days.

Therefore, no conclusions can be drawn. When looking at the results, most studies with xenografts only described healing in parts of the patients after thirty days.

Other components like clinical practice might influence the results: Elmasry had a grafting rate of 30%. Nevertheless, in TBSA and burn depth analysis, superficial second-degree burns in his study had a mean TBSA of 5%, and deep second- and third-degree burns only had a TBSA range from 0 to 0.1%, so the depth of wounds could not be the reason for the higher grafting rate.

The healing time in deep partial-thickness burns with completed healing within 218 patients. 30 days as demonstrated by Keck et al. with ST® compared to that of PX, as reported by Hosseini et al. [21] revealed that after one week, stage four granulation tissue was found in 13% of the PX patients (see Table 7). The results are lacking statistical validity.

4.3.2. Burn Wound Progression

In some studies, wounds were covered in mixed and deep burns until definitive healing or grafting [4,18,37,80]. As shown in longitudinal and comparative ST® studies, a temporary covering predisposes to partial spontaneous healing and limits the areas that must be grafted.

ST® is possibly causing less irritation and positive healing effects [29,55]. Both ST and PXs trigger faster epithelialization than does silver sulfadiazine and povidone-iodine cream [21,53]. Healey et al. described no significant difference in healing time between PX and paraffin gauze [40]. The reduced grafting rate in ST studies might indicate a reduction of burn wound conversion.

The reduction of oxidative stress is an essential prerequisite in ongoing wound healing. Dressings can have systemic effects, as demonstrated by occlusive dressings [81]. Karlsson et al. found lower CRP levels, indicating reduced oxidative stress when comparing PX efficacy with that of silver foam in partial-thickness burns; however, PX will trigger an immune response in wounds.

Ogawa found chronic inflammation as an essential trigger of hypertrophic scarring [82]. Gürünlüoglu et al. demonstrated that polylactide epidermal substitutes exert positive systemic effects on oxidative stress in burns' pathophysiology [29,30,55]. These positive effects were explained with a new understanding of lactate's role in energy distribution, utilization, and radical scavenging. The rate of hypertrophic scarring was not investigated in a direct comparison of PXs, and therefore only personal impressions about a better scar outcome in ST® treated are reported [4,29,83].

4.3.3. Temporary Cover of Full Thickness Burns

Both products have been used for the temporary closure of full-thickness burns. Middelkoop, Grigg et al., and others described the use of PX for this indication [80,84]. However, they provide no information about the maximum duration of the temporary closure. Heimbach et al. described PX use as limited to 7 days due to a reduced resistance against infection [85,86]. Saffle concluded that PX was less effective than allograft in excised burn wounds [87].

Chiu et al. did not include full-thickness burns as an indication for PX in their review [34]; nevertheless, it is used with frequent material changes. Notwithstanding, a previous study reported partial healing of full thickness wounds in very young pigs after applying freshly harvested PX only [88].

Small full-thickness areas can be covered with ST® until complete wound healing [75]. Case reports describe the temporary closure of excised burn wounds for up to 218 patients. 3 weeks [89,90] under the same surgical conditions as temporary dermal templates. So far, ST® has been used as a temporization product, although with insufficient evidence.

4.3.4. Use as a Dermal Template in Supporting Tissue Replacement and to Bridge Time to Availability of Donor Skin or CEA

In deep dermal burns, where there is limited availability of donor areas, mono- and bilayer dermal regeneration templates [91–93] of biological or biosynthetic or fully synthetic origin [94] can help bridge the time until skin grafts or cultured epithelial autografts or dermal–epidermal substitutes [8,95–98] are available again. Other methods use pathogen-free human keratinocyte progenitor cells to replace autologous epidermal cells [99] and can be used immediately, as demonstrated in traumatic wounds [100].

Dermal templates can help to improve the stability of the new dermo-epidermal constructs and the cosmetical outcome [92]. The use of Suprathel as a dermal template or in covering full thickness wounds temporarily has been demonstrated in single cases but not described in studies [89,101].

Polylactic membranes might even have a positive effect on osteogenicity [102] and might be helpful to support techniques like the "induced membrane technique" for replacement of bone loss [103] or in maxillofacial surgery, porcine bone xenografts were tested in a non-inferiority study to bovine-derived xenografts in rat calvaria with good results.

4.4. Pain Reduction

Reduced pain and workload are essential features during wound healing and enable early mobilization and early weaning from the ventilator with reduced stress for patients and staff. Pain reduction might even help to reduce opioid dependency after burns treatment. Both products were shown to reduce pain [7,31,41,73]. The only direct study comparing ST® and PX efficacies on pain control was conducted on TENS and not on burns. Lindford [104], in a case report, found no pain in the ST®- and xenograft treated areas; however, the allograft-treated areas were painful during movement.

In the xenograft studies, Burkey et al. [31] evaluated the effect of PX on pain using the need for intravenous narcotics and moderate sedation in each patient. They found less use of intravenous narcotics in 32%, unchanged in 61%, and increased by 6.7%. Therefore, positive effects on pain could be seen in 32% and no or adverse effects in the rest. The sedation reduction effect was more pronounced, as only 35% did not show a positive effect. Sixty-four percent of patients no longer received sedation. In 29.9% of patients, no change in use was found, and 6.1% of patients who did not receive preoperative sedation received it postoperatively.

Elmasry found a significant reduction in the Face, Legs, Activity, Cry, and Consolability (FLACC) scores, initially ranging from 3 to 7 and decreased after day 3 to <3, which could be interpreted as mild discomfort [20]. Karlsson et al. found no difference in pain at any time when comparing the efficacies of xenografts and silver foam [22]. However, the dressing was applied with Safetac, which might reduce pain by itself [105]. Dressing changes were conducted under ketamine and midazolam, propofol and fentanyl, and, in some cases, even under sevoflurane [22]. Zajicek needed analgesics in 90% of his pediatric patients and 100% of his adult patients during the first seven days of dressing changes [45]. Bukovcan et al. [38], Hobby et al. [106], Priebe et al. [41], and Troy et al. [32] found a positive effect on pain reduction.

In the ST® group, Everet et al. [5] reported delivery of intravenous narcotic doses with 1.5 before ST® and 0.1 shortly after ST® application. The average pain score at the first follow-up visit was 1.2/10, comparable to Blome-Eberwein et al., who reported an average pain scale score of 1.9/10, both without describing variance interpreted as a moderate pain the study in partial-thickness burns over the entire period [4]. Glat et al. [7] used the Wong–Baker face pain scale score and calculated a pain score of 1.2/10 shortly after debridement and ST® application. Schwarze et al. [72] reported a median pain VAS score of 0.9/10, compared to that using Omiderm of 1.59. Hundeshagen et al. [11] showed a significant reduction in pain during the first 20 days compared to Mepilex Ag®, especially in children. Rashaan et al. [16], using Comfort B scores, described only minimal background pain and procedural pain changes. Fischer et al. [6] reported positive side effects: the avoidance of secondary pain killers and sedative drugs during dressing changes contributed to stability. Only Glik et al. [8] found inferiority in pain reduction measured by VAS on day 5 with ST® than with Oasis, without statistical significance; however, all studies comparing pain reduction seemed to show a more substantial ST® effect, where no statistical comparisons could be made.

4.5. Infection Rates

Infections are serious adverse effects in burns treatment. Infections, premature detachment, wound colonization, and possibly unexpected grafting are critical irritations in wound healing, which are only partially described. Infection rates seemed to be higher in deeper wounds, extensive burns, and burns treated later after injury.

Infections and the number of early dissolutions of ST® and PX might be reflected in the number of external dressing changes. Infections prolonged the healing time with ST®.

In weighted cases, a statistical difference between the treatment groups could be identified with a *p*-value of <0.001. Nevertheless, efficiency measured by Cohen's d only showed a small effect on infection reduction of ST compared to PXs.

A higher infection rate indicated deeper burns or necrotic tissue persistence. Closure with an epidermal template might influence the infection rate. Iqbal et al., who initially washed and debrided the wound from dead tissue in superficial, mid-dermal, and deep dermal burns, had 20 patients (31%) with healing >21 days and a strong association of longer healing time with infections. Similarly, Rashaan et al. found that only patients with wound infection had prolonged wound healing.

Xenografts are described as limiting bacterial growth [52,107], whereas ST® forms a bacterial tight barrier [108]. Karlsson found no differences in C-reactive protein or core temperature between PX and silver foam use [22] as indicators for reduced inflammatory response. ST® has the feature of bacterial impermeability and reducing systemic oxidative stress compared to a silver product [29].

4.6. Grafting Rates in Partial Thickness Burns

One of the indications of skin substitutes in burns is the intention to reduce burn wound conversion. Some have different definitions of burn wound conversion; therefore, it is a pragmatic approach to evaluating the unexpected grafting rate in partial thickness burns after a specific time. Grafting should generally be performed within three weeks in order to avoid hypertrophic scarring [109].

The studies' different grafting frequency demonstrates varying evaluation modalities of the grafting necessity and reflects different patient inclusion criteria and different ways of classifying partial-thickness burns. Wounds not entirely healed with minimal residual defects after detachment of ST® or PX were treated conservatively in both groups until healing was attained.

In PX studies, Burkey et al. [31] (superficial partial-thickness as inclusion criterion) reported that 14% of patients needed unexpected autografting, Duteille et al., (undetermined face burns as inclusion criterion) reported this in 3/20 patients [35], Elmasry et al. [20] (superficial and deep partial-thickness as inclusion criterion) needed an operation in 20% of patients. However, his study contained nearly no full thickness burns. Klosova et al. [36] (partial-thickness as inclusion criterion) reported early dissolution in 19% of patients.

Troy et al. [32] (charge codes as inclusion criteria) reported premature graft separation in 6.8% of patients.

Grafting after application in the ST® studies in partial-thickness burns was 0% in the Everett et al. study ($n = 17$); Blome-Eberwein et al. ($n = 227$) found no areas to be grafted, 2.4% were treated topically due to minimal size of residual defects. Patients in the Hundeshagen et al. study ($n = 31$), in 3%, needed grafting; Schwarze et al., ($n = 30$) excluded patients with Abbreviated Burn Severity Index >10 and showed a skin grafting rate of 0%. Rashaan et al., ($n = 21$) found problems with ST® adherence attributed to insufficient debridement with a grafting rate of 14%.

The average grafting rates derived from single studies were 2.5 ± 4.06 and 8.63 ± 13.14 demonstrating the difference, supporting the calculated efficiency of 0.52 with a p-value < 0.001 and a power of 0.99.

4.7. The Frequency of Outer Dressing Changes

The frequency of outer dressing changes might be a summative effect of undisturbed wound healing, as it reflects infections, unexpected dissolution of the epidermal skin substitute, and unwanted effects derived from dressings, and the number of controls estimated as necessary. It also reflects the workload for the staff.

It was calculated as the number of dressing changes until the wounds were healed. On average, the ST® treated patients had 4.38 ± 1.83 dressing changes, and the PX treated patients 4.79 ± 4.28. However, the difference is not significant ($p = 0.139$ Wilcoxon Test). As the data might be derived on study schedules, this limits the meaning. Nevertheless, the difference might mean fewer unwanted situations and a lower workload in the ST® group.

Elmasry et al. performed daily dressing changes [20]; this frequency seemed predetermined by the study protocol. In the study by Karlsson et al. [22], up to three outpatient visits and external dressing controls were performed weekly. Troy et al. [32] performed weekly wound surveillance. Duteille et al. [35] scheduled follow-up visits on day 14 after the facial treatment. Hosseini et al. reported a mean hospital LOS after PX of 4.69 days and a mean number of dressing changes of 1.5 after PX application. Patients were discharged after ST® Treatment the same day or the next day by Glat et al. [7].

4.8. Hospital LOS

Depending on the burn severity, the procedures applied in the different burn units, and complications, and the number of outpatients visits heretofore may reflect the study protocol. The average patient hospital LOS ranged from one day to 16 days in the PX studies and 0 to 23 days. Two studies were excluded from this report: an 81-year-old patient with a 51% TBSA burn and 55 days LOS [8] and a 40 days average in a comparison study with OASIS in the ST® [39] studies. It has to be considered that LOS can be reduced substantially when the outpatient treatment infrastructure is adapted to the needs.

4.9. Use of Both Product Categories in Other Fields of Trauma

In other indications as mechanical trauma, partial thickness wounds, donor areas for skin grafting, and temporary cover of skin defects might indicate both products. To reduce the consequences of surgical trauma, Suprathel also was used successfully as a peritoneal adhesion barrier in abdominal surgery [110] and as a pericardial adhesion barrier in cardiac surgery [111].

Many other products are in use for superficial and partial thickness burns and donor sites, but a comparison to Suprathel was not the paper's topic.

5. Conclusions

ST has a broad range of indications and has become the dressing of choice in many burn centers to treat partial thickness burns and donor areas, and it can be used successfully to cover sprayed keratinocytes. It appears to enable undisturbed wound healing at a substantially higher rate than PX. With an equal healing time, fewer infections, and a significantly lower transplantation rate, a lower number of dressing changes that were not statistically significant and may be based on study protocols during treatment of partial thickness burns supports wound healing even in more extensive burns. It reduces burn wound progression better than PX. Although no direct comparison was possible, there are strong indicators of more significant pain reduction and increased treatment comfort for patients and the team under ST treatment, as visible in the comparison of effectiveness data.

Although limitations exist regarding comparability, ST® treatment appears to be the right choice for PX replacement in the above-outlined indications. The fully synthetic and biocompatible off-the-shelf product is safe and cannot transmit viral or bacterial diseases, unlike other biological products. We hope to evaluate the ongoing results as ST® entirely moves to replace PXs. We suspect ST® will be superior to PXs, but this will need to be rigorously studied.

6. Limitations

In nearly all the studies, the diagnosis of partial thickness burn was solely based on clinical assessment. No study has objectively evaluated burn depth, for example, by laser Doppler imaging. Therefore, the differentiation of superficial partial-thickness and deep partial-thickness burns or partial full-thickness burns remains somewhat questionable. Many PX studies were retrospective investigations based on current procedural codes; thus, the primary indications may have differed.

The studies were based on an average TBSA in the groups, which were approximately only one-sixth of the ST studies in the PX studies.

A definitive treatment intention or a diagnostic evaluation of wound healing potential might have been the indication for PX use; however, this was not defined in the studies. The same applies to some ST® studies, where the progress of wound healing up to a specific day was observed to minimize the grafted area. The low rate of PX studies with a definitive time of healing reduced the comparability and the incompleteness of the description. The study misses result on parameters, as pliability of the skin and functional impairment, and a long-time outcome that was not described sufficiently and in the numbers to be comparable.

This comparison was based on partial thickness burns and wounds, as ST® was mainly used for this purpose. In a few cases, however, ST® was placed on small full-thickness areas. Although some centers have successfully used ST® to temporize excised full-thickness burns, there are no studies on this topic. Therefore, this review's level of evidence is reduced by the small number of studies and non-standardized methods.

To date, there is no side-by-side comparison of ST to Xenograft, and likely will not be one given one as PX is no longer available. Nonetheless, this manuscript describes the advantages of utilizing a safe, allogenic alternative for burn care as PX's old technology phases out. Data quality limited the statistical evaluation, and the results should be seen with caution.

Author Contributions: Conceptualization and methodology and reviewing: H.L.H., S.E.B.-E., L.P.K., S.E.W. and W.L.H.; writing—original draft preparation, review and editing: H.L.H., L.K.B., J.S.C., R.E.C., B.T.K., S.P.N., J.W.S. and D.P. All authors have read and agreed to the published version of the manuscript.

Funding: Editing costs were paid by Polymedics Innovations GmbH, Denkendorf. The company had no role in the design of the study; in the collection, analyses, or interpretation of data; in the writing of the manuscript, and in the decision to publish the results.

Institutional Review Board Statement: Not applicable.

Informed Consent Statement: Not applicable.

Data Availability Statement: Data are publicly available, as cited in the references.

Conflicts of Interest: Herbert Haller is a consultant for Polymedics Innovations GmbH for training and teaching, and other companies not dealing with the paper's topic. The other authors declare no conflicts of interest.

Abbreviations

ST:	Suprathel®
PX:	Porcine xenograft
TNF-α:	Tumor Necrosis Factor Alpha
TEN:	Toxic Epidermal Necrolysis
LOS:	Length of stay
VAS:	Visual Analogue Scale
PPPM:	Parents Postoperative Pain Measurement
ns:	not significant

References

1. Hozo, S.P.; Djulbegovic, B.; Hozo, I. Estimating the mean and variance from the median, range, and the size of a sample. *BMC Med. Res. Methodol.* **2005**, *5*, 13. [CrossRef] [PubMed]
2. Bravata, D.M.; Olkin, I. Simple pooling versus combining in meta-analysis. *Eval. Health Prof.* **2001**, *24*, 218–230.
3. Two Sample T-Test (Welch's T-test) n.d. Available online: https://www.statskingdom.com/150MeanT2uneq.html (accessed on 15 March 2021).
4. Blome-Eberwein, S.A.A.; Amani, H.; Lozano, D.D.D.; Gogal, C.; Boorse, D.; Pagella, P. A bio-degradable synthetic membrane to treat superficial and deep second degree burn wounds in adults and children—4 year experience. *Burns* **2020**, *46*, 1571–1584. [CrossRef] [PubMed]
5. Everett, M.; Massand, S.; Davis, W.; Burkey, B.; Glat, P. Use of a copolymer dressing on superficial and partial-thickness burns in a paediatric population. *J. Wound Care* **2015**, *24*, S4–S8. [CrossRef]
6. Fischer, S.; Kremer, T.; Horter, J.; Schaefer, A.; Ziegler, B.; Kneser, U.; Hirche, C. Suprathel® for severe burns in the elderly: Case report and review of the literature. *Burns* **2016**, *42*, e86–e92. [CrossRef]
7. Glat, P.M.; Burkey, B.; Davis, W. The use of Suprathel in the treatment of pediatric burns: Retrospective review of first pilot trial in a burn unit in the United States. *J. Burn Care Res.* **2014**, *35*, S159.
8. Glik, J.; Kawecki, M.; Kitala, D.; Klama-Baryła, A.; Łabuś, W.; Grabowski, M.; Durdzińska, A.; Nowak, M.; Misiuga, M.; Kasperczyk, A. A new option for definitive burn wound closure-pair matching type of retrospective case-control study of hand burns in the hospitalised patients group in the Dr Stanislaw Sakiel Centre for Burn Treatment between 2009 and 2015. *Int. Wound J.* **2017**, *14*, 849–855. [CrossRef]
9. Gürünlüoğlu, K.; Demircan, M.; Koç, A.; Koçbıyık, A.; Taşçi, A.; Durmuş, K.; Gürünlüoğlu, S.; Bağ, H.G.; Taşçı, A.; Koçbiyik, A. The effects of different burn dressings on length of telomere and expression of telomerase in children with thermal burns. *J. Burn Care Res.* **2019**, *40*, 302–311. [CrossRef]
10. Highton, L.; Wallace, C.; Shah, M. Use of Suprathel® for partial thickness burns in children. *Burns* **2012**, *39*, 2–7. [CrossRef]
11. Hundeshagen, G.; Collins, V.N.; Wurzer, P.; Sherman, W.; Voigt, C.D.; Cambiaso-Daniel, J.; Nunez-Lopez, O.; Sheaffer, J.; Herndon, D.N.; Finnerty, C.C.; et al. A prospective, randomized, controlled trial comparing the outpatient treatment of pediatric and adult partial-thickness burns with Suprathel or Mepilex Ag. *J. Burn Care Res.* **2017**, *39*, 261–267. [CrossRef]
12. Iqbal, T.; Ali, U.; Iqbal, Z.; Fatima, Z.J.; Rehan, M.; Khan, M.S. Role of Suprathel in dermal burns in children. *Emerg. Med. Investig.* **2018**, *6*, 2–5. [CrossRef]
13. Kukko, H.; Kosola, S.; Pyorala, S.; Vuola, J. Suprathel® in treatment of children's scald injuries. *Burns* **2009**, *35*, S22. [CrossRef]
14. Mądry, R.; Strużyna, J.; Stachura-Kułach, A.; Drozdz, Ł.; Bugaj, M. Effectiveness of Suprathel® application in partial thickness burns, frostbites and Lyell syndrome treatment. *Pol. J. Surg.* **2011**, *83*, 541–548. [CrossRef]
15. Radu, C.; Gazyakan, E.; Germann, G.; Riedel, K.; Reichenberger, M.; Ryssel, H. Optimizing Suprathel®—Therapy by the use of Octenidine-Gel®. *Burns* **2011**, *37*, 294–298. [CrossRef]
16. Rashaan, Z.M.; Krijnen, P.; Allema, J.H.; Vloemans, A.F.; Schipper, I.B.; Breederveld, R.S. Usability and effectiveness of Suprathel in partial thickness burns in children. *Eur. J. Trauma Emerg. Surg.* **2017**, *43*, 1–8. [CrossRef]
17. Schulz, A.; Perbix, W.; Shoham, Y.; Daali, S.; Charalampaki, C.; Fuchs, P.; Schiefer, J. Our initial learning curve in the enzymatic debridement of severely burned hands—Management and pit falls of initial treatments and our development of a post debridement wound treatment algorithm. *Burns* **2017**, *43*, 326–336. [CrossRef]
18. Schriek, K.S.; Sinnig, M.M. 473 The use of caprolacton dressings in pediatric burns—A gold standard? *J. Burn Care Res.* **2018**, *39*, S209. [CrossRef]
19. Schwarze, H.; Küntscher, M.; Uhlig, C.; Hierlemann, H.; Prantl, L.; Ottomann, C.; Hartmann, B. Suprathel, a new skin substitute, in the management of partial-thickness burn wounds. *Ann. Plast. Surg.* **2008**, *60*, 181–185. [CrossRef]
20. Elmasry, M.; Steinvall, I.; Thorfinn, J.; Abbas, A.H.; Abdelrahman, I.; Adly, O.A.; Sjöberg, F. Treatment of children with scalds by xenografts. *J. Burn Care Res.* **2016**, *37*, e586–e591. [CrossRef]

21. Hosseini, S.N.; Mousavinasab, S.N.; Fallahnezhat, M. Xenoderm dressing in the treatment of second degree burns. *Burns* **2007**, *33*, 776–781. [CrossRef]
22. Karlsson, M.; Elmasry, M.; Steinvall, I.; Sjöberg, F.; Olofsson, P.; Thorfinn, J. Superiority of silver-foam over porcine xenograft dressings for treatment of scalds in children: A prospective randomised controlled trial. *Burns* **2019**, *45*, 1401–1409. [CrossRef] [PubMed]
23. Hunt, T.K.; Conolly, W.B.; Aronson, S.B.; Goldstein, P. Anaerobic metabolism and wound healing: An hypothesis for the initiation and cessation of collagen synthesis in wounds. *Am. J. Surg.* **1978**, *135*, 328–332. [CrossRef]
24. Wahl, P.; Bloch, W.; Mester, J. Moderne Betrachtungsweisen des Laktats: Laktat ein überschätztes und zugleich unter-schätztes Molekül. *Schweiz. Z. Sportmed. Sporttraumatol.* **2009**, *57*, 100–107.
25. Philp, A.; Macdonald, A.L.; Watt, P.W. Lactate—A signal coordinating cell and systemic function. *J. Exp. Biol.* **2005**, *208*, 4561–4575. [CrossRef]
26. Milovanova, T.N.; Bhopale, V.M.; Sorokina, E.M.; Moore, J.S.; Hunt, T.K.; Hauer-Jensen, M.; Velazquez, O.C.; Thom, S.R. Lactate Stimulates Vasculogenic Stem Cells via the Thioredoxin System and Engages an Autocrine Activation Loop Involving Hypoxia-Inducible Factor 1. *Mol. Cell. Biol.* **2008**, *28*, 6248–6261. [CrossRef]
27. Cruz, R.S.D.O.; De Aguiar, R.A.; Turnes, T.; Penteado Dos Santos, R.; Fernandes Mendes De Oliveira, M.; Caputo, F. Intracellular shuttle: The lactate aerobic metabolism. *Sci. World J.* **2012**, *2012*. [CrossRef]
28. Groussard, C.; Morel, I.; Chevanne, M.; Monnier, M.; Cillard, J.; Delamarche, A. Free radical scavenging and antioxidant effects of lactate ion: An in vitro study. *J. Appl. Physiol.* **2000**, *89*, 169–175. [CrossRef]
29. Gürünlüoğlu, K.; Demircan, M.; Taşçı, A.; Üremiş, M.M.; Türköz, Y.; Bağ, H.G.; Ercan, B. The effects of two different burn dressings on serum oxidative stress indicators in children with partial burn. *J. Burn Care Res.* **2019**, *40*, 444–450. [CrossRef]
30. Demircan, M.; Gürünlüoğlu, K.; Bayrakçı, E.; Taşçı, A. Effects of Suprathel®, Aquacel® Ag or auto-grafting on human telomerase reverse transcriptase expression in the healing skin in children with partial thickness burn. *Ann. Burn. Fire Disasters* **2017**, *48*, 49.
31. Burkey, B.; Davis, W.; Glat, P.M. Porcine xenograft treatment of superficial partial-thickness burns in paediatric patients. *J. Wound Care* **2016**, *25*, 10–15. [CrossRef]
32. Troy, J.; Karlnoski, R.; Downes, K.; Brown, K.S.; Cruse, C.W.; Smith, D.J.; Payne, W.G. The use of EZ Derm® in partial-thickness burns: An institutional review of 157 patients. *Eplasty* **2013**, *13*, 14.
33. Fabia, R.; Groner, J.I. Advances in the care of children with burns. *Adv. Pediatr.* **2009**, *56*, 219–248. [CrossRef]
34. Chiu, T.; Burd, A. "Xenograft" dressing in the treatment of burns. *Clin. Dermatol.* **2005**, *23*, 419–423. [CrossRef]
35. Duteille, F.; Perrot, P. Management of 2nd-degree facial burns using the Versajet® hydrosurgery system and xenograft: A prospective evaluation of 20 cases. *Burns* **2012**, *38*, 724–729. [CrossRef]
36. Klosová, H.; Klein, L.; Bláha, J. Analysis of a retrospective double-centre data-collection for the treatment of burns using biological cover xe-derma. *Ann. Burn. Fire Disasters* **2014**, *27*, 171–174.
37. Keck, M.; Selig, H.; Lumenta, D.; Kamolz, L.; Mittlbock, M.; Frey, M. The use of Suprathel® in deep dermal burns: First results of a prospective study. *Burns* **2012**, *38*, 388–395. [CrossRef]
38. Bukovčan, P.; Koller, J. Treatment of partial-thickness scalds by skin xenografts—A retrospective study of 109 cases in a three-year period. *Acta Chir. Plast.* **2010**, *52*, 7–12. [CrossRef]
39. Diegidio, P.; Hermiz, S.J.; Ortiz-Pujols, S.; Jones, S.W.; Van Duin, D.; Weber, D.J.; Cairns, B.A.; Hultman, C.S. Even better than the real thing? Xenografting in pediatric patients with scald injury. *Clin. Plast. Surg.* **2017**, *44*, 651–656. [CrossRef]
40. Healy, C.; Boorman, J. Comparison of E-Z Derm and Jelonet dressings for partial skin thickness burns. *Burns* **1989**, *15*, 52–54. [CrossRef]
41. Priebe, C.; Friedman, R.; Noble, G.; Martucci, G.; Driessnack, M.; Soroff, H. Treatment of second-degree burns with porcine xenografts versus silver sulfadiazine cream: A study of pain and wound healing. *J. Pediatr. Surg.* **1992**, *27*, 390–391. [CrossRef]
42. Rodriguez-Ferreyra, P. The use of xenograft to manage extensive but superficial burns. *Burns* **2007**, *33*, S91. [CrossRef]
43. Burleson, R.; Eiseman, B. Nature of the bond between partial-thickness skin and wound granulations. *Plast. Reconstr. Surg.* **1973**, *51*, 353. [CrossRef]
44. Rappaport, I.; Pepino, A.; Dietrick, W. Early use of xenografts as a biologic dressing in burn trauma. *Am. J. Surg.* **1970**, *120*, 144–148. [CrossRef]
45. Zajicek, R.; Matouskova, E.; Broz, L.; Kubok, R.; Waldauf, P.; Königova, R. New biological temporary skin cover Xe-Derma® in the treatment of superficial scald burns in children. *Burns* **2011**, *37*, 333–337. [CrossRef]
46. Esteban-Vives, R.; Young, M.T.; Ziembicki, J.; Corcos, A.; Gerlach, J.C. Effects of wound dressings on cultured primary keratinocytes. *Burns* **2016**, *42*, 81–90. [CrossRef]
47. Hartmann, B.; Ekkernkamp, A.; Johnen, C.; Gerlach, J.C.; Belfekroun, C.; Küntscher, M.V. Sprayed cultured epithelial autografts for deep dermal burns of the face and neck. *Ann. Plast. Surg.* **2007**, *58*, 70–73. [CrossRef]
48. Sander, F.; Haller, H.; Belfekroun, C.; Hartmann, B. Suprathel und gesprühte Keratinozyten—Eine retrospektive Qualitätssicherungsstudie. *Ger. Med. Sci.* **2019**, 36–37. [CrossRef]
49. Wood, F.; Martin, L.; Lewis, D.; Rawlins, J.; McWilliams, T.; Burrows, S.; Rea, S. A prospective randomised clinical pilot study to compare the effectiveness of Biobrane® synthetic wound dressing, with or without autologous cell suspension, to the local standard treatment regimen in paediatric scald injuries. *Burns* **2012**, *38*, 830–839. [CrossRef]

50. Wood, F.; Kolybaba, M.; Allen, P. The use of cultured epithelial autograft in the treatment of major burn wounds: Eleven years of clinical experience. *Burns* **2006**, *32*, 538–544. [CrossRef]
51. Tan, A.; Whybro, N.; Frew, Q.; Barnes, D.; Philp, B.; Dziewulski, P. The use of Recell® in a regional burn service. *Ann. Burn. Fire Disasters* **2015**, *28*, 1–2.
52. Rapp, M.; Schappacher, R.; Liener, U. Zweizeitige Deckung von Spalthaut-Meek-Inseln nach 7–10 Tagen mit einer Polylactid-Membran (Suprathel). In Proceedings of the DAV 2020, Schladming, Austria, 15–18 January 2020. [CrossRef]
53. Feng, X.S.; Pan, Y.G.; Tan, J.J.; Wu, Q.H.; Shen, R.; Ruan, S.B.; Chen, X.D.; Zhang, F.G.; Lin, Z.P.; Du, Y.L. Treatment of deep partial thickness burns by a single dressing of porcine acellular dermal matrix. *Chin. J. Surg.* **2006**, *44*, 467–470. [PubMed]
54. Iwase, H.; Ekser, B.; Zhou, H.; Liu, H.; Satyananda, V.; Humar, R.; Humar, P.; Hara, H.; Long, C.; Bhama, J.K.; et al. Further evidence for sustained systemic inflammation in xenograft recipients (SIXR). *Xenotransplantation* **2015**, *22*, 399–405. [CrossRef] [PubMed]
55. Demircan, M.; Gürünlüoğlu, K.; Bag, H.G.G.; Koçbıyık, A.; Gül, M.; Uremis, N.; Gul, S.; Gürünlüoğlu, S.; Türköz, Y.; Taşçı, A. Impaction of the polylactic membrane or hydrofiber with silver dressings on the Interleukin-6, Tumor necrosis factor-α, Transforming growth factor-3 levels in the blood and tissues of pediatric patients with burns. *Turk. J. Trauma Emerg. Surg.* **2021**, *27*, 122–131. [CrossRef]
56. Wurzer, P.; Keil, H.; Branski, L.K.; Parvizi, D.; Clayton, R.P.; Finnerty, C.C.; Herndon, D.N.; Kamolz, L.P. The use of skin substitutes and burn care—A survey. *J. Surg. Res.* **2016**, *201*, 293–298. [CrossRef]
57. Jin, R.; Greenwald, A.; Peterson, M.D.; Waddell, T.K. Human Monocytes Recognize Porcine Endothelium via the Interaction of Galectin 3 and α-GAL. *J Immunol.* **2006**, *177*, 1289–1295. [CrossRef]
58. Schechter, I. Prolonged retention of glutaraldehyde-treated skin allografts and xenografts. *Ann. Surg.* **1975**, *182*, 699–704. [CrossRef]
59. Cooke, A.; Oliver, R.F.; Edward, M. An in vitro cytotoxicity study of aldehyde-treated pig dermal collagen. *Br. J. Exp. Pathol.* **1983**, *64*, 172–176.
60. El-Khatib, H.A.; Hammouda, A.; Al-Ghol, A.; Habib, B. Aldehyde-treated porcine skin versus biobrane as biosynthetic skin substitutes for excised burn wounds: Case series and review of the literature. *Ann. Burn. Fire Disasters* **2007**, *20*, 78–82.
61. Yamamoto, T.; Iwase, H.; King, T.W.; Hara, H.; Cooper, D.K. Skin xenotransplantation: Historical review and clinical potential. *Burns* **2018**, *44*, 1738–1749. [CrossRef]
62. Salisbury, R.E.; Wilmore, D.W.; Silverstein, P.; Pruitt, B.A. Biological dressings for skin graft donor sites. *Arch. Surg.* **1973**, *106*, 705–706. [CrossRef]
63. Vanstraelen, P. Comparison of calcium sodium alginate (KALTOSTAT) and porcine xenograft (E-Z DERM) in the healing of split-thickness skin graft donor sites. *Burns* **1992**, *18*, 145–148. [CrossRef]
64. Barone, A.A.L.; Mastroianni, M.; Farkash, E.A.; Mallard, C.; Albritton, A.; Torabi, R.; Leonard, D.A.; Kurtz, J.M.; Sachs, D.H.; Cetrulo, C.L., Jr. Genetically modified porcine split-thickness skin grafts as an alternative to allograft for provision of temporary wound coverage: Preliminary characterization. *Burns* **2015**, *41*, 565–574. [CrossRef]
65. Leonard, D.; Mallard, C.; Albritton, A.; Torabi, R.; Mastroianni, M.; Sachs, D.; Kurtz, J.; Cetrulo, C. Skin grafts from genetically modified α-1,3-galactosyltransferase knockout miniature swine: A functional equivalent to allografts. *Burns* **2017**, *43*, 1717–1724. [CrossRef]
66. Janich, E.J. Safety of Xenotransplantation: Development of Screening Methods and Testing for Porcine Viruses. Ph.D. Thesis, Freie Universität, Berlin, Germany, 2017.
67. Hume, A.J.; Ames, J.; Rennick, L.J.; Duprex, W.P.; Marzi, A.; Tonkiss, J.; Mühlberger, E. Inactivation of RNA viruses by gamma irradiation: A study on mitigating factors. *Viruses* **2016**, *8*, 204. [CrossRef]
68. Feng, X.; Shen, R.; Tan, J.; Chen, X.; Pan, Y.; Ruan, S.; Zhang, F.; Lin, Z.; Zeng, Y.; Wang, X.; et al. The study of inhibiting systematic inflammatory response syndrome by applying xenogenic (porcine) acellular dermal matrix on second-degree burns. *Burns* **2007**, *33*, 477–479. [CrossRef]
69. Eriksson, A.; Burcharth, J.; Rosenberg, J. Animal derived products may conflict with religious patients' beliefs. *BMC Med. Ethics* **2013**, *14*, 48. [CrossRef]
70. Jenkins, E.D.; Yip, M.; Melman, L.; Frisella, M.M.; Matthews, B.D. Informed consent: Cultural and religious issues associated with the use of allogeneic and xenogeneic mesh products. *J. Am. Coll. Surg.* **2010**, *210*, 402–410. [CrossRef]
71. Brady, S.C.; Snelling, C.F.T.; Chow, G. Comparison of donor site dressings. *Ann. Plast. Surg.* **1980**, *5*, 238–245. [CrossRef]
72. Schwarze, H.; Küntscher, M.; Uhlig, C.; Hierlemann, H.; Prantl, L.; Noack, N.; Hartmann, B. Suprathel®, a new skin substitute, in the management of donor sites of split-thickness skin grafts: Results of a clinical study. *Burns* **2007**, *33*, 850–854. [CrossRef] [PubMed]
73. Kaartinen, I.S.; Kuokkanen, O.H. Suprathel® causes less bleeding and scarring than Mepilex® Transfer in the treatment of donor sites of split-thickness skin grafts. *J. Plast. Surg. Hand Surg.* **2011**, *45*, 200–203. [CrossRef] [PubMed]
74. Grigg, M.; Brown, J.T.C. Donor Site Dressings: How Much Do They Affect Pain? *EJCB* **2020**, *1*, 88. Available online: www.mendeley.com/reference-manager/reader/8ea85f41-059c-3096-ab92-ee76clf2b04e4/1e556e1f-5932-1173-6f10-287641fb2542/ (accessed on 15 May 2020).
75. Uhlig, C.; Rapp, M.; Hartmann, B.; Hierlemann, H.; Planck, H.; Dittel, K.-K. Suprathel®—An innovative, resorbable skin substitute for the treatment of burn victims. *Burns* **2007**, *33*, 221–229. [CrossRef]

76. Markl, P.; Prantl, L.; Schreml, S.; Babilas, P.; Landthaler, M.; Schwarze, H. Management of split-thickness donor sites with synthetic wound dressings. *Ann. Plast. Surg.* **2010**, *65*, 490–496. [CrossRef]
77. Griggs, C.; Goverman, J.; Bittner, E.A.; Levi, B. Sedation and Pain Management in Burn Patients. *Clin. Plast. Surg.* **2017**, *44*, 535–540. [CrossRef]
78. Lamy, J.; Yassine, A.-H.; Gourari, A.; Forme, N.; Zakine, G. Place des substituts cutanés dans le traitement chirurgical des grands brûlés sur plus de 60% de la Surface corporelle. Revue de patients sur 11 ans dans le centre des brûlés adultes du CHRU de Tours. *Ann. Chir. Plast. Esthét.* **2015**, *60*, 131–139. [CrossRef]
79. Shubitidze, D.K. Prospektive Multicenterstudie für Eine Neue Lokaltherapie des Ulcus Cruris Mit Einer Resorbierbaren Wundabdeckung (Suprathel®). Ph.D. Thesis, Eberhard Karls Universität, Tubingen, Germany, 2016.
80. Uhlig, C.; Rapp, M.; Dittel, K.-K. Neue Strategien zur Behandlung thermisch geschädigter Hände unter Berücksichtigung des Epithelersatzes Suprathel®. *Handchir. Mikrochir. Plast. Chir.* **2007**, *39*, 314–319. [CrossRef]
81. Kloeters, O.; Schierle, C.; Tandara, A.; Mustoe, T.A. The use of a semiocclusive dressing reduces epidermal inflammatory cytokine expression and mitigates dermal proliferation and inflammation in a rat incisional model. *Wound Repair Regen.* **2008**, *16*, 568–575. [CrossRef]
82. Ogawa, R. Keloid and hypertrophic scars are the result of chronic inflammation in the reticular dermis. *Int. J. Mol. Sci.* **2017**, *18*, 606. [CrossRef]
83. Ziegler, B.; Hundeshagen, G.; Cordts, T.; Kneser, U.; Hirche, C. State of the art in enzymatic debridement. *Plast. Aesthet. Res.* **2018**, *5*, 33. [CrossRef]
84. Blome-Eberwein, S.; Pagella, P.; Boorse, D.; Amani, H. Results from Application of an Absorbable Synthetic Membrane to Superficial and Deep Second Degree Burn Wounds. In Proceedings of the 7th World Congress on Pediatric Burns, Boston, MA, USA, 29 August–1 September 2014; Available online: http://www.silon.com/wp-content/uploads/2014/09/ECPB2014-Results-from-Application-of-an-Absorbable-Synthetic-Membrane.pdf (accessed on 20 December 2020).
85. Mu, X.X. Treatment of full-thickness burn by planned replacement using glutaraldehyde porcine skin with an autograft. *Chin. J. Plast. Surg. Burn.* **1989**, *5*, 193–196.
86. Middelkoop, E.; Sheridan, R.L. Skin substitutes and 'the next level'. In *Total Burn Care*, 5th ed.; Elsevier: Amsterdam, The Netherlands, 2018.
87. Saffle, J.R. Closure of the Excised Burn Wound: Temporary Skin Substitutes. *Clin. Plast. Surg.* **2009**, *36*, 627–641. [CrossRef]
88. Zuo, H.; Song, G.; Shi, W.; Jia, J.; Zhang, Y. Observation of viable alloskin vs. xenoskin grafted onto subcutaneous tissue wounds after tangential excision in massive burns. *Burn. Trauma* **2016**, *4*, 23. [CrossRef]
89. Reumuth, G.; Schulz, T.; Reichelt, B.; Corterier, C.; Siemers, F. Die Temporäre Anwendung Eines Alloplastischen Hautersatzes—SUPRATHEL®—Bei Drittgradiger Verbrennung Fallbericht. In Proceedings of the DAV 2019, Schladming, Austria, 9–12 January 2019; Available online: https://www.egms.de/static/en/meetings/dav2019/19dav51.shtml (accessed on 4 December 2020).
90. Haller, L.H.; Hafner, R.; Giretzlehner, M.; Thumfart, S.; Ottomann, C.; Hartmann, B.; Rapp, M.; Sander, F.; Lumenta, D.; Katzensteiner, K. Suprathel More Than a Dressing?! *Ann. Burn. Fire Disasters* **2015**, *28*, 173.
91. Schneider, J.; Biedermann, T.; Widmer, D.; Montano, I.; Meuli, M.; Reichmann, E.; Schiest, C. Matriderm® versus Integra®: A comparative experimental study. *Burns* **2009**, *35*, 51–57. [CrossRef]
92. Phillips, G.S.A.; Nizamoglu, M.; Wakure, A.; Barnes, D.; El-Muttardi, N.; Dziewulski, P. The use of dermal regeneration templates for primary burns surgery in a UK regional burns centre. *Ann. Burn. Fire Disasters* **2020**, *33*, 245–252.
93. Baur, J.O.; Rahmanian-Schwarz, A.; Held, M.; Schiefer, J.; Daigeler, A.; Eisler, W. Evaluation of a cross-linked versus non-cross-linked collagen matrix in full-thickness skin defects. *Burns* **2021**, *47*, 150–156. [CrossRef]
94. Greenwood, J.E.; Wagstaff, M.J. Changing Practice in the Surgical Management of Major Burns—Delayed Definitive Closure. *J. Burn Care Res.* **2018**, *39* (Suppl. S1), S231–S232. [CrossRef]
95. SkinTE For Providers: PolarityTE, Inc. (PTE): PolarityTE, Inc. (PTE) n.d. Available online: https://www.polaryte.com/products/skinte-providers (accessed on 13 May 2020).
96. ClinicalTrials.gov. Study with an Autologous Dermo-epidermal Skin Substitute for the Treatment of Full-Thickness Skin Defects in Adults and Children—Full Text View—ClinicalTrials.gov n.d. Available online: https://clinicaltrials.gov/ct2/show/NCT03394612?term=denovoSkin&draw=2&rank=2 (accessed on 13 May 2020).
97. Martinson, M.; Martinson, N. A comparative analysis of skin substitutes used in the management of diabetic foot ulcers. *J. Wound Care* **2016**, *25*, S8–S17. [CrossRef]
98. Boyce, S.T.; Simpson, P.S.; Rieman, M.T.; Warner, P.M.; Yakuboff, K.P.; Bailey, J.K.; Nelson, J.K.; Fowler, L.A.; Kagan, R.J. Randomized, Paired-Site Comparison of Autologous Engineered Skin Substitutes and Split-Thickness Skin Graft for Closure of Extensive, Full-Thickness Burns. *J. Burn Care Res.* **2017**, *38*, 61–70. [CrossRef] [PubMed]
99. Roy, M.; King, T.W. Epidermal growth factor regulates NIKS keratinocyte proliferation through Notch signaling. *J. Surg. Res.* **2013**, *185*, 6–11. [CrossRef] [PubMed]
100. Centanni, J.M.; Straseski, J.A.; Wicks, A.; Hank, J.A.; Rasmussen, C.A.; Lokuta, M.A.; Schurr, M.J.; Foster, K.N.; Faucher, L.D.; Caruso, D.M.; et al. Stratagraft skin substitute is well-tolerated and is not acutely immunogenic in patients with traumatic wounds: Results from a prospective, randomized, controlled dose escalation trial. *Ann. Surg.* **2011**, *253*, 672–683. [CrossRef] [PubMed]

101. Rapp, M.; Al-Shukur, F.-F.; Liener, U.C. Der Einsatz des Alloplastischen Epithelersatzes Suprathel®bei Großflächigen Gemischt 2.-Gradigen Verbrennungen Über 25% KOF—Das Stuttgarter Konzept. (DAV 2010). 2010. Available online: https://www.egms.de/static/en/meetings/dav2010/10dav18.shtml (accessed on 27 November 2020).
102. Tsuchiya, S.; Ohmori, M.; Hara, K.; Fujio, M.; Ikeno, M.; Hibi, H.; Ueda, M. An Experimental Study on Guided Bone Regeneration Using a Polylactide-co-glycolide Membrane–Immobilized Conditioned Medium. *Int. J. Oral Maxillofac. Implant.* **2015**, *30*, 1175–1186. [CrossRef]
103. Ronga, M.; Cherubino, M.; Corona, K.; Fagetti, A.; Bertani, B.; Valdatta, L.; Mora, R.; Cherubino, P. Induced membrane technique for the treatment of severe acute tibial bone loss: Preliminary experience at medium-term follow-up. *Int. Orthop.* **2019**, *43*, 209–215. [CrossRef]
104. Lindford, A.J.; Kaartinen, I.S.; Virolainen, S.; Vuola, J. Comparison of Suprathel® and allograft skin in the treatment of a severe case of toxic epidermal necrolysis. *Burns* **2011**, *37*, e67–e72. [CrossRef]
105. Morris, C.; Emsley, P.; Meuleneire, F.; White, R.; Marland, E. Use of wound dressings with soft silicone adhesive technology. *Paediatr. Nurs.* **2009**, *21*, 38–43. [CrossRef]
106. Hobby, J.A.; Levick, P.L. Clinical evaluation of porcine xenograft dressings. *Burns* **1978**, *4*, 188–192. [CrossRef]
107. Sun, T.; Han, Y.; Chai, J.; Yang, H. Transplantation of microskin autografts with overlaid selectively decellularized split-thickness porcine skin in the repair of deep burn wounds. *J. Burn Care Res.* **2011**, *32*, e67–e73. [CrossRef]
108. Haller, H.; Held-Föhn, E. 654 Investigation of germ patency of a polylactic acid-based membrane for the treatment of burns. *J. Burn Care Res.* **2020**, *41*, S173. [CrossRef]
109. Deitch, E.A.; Wheelahan, T.M.; Rose, M.P.; Clothier, J.; Cotter, J. Hypertrophic burn scars. *J. Trauma Inj. Infect. Crit. Care* **1983**, *23*, 895–898. [CrossRef]
110. Kraemer, B.; Wallwiener, M.; Brochhausen, C.; Planck, C.; Hierlemann, H.; Isaacson, K.B.; Rajab, T.K.; Wallwiener, C. A Pilot Study of Laparoscopic Adhesion Prophylaxis after Myomectomy with a Copolymer Designed for Endoscopic Application. *J. Minim. Invasive Gynecol.* **2010**, *17*, 222–227. [CrossRef]
111. Al-Saidi, A.A.M. Myokardiale Adhäsionsprophylaxe am Schweinemodell Mittels Antiadhäsiver Bioresorbierbarer Polymerfolien. Ph.D. Thesis, Eberhard Karls Universität zu Tübingen, Tuebingen, Germany, 2018.

MDPI
St. Alban-Anlage 66
4052 Basel
Switzerland
Tel. +41 61 683 77 34
Fax +41 61 302 89 18
www.mdpi.com

Medicina Editorial Office
E-mail: medicina@mdpi.com
www.mdpi.com/journal/medicina

MDPI
St. Alban-Anlage 66
4052 Basel
Switzerland
Tel. +41 61 683 77 34
Fax +41 61 302 89 18
www.mdpi.com

Medicina Editorial Office
E-mail: medicina@mdpi.com
www.mdpi.com/journal/medicina

www.ingramcontent.com/pod-product-compliance
Lightning Source LLC
LaVergne TN
LVHW070728100526
838202LV00013B/1192